theclinics.com

CARDIOLOGY CLINICS

Thromboembolic Disease and Antithrombotic Agents in the Elderly

GUEST EDITOR
Laurie G. Jacobs, MD, FACP, AGSF

CONSULTING EDITOR
Michael H. Crawford, MD

May 2008 • Volume 26 • Number 2

SAUNDERS

An Imprint of Elsevier, Inc.
PHILADELPHIA   LONDON   TORONTO   MONTREAL   SYDNEY   TOKYO

W.B. SAUNDERS COMPANY
A Division of Elsevier Inc.

Elsevier Inc. • 1600 John F. Kennedy Blvd., Suite 1800 • Philadelphia, Pennsylvania 19103-2899

http://www.theclinics.com

CARDIOLOGY CLINICS
May 2008
Editor: Barbara Cohen-Kligerman

Volume 26, Number 2
ISSN 0733-8651
ISBN-13: 978-1-4160-5889-2
ISBN-10: 1-4160-5889-3

The ideas and opinions expressed in *Cardiology Clinics* do not necessarily reflect those of the Publisher. The Publisher does not assume any responsibility for any injury and/or damage to persons or property arising out of or related to any use of the material contained in this periodical. The reader is advised to check the appropriate medical literature and the product information currently provided by the manufacturer of each drug to be administered to verify the dosage, the method and duration of administration, or contraindications. It is the responsibility of the treating physician or other health care professional, relying on independent experience and knowledge of the patient, to determine drug dosages and the best treatment for the patient. Mention of any product in this issue should not be construed as endorsement by the contributors, editors, or the Publisher of the product or manufacturers' claims.

Cardiology Clinics (ISSN 0733-8651) is published quarterly by Elsevier Inc., 360 Park Avenue South, New York, NY 10010-1710. Months of issue are February, May, August, and November. Business and editorial Offices: 1600 John F. Kennedy Blvd., Suite 1800, Philadelphia, PA 19103-2899. Customer Service Office: 6277 Sea Harbor Drive, Orlando, FL 32887-4800. Periodicals postage paid at New York, NY, and additional mailing offices. Subscription prices are $226.00 per year for US individuals, $344.00 per year for US institutions, $113.00 per year for US students and residents, $276.00 per year for Canadian individuals, $418.00 per year for Canadian institutions, $301.00 per year for international individuals, $418.00 per year for international institutions and $150.00 per year for Canadian and foreign students/residents. To receive student/resident rate, orders must be accompanied by name of affiliated institution, data of term, and the *signature* of program/residency coordinator on institution letterhead. Orders will be billed at individual rate until proof of status is received. Foreign air speed delivery is included in all *Clinics* subscription prices. All prices are subject to change without notice. POSTMASTER: Send address changes to *Cardiology Clinics*, Elsevier Periodicals Customer Service, 6277 Sea Harbor Drive, Orlando, FL 32887-4800. **Customer Service: 1-800-654-2452 (US). From outside of the US, call 1- 407-563-6020. Fax: 1-407-363-9661. E-mail: JournalsCustomerService-usa@elsevier.com.**

Cardiology Clinics is also published in Spanish by McGraw-Hill Interamericana Editores S. A., P.O. Box 5-237, 06500, Mexico D. F., Mexico; in Portuguese by Reichmann and Alfonso Editores Rio de Janeiro, Brazil; and in Greek by Dimitrios P. Lagos, 8 Pondon Street, GR115-28 Ilissia, Greece.

Cardiology Clinics is covered in *Index Medicus, Excerpta Medica, The Cumulative Index to Nursing and Allied Health Literature* (CINAHL).

Printed in the United States of America.

CONSULTING EDITOR

MICHAEL H. CRAWFORD, MD, Professor of Medicine, University of California San Francisco; Lucie Stern Chair in Cardiology, and Interim Chief of Cardiology, University of California San Francisco Medical Center, San Francisco, California

GUEST EDITOR

LAURIE G. JACOBS, MD, Professor of Clinical Medicine; Division Head, Geriatrics; Director, Resnick Gerontology Center, Albert Einstein College of Medicine and Montefiore Medical Center, Bronx, New York

CONTRIBUTORS

JACK E. ANSELL, MD, Department of Medicine, Lenox Hill Hospital, New York, New York

HENNY H. BILLETT, MD, Professor of Clinical Medicine and Pathology, Albert Einstein College of Medicine; Director, Thrombosis Prevention and Treatment Program, Department of Medicine, Division of Hematology, Montefiore Medical Center, Bronx, New York

DANIEL J. BROTMAN, MD, Director and Assistant Professor of Medicine, Hospitalist Program, The Johns Hopkins Hospital, Baltimore, Maryland

AIMEE CHEVALIER, PharmD, Clinical Assistant Professor, Department of Pharmacy Practice; Clinical Pharmacist, Antithrombosis Center, University of Illinois at Chicago, College of Pharmacy and Medical Center, Chicago, Illinois

ORIANA CORNETT, MD, Department of Neurology, SUNY Downstate, Brooklyn, New York

DANYA L. DINWOODEY, MD, Section of Cardiology, Boston University School of Medicine, Boston, Massachusetts

MICHAEL EZEKOWITZ, MB ChB, PhD, Vice President, Lankenau Institute for Medical Research, Wynnewood, Pennsylvania

DAVID A. GARCIA, MD, Associate Professor, Department of Internal Medicine, University of New Mexico, Albuquerque, New Mexico

JEFFREY GINSBERG, MD, FRCPC, Professor of Medicine, McMaster University Medical Centre, Hamilton, Ontario, Canada

ELAINE HYLEK, MD, MPH, Associate Professor, Department of Medicine, General Internal Medicine Research Unit, Boston University School of Medicine, Boston, Massachusetts

LAURIE G. JACOBS, MD, Professor of Clinical Medicine; Division Head, Geriatrics; Director, Resnick Gerontology Center, Albert Einstein College of Medicine and Montefiore Medical Center, Bronx, New York

AMIR K. JAFFER, MD, Associate Professor of Medicine; Chief, Service of Medicine, University of Miami Hospital; and Division Chief, Hospital Medicine, Department of Medicine, University of Miami, Miami, Florida

CLIVE KEARON, MB, MRCP(I), FRCP(C), PhD, Professor, Department of Medicine, McMaster University and Henderson Research Centre, Ontario, Canada

SOO KIM, MD, Fellow, Vascular Surgery, University of Medicine and Dentistry of New Jersey, New Jersey Medical School, Newark, New Jersey

ROBERT LEE, MD, Department of Medicine, Harbor-UCLA Medical Center, Torrance, California

EVAN C. LIPSITZ, MD, FACS, Associate Professor of Surgery, Acting Chief, Division of Vascular and Endovascular Surgery, Medical Director, Vascular Diagnostic Laboratory Services, Albert Einstein College of Medicine and Montefiore Medical Center, Bronx, New York

SAMIT MALHOTRA, MD, Department of Neurology, SUNY Downstate, Brooklyn, New York

SIMON MCRAE, MB, ChB, FRACP, FRCPA, Research Fellow, McMaster University Medical Centre, Hamilton, Ontario, Canada

GENO J. MERLI, MD, Professor of Medicine, Chief Medical Officer, Director, Jefferson Center for Vascular Diseases, Jefferson Medical College, Thomas Jefferson University Hospital, Philadelphia, Pennsylvania

RANGADHAM NAGARAKANTI, MD, Lankenau Institute for Medical Research, Wynnewood, Pennsylvania

EDITH A. NUTESCU, PharmD, FCCP, Clinical Associate Professor, Department of Pharmacy Practice; Director, Antithrombosis Center, University of Illinois at Chicago, College of Pharmacy and Medical Center, Chicago, Illinois

MARTIN O'DONNELL, MB, MRCP(I), Assistant Professor, Department of Medicine, McMaster University and Henderson Research Centre, Ontario, Canada

LENORE C. OCAVA, MD, Department of Neurology, Kennedy Center, Albert Einstein College of Medicine, Bronx, New York; and Stroke Center, Jacobi Medical Center, Bronx, New York

DANIEL M. ROSENBAUM, MD, Professor and Chair, Department of Neurology, SUNY Downstate, Brooklyn, New York

NANCY L. SHAPIRO, PharmD, Clinical Assistant Professor, Department of Pharmacy Practice; Clinical Pharmacist, Antithrombosis Center, University of Illinois at Chicago, College of Pharmacy and Medical Center, Chicago, Illinois

MANJEET SINGH, MD, Department of Neurology, Kennedy Center, Albert Einstein College of Medicine, Bronx, New York

SANDEEP SODHI, MD, Academic Office, Drexel University College of Medicine, Philadelphia, Pennsylvania

HUYEN TRAN, MBBS, FRACP, FRCPA, Research Fellow, McMaster University Medical Centre, Hamilton, Ontario, Canada

CONTENTS

thrombin; a more predictable anticoagulant response, because they do not bind to plasma proteins and are not neutralized by platelet factor 4; lack of required cofactors, such as antithrombin or heparin cofactor II; inhibiting thrombin-induced platelet aggregation; and absence of induction of immune-mediated thrombocytopenia. Various injectable DTIs are currently available and used for many indications. In addition, research is now focusing on oral DTIs that seem promising and offer various advantages, such as oral administration, predictable pharmacokinetics and pharmacodynamics, a broad therapeutic window, no routine monitoring, no significant drug interactions, and fixed-dose administration.

morbidity and mortality. When considering long-term oral anticoagulant therapy in older patients, however, careful ongoing evaluation is imperative to ensure that the risk of bleeding does not outweigh the antithrombotic benefits.

Antithrombotic and Thrombolytic Therapy for Ischemic Stroke

Oriana Cornett, Lenore C. Ocava, Manjeet Singh, Samit Malhotra, and Daniel M. Rosenbaum

Thrombolytic and antithrombotic agents form the cornerstone of stroke treatment and prevention. Recombinant tissue plasminogen activation (rt-PA) improves the outcome in patients treated within 3 hours of stroke onset. The risk-benefit ratio is narrow because of an increased risk for bleeding, but studies do not support a higher risk in the geriatric population. Emerging trials are directed at extending the therapeutic window and identifying agents that could provide better safety profiles. Large randomized trials have also highlighted the effectiveness and safety of early and continuous antiplatelet therapy in reducing atherothrombotic stroke recurrence. Aspirin has become the antiplatelet treatment standard against which several other antiplatelet agents have been shown to be more effective. The prevention of cardioembolic stroke is best accomplished with oral anticoagulation, barring any contraindications.

Reducing the Risk for Stroke in Patients Who Have Atrial Fibrillation

David A. Garcia and Elaine Hylek

Warfarin is highly effective at reducing the risk of stroke in AF. The benefit of oral anticoagulant therapy strongly outweighs the risk in most patients who have AF. More data are needed to define the overall risk-to-benefit ratio better for patients aged 80 years and older. Because a significant proportion of elderly individuals may not be optimal candidates for anticoagulant therapy, we must continue to evaluate alternative stroke prevention strategies while redoubling our efforts to understand the mechanisms underlying AF and thrombogenesis.

Chronic Antithrombotic Therapy in Post–Myocardial Infarction Patients

Rangadham Nagarakanti, Sandeep Sodhi, Robert Lee, and Michael Ezekowitz

Because 1.1 million myocardial infarctions occur in the United States alone each year, and 450,000 of them are recurrent infarctions, which carry an inherently greater risk of death and disability than first events, the importance of secondary prevention strategies that can be implemented widely is unparalleled in health care. Antithrombotic therapies, both antiplatelet and anticoagulant, have become the mainstays of these strategies. This article covers the use of chronic antiplatelet and anticoagulation agents after myocardial infarction. It does not include the management of these patients in the acute phase.

Antithrombotic Therapy in Peripheral Arterial Disease

Evan C. Lipsitz and Soo Kim

The management of elderly patients with peripheral arterial disease requires a multidisciplinary and individualized approach, especially for patients requiring intervention and for those on antithrombotic therapy. Communication between the patient's primary physician, consulting medical specialists, and vascular surgeon is essential because all may contribute synergistically to deliver optimal care to the patient. This article reviews the pathophysiology of peripheral arterial disease and data regarding the use of antiplatelet and anticoagulant agents.

FORTHCOMING ISSUES

RECENT ISSUES

VISIT OUR WEB SITE

The Clinics are now available online!
Access your subscription at www.theclinics.com

ELSEVIER
SAUNDERS

Cardiol Clin 26 (2008) xi

CARDIOLOGY
CLINICS

Foreword

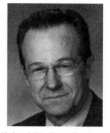

Michael H. Crawford, MD
Consulting Editor

Dr. Jacobs and an international group of experts in thromboembolic disease and antithrombic therapy originally published a version of this issue in *Clinics in Geriatric Medicine*. I thought the topics covered and the focus on elderly patients was highly appropriate for *Cardiology Clinics*; therefore, I was delighted when this group agreed to update and revise their articles for this issue of *Cardiology Clinics*. The first four articles focus on the most commonly used antithrombic agents. The next three focus on the pathophysiology, prevention, and treatment of deep venous thrombosis and pulmonary embolism, highly lethal diseases in elderly cardiac patients. The final five articles describe the treatment of specific cardiovascular diseases.

Considerable practical information may be found in this issue. Particularly valuable are the discussions of the treatment of diseases less commonly managed by cardiologists, such as ischemic stroke and peripheral arterial disease.

Other valuable discussions include the perioperative management of oral anticoagulation and prevention of deep venous thrombosis. The focus on the elderly is important because antithrombic treatment is a double-edged sword in this group. Antithrombic therapy can provide large benefits in these higher risk patients but also carries higher risks. Balancing these aspects is critical to the successful management of thrombotic diseases in the elderly. I found the articles in this issue very useful and plan on keeping my copy handy.

Michael H. Crawford, MD
Division of Cardiology
Department of Medicine
University of California
San Francisco Medical Center
505 Parnassus Avenue, Box 0124
San Francisco, CA 94143-0124, USA

E-mail address: crawfordm@medicine.ucsf.edu

ELSEVIER
SAUNDERS

Cardiol Clin 26 (2008) xiii–xiv

CARDIOLOGY
CLINICS

Preface

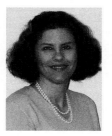

Laurie G. Jacobs, MD
Guest Editor

There has been an explosion in the study of thromboembolic disorders heralded by the development of new antiplatelet and anticoagulant agents. Venous and arterial thromboembolic diseases have historically been considered clinically silent until an event associated with considerable morbidity or mortality occurs. Elucidation of the role of antiplatelet and anticoagulant agents in the pathophysiology of clotting and disease in the venous and arterial systems has led to important opportunities for prevention and advances in the treatment of thromboembolic disease.

Increased longevity caused by a reduction in cardiovascular disease and other factors has led to a rapid demographic expansion of the adult population older than 65 years of age, particularly those older than 85 years. Age alone has emerged as one of the key risk factors for venous thromboembolic disease, encompassing deep and superficial venous thrombosis and pulmonary embolism. Age is also highly associated with arterial thromboembolic disease, such as myocardial infarction and coronary artery disease, ischemic stroke, atrial fibrillation, and peripheral arterial disease. In addition to an increase in risk, prevalence, and mortality of thromboembolic disease in older adults, the morbidity of events is

increased. This issue of *Cardiology Clinics* is dedicated to a discussion of the identification, prevention, and management of venous and arterial thromboembolic disease in older adults with the goal of at least improving morbidity and perhaps delaying mortality for this population.

A discussion is not complete, however, without a careful examination of the efficacy and risk of antithrombotic agents in this population. Antiplatelet and anticoagulant agents are associated with an increased risk for bleeding associated with age alone. It is essential that health care providers understand the pharmacology of these agents, be familiar with estimates of their efficacy in clinical trials and practice, and be adept at their management.

The identification of risk factors associated with deep venous thrombosis has altered the view of venous thromboembolic disease from a cause of unexpected mortality to one requiring anticipation and prevention, particularly in patients undergoing surgery or those who have underlying malignancies. The development of institutional guidelines for prevention of venous thromboembolic disease in the elderly is on the horizon. Patients who have idiopathic deep venous thrombosis are now considered to have a chronic disease, transforming their management from an episodic treatment to consideration of lifelong anticoagulation. In addition, advances in the clinician's ability to determine

A version of this Preface originally appeared in *Clinics in Geriatric Medicine*, volume 22, issue 1.

0733-8651/08/$ - see front matter © 2008 Elsevier Inc. All rights reserved.
doi:10.1016/j.ccl.2007.12.018

cardiology.theclinics.com

pretest probability and apply that information to results from diagnostic testing, such as the D-dimer test and duplex ultrasonography of the leg, have considerably improved decision making around the diagnosis of deep venous thrombosis. With the advent of low molecular weight heparins, prevention and treatment can be provided outside of the hospital, with important opportunities to improve care, cost, and outcomes.

The prevalence of arterial thromboembolic disease (stroke, myocardial infarction, and peripheral vascular disease) continues to plague the elderly. The functional and cognitive loss caused by disability from stroke, congestive heart failure, dementia, and vascular disease has a profound impact on quality of life. An understanding of the pathophysiology of disease and the efficacy and risk of antiplatelet agents and anticoagulant agents promises to provide considerable benefit to the population of older adults.

Laurie G. Jacobs, MD
Resnick Gerontology Center
Albert Einstein College of Medicine
Montefiore Medical Center
111 East 210 Street, Bronx, NY 10467

E-mail address: lajacobs@montefiore.org

ELSEVIER
SAUNDERS

CARDIOLOGY
CLINICS

Cardiol Clin 26 (2008) 145–155

Heparins, Low-Molecular-Weight Heparins, and Pentasaccharides: Use in the Older Patient

Danya L. Dinwoodey, MD[a], Jack E. Ansell, MD[b],*

[a]Section of Cardiology, Boston University School of Medicine, 88 East Newton Street, C-8, Boston, MA 02118, USA
[b]Department of Medicine, Lenox Hill Hospital, 100 East 77th Street, New York, NY 10075, USA

Anticoagulation in the elderly is a growing concern as patients live longer and have an increasing number of co-morbid illnesses. Given the increased risk of venous thromboembolism (VTE) with normal aging, it is important to understand the therapeutic and prophylactic options available to clinicians. This article reviews the use of anticoagulants, specifically unfractionated heparin (UFH), low-molecular-weight heparin (LMWH), and the newer synthetic pentasaccharides for the treatment and prophylaxis of VTE as well as their use in acute coronary syndromes (ACS). Furthermore, heparin- induced thrombocytopenia (HIT) is addressed as it relates to each of the previously mentioned medications.

Aging is a well-established risk factor for VTE, and elderly patients experience higher morbidity and mortality with this disease [1]. In a large community-based study in France, the incidence of symptomatic VTE was 1.83 per 1000 persons. This figure rises to 10 per 1000 persons for those over the age of 75 [2]. A study examining the incidence of asymptomatic deep venous thrombosis (DVT) in geriatric patients admitted to a medical service showed that 4% of patients aged 70 to 80 and nearly 18% of patients aged over 80 had evidence of DVT [3].

In addition to aging, numerous other factors are noted to increase the risk of thrombosis. These include hospital or nursing home stay, surgery, central venous access catheters, pacemakers, chemotherapy, and hormone therapy [4]. Patient specific risk factors include congestive heart failure, myocardial infarction, stroke, and malignancy within the preceding 6 months of an event. Also included as risk factors are prior thrombosis, hypercoagulable states, chronic obstructive pulmonary disease, hip fractures, trauma, varicose veins, paralysis of lower limbs, obesity, nephrotic syndrome, and severe infection [1,4–6].

Despite these multiple risk factors, anticoagulation is underused in the prevention of VTE in the United States [4]. A retrospective study investigating the use of anticoagulant prophylaxis among hospitalized patients showed that 183 (48%) of 384 patients who subsequently developed VTE were not on prophylactic anticoagulation [7]. Given the higher propensity of the elderly to experience VTE, clinicians caring for these patients need to be cognizant of the mechanisms, monitoring, and adverse effects of anticoagulation for both treatment and prophylaxis of VTE.

The elderly also represent a distinct subgroup with respect to the pharmacokinetics of many drugs, notably because of decreases in creatinine clearance with advancing age. Aging is associated with alterations in drug-binding proteins, but the significance of these alterations is unclear with respect to anticoagulant drugs [4].

Hemostasis involves a sequence of interactions of coagulation factor interactions in two pathways called the intrinsic and extrinsic coagulation cascades (Fig. 1). The final common pathway involves the transformation of prothrombin to thrombin by factor Xa. Thrombin (factor IIa) then serves to catalyze the activation of fibrinogen to fibrin, in addition to its role in feedback

A version of this article originally appeared in *Clinics in Geriatric Medicine*, volume 22, issue 1.

* Corresponding author.

E-mail address: jansell@lenoxhill.net (J.E. Ansell).

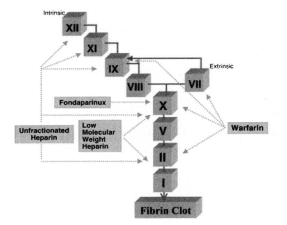

Fig. 1. The clotting cascade and sites of action of anticoagulant medications.

activation of several other clotting factors. UFH, LMWH, and fondaparinux all exert their anticoagulant effect in a similar fashion, by binding to and activating antithrombin that then neutralizes selected coagulation factors.

Unfractionated heparin

Pharmacology

UFH is a glycosaminoglycan first used clinically in the 1930s [8]. It is derived from animal tissue (porcine or bovine), with molecular weight ranging from 3000 to 30,000 d [9,10]. The mechanism of action is through binding to and activation of antithrombin, which then binds to and neutralizes the serine protease coagulation factors, particularly factors Xa and thrombin [11]. Only 30% of UFH chains contain the sequence necessary for activating antithrombin. The remaining chains are inactive, but bind nonspecifically to other plasma proteins, endothelial cells, and platelet factor 4. Because of nonspecific protein binding, the pharmacokinetics of UFH are unpredictable, and monitoring is necessary [10–12]. Additionally, UFH binds to heparin cofactor II that serves to further reduce the activity and availability of thrombin [11,13].

The half-life of UFH is approximately 1 hour after an intravenous bolus, and longer with subcutaneous administration. For this reason, subcutaneous initial doses should be increased by 10% compared with intravenous doses [14]. UFH is metabolized in part by the liver and is excreted

through the kidneys, but does not need to be dosed specifically for renal insufficiency or hepatic dysfunction [11]. Only free heparin is active, and patients with renal or hepatic dysfunction have varied protein binding. Because protein binding can either be increased or decreased, a standard dose of UFH is given and subsequent dosing is based on results of an activated partial thromboplastin time (aPTT), aiming for a predetermined therapeutic range.

Dosing

UFH dosing for VTE prophylaxis is 5000 IU administered subcutaneously every 8 hours [4]. When UFH is used for treatment of VTE or ACS, a weight-based nomogram is the safest and most effective method to anticoagulate patients (Table 1). A retrospective analysis of 355 patients with treatment guided by either a weight-based nomogram or with a standard bolus and physician choice for dose adjustment found that the weight-based nomogram patients experienced fewer bleeding episodes and had

Table 1
Heparin dosing nomogram

aPTT[a]	Dose adjustment
<35 s	80 units/kg bolus; increase drip by 4 units/kg/h
35–50 s	40 units/kg bolus; increase drip by 2 units/kg/h
51–70 s	No change
71–90 s	Reduce drip by 2 units/kg/h
>90 s	Hold heparin for 1 hour; reduce drip by 3 units/kg/h

Check baseline aPTT, INR, CBC-platelet count.

Give heparin bolus, 80 units/kg IV.

Begin IV heparin infusion, 18 units/kg/h.

Each laboratory must perform its own in vitro heparin titration curve to establish the therapeutic range for the specific aPTT reagent in use, which is equivalent to a heparin concentration of 0.3–0.7 anti Xa U/mL (by anti Xa assay) or 0.2–0.4 U/mL (by protamine titration assay). The therapeutic range varies depending on the aPTT reagent in use.

Abbreviations: aPTT, activated partial thromboplastin time; CBC, complete blood count; INR, international normalized ratio; IV, intravenous.

[a] Target aPTT for institution-specific therapeutic range.

Data from Raschke RA, Reilly BM, Guidry JR, et al. The weight-based heparin dosing nomogram compared with a standard care nomogram: a randomized controlled trial. Ann Intern Med 1993;119:874–81.

more frequent aPTT values in the target range [15]. A meta-analysis of 16 studies revealed that a higher percentage of patients treated with weight-based nomograms reached therapeutic levels within 24 hours when compared with patients administered heparin in the traditional method. There were no statistically significant differences in bleeding rates [16].

Even in hospitals with heparin nomograms, however, doses vary widely and anticoagulation is often subtherapeutic or supratherapeutic. In a retrospective study examining patients receiving UFH for treatment of VTE and as a bridge to warfarin therapy, the difficulty in achieving therapeutic heparin levels was demonstrated. After a therapeutic aPTT range was reached, only 29% of patients remained in the therapeutic range on subsequent measurements. Several dose changes and boluses were often required to provide adequate anticoagulation [17].

Monitoring

As a result of the unpredictable binding of UFH to plasma proteins, its anticoagulant effect needs to be monitored to maintain a therapeutic level. Numerous tests have been suggested for heparin monitoring including the aPTT, the activated clotting time (ACT), anti–factor Xa levels, plasma heparin levels, and thrombin clotting time [13]. In the United States, the aPTT is the most widely used test.

In general, the recommended range of an aPTT for therapeutic heparin levels is 1.5 to 2.5 times the control aPTT. Reagents used in various laboratories have different sensitivities to heparin, however, and must be calibrated based on therapeutic heparin levels to a reagent-specific range. Laboratories using different reagents have different therapeutic aPTT ranges, and heparin should be dosed according to their range [12,18]. Blood is usually collected 4 to 6 hours after initial infusion. Although widely used, the aPTT lacks specificity in several circumstances, and the relation to heparin level is often poor. This may occur in the presence of the antiphospholipid antibody, clotting factor deficiencies, thrombolytics, or even warfarin use [18]. Warfarin affects clotting factors II, IX, and X that can alter the aPTT.

Heparin-resistant patients also have been described. These patients require an unusually high dose of heparin to reach a therapeutic aPTT. For these patients, measuring the anti–factor Xa level is recommended [10,18].

The ACT is used commonly when very high doses of heparin are needed, such as percutaneous angioplasty and cardiopulmonary bypass. At high levels of heparin the aPTT loses sensitivity [19,20]. The ACT has the advantage of being a rapid bedside assay, but does not correlate well with aPTT levels. Studies directly comparing the two tests are lacking, and the ACT is not used routinely outside of cardiac procedures [19].

Adverse effects

The most common adverse effect of UFH is bleeding. This risk is further accentuated in the setting of concomitant aspirin use [21]. In the elderly population extra caution must be given to heparin treatment, because older patients are more likely to have serious bleeding. Elderly patients require a generally lower heparin dose to achieve therapeutic levels. It is for this reason that lower initial bolus doses of UFH are recommended for elderly patients [22]. No studies, however, have directly compared different doses of UFH to assess for bleeding risk [23].

In cases of heparin-related bleeding, supportive care and transfusion therapy should be initiated once heparin has been discontinued. In the setting of severe bleeding, protamine sulfate can be used to rapidly reverse the effect of heparin. One milligram of protamine neutralizes approximately 100 units of UFH [10].

Apart from bleeding, heparin can cause thrombocytopenia, as discussed later. Heparin has also been reported to cause three types of skin lesions infrequently: (1) urticarial lesions, (2) skin necrosis, and (3) erythematous papules and plaques [20]. Finally, heparin can activate osteoclasts in bone, causing osteopenia [10,20]. This is a concern with long-term heparin use, particularly when used for prophylaxis in chronically bed-bound patients. The resulting osteopenia can be devastating for the many elderly patients with underlying osteoporosis and osteopenia, putting them at even greater risk for fractures.

Indications

As the oldest anticoagulant with the most experience, UFH is used for a wide variety of indications. UFH is used for primary prophylaxis of VTE for hospitalized patients at increased risk. Additionally, UFH is indicated for the initial treatment of DVT, pulmonary embolism (PE), ACS, stroke, and during cardiac procedures [12]. Other recent clinical applications include UFH as a surface coating for biomedical devices, as a modulatory agent for growth factors, and as an adjunct to both chemotherapeutic and anti-inflammatory agents [9].

Low-molecular-weight heparin

Pharmacology

LMWH, as its name suggests, is a glycosaminoglycan that is approximately one third the molecular weight of UFH. It is derived from UFH through various depolymerization processes. LMWH binds to antithrombin, which in turn neutralizes factors Xa and IIa. Because LMWH lacks many of the longer chains required for binding to thrombin, it has less ability to neutralize thrombin relative to its ability to neutralize factor Xa [10,24].

LMWH also has less nonspecific binding to other proteins. There is greater bioavailability with more predictable pharmacokinetics that eliminates the need for monitoring. The smaller size also allows for enhanced subcutaneous absorption when compared with UFH.

Dosing

Three LMWH preparations are currently approved for use in the United States: (1) enoxaparin, (2) dalteparin, and (3) tinzaparin. They are all administered subcutaneously at intervals of either once or twice daily for both prophylaxis and treatment doses. A meta-analysis of six studies found that there was no increase in bleeding in once-daily versus twice-daily dosing of LMWH [25]. Because LMWH is renally excreted, administration for treatment of VTE or ACS is not recommended in patients who have a creatinine clearance of less than 30 mL/min. Dose finding trials have yet to be completed for these patients. For thromboprophylaxis, however, enoxaparin can be used in patients with renal failure, at a dose of 40 mg once daily [10,13]. Another group of patients for whom LMWH dosing is unclear is obese patients with weights over 150 kg [10]. For these two groups of patients, monitoring by the anti Xa assay is recommended if LMWH is used.

In the elderly, a population with increased bleeding risks and age-related renal insufficiency, three approaches have been recommended to ensure safety. First, is to use UFH in patients with severe renal disease. Second, is to use reduced dosages in the elderly. This practice has not yet been validated by any studies. Third, LMWH can be monitored by an anti-Xa assay in patients who are deemed to be at higher risk of bleeding or thrombosis [26].

Monitoring

Because LMWH has more predicable pharmacokinetics than UFH, routine monitoring is not performed. The aPTT is not used in monitoring LMWH because the aPTT predominantly measures anti–factor II activity. The more clinically relevant activity to measure in LMWH is anti–factor Xa activity, which is not measured well with the aPTT [10].

Assays for anti–factor Xa activity have been developed and are now available at most clinical laboratories. The question of exactly who should be monitored remains controversial. Many agree that monitoring with anti Xa levels should be considered for the following patient groups: severe obesity, renal insufficiency, and very low body weight [10,18,27].

Adverse effects

The risks of age-related increases in bleeding have not been directly investigated in clinical trials with LMWH [28]. A meta-analysis of 4669 medical patients, however, found that the risk of major bleeding in the setting of prophylactic doses was 52% lower with LMWH when compared with UFH [29]. When used in higher doses in the setting of ACS, consensus from the Seventh American College of Chest Physicians Conference on Antithrombotic and Thrombolytic Therapy was that there was no higher risk of major bleeding with LMWH when compared with UFH [23]. LMWH seems to have a similar, if not improved, safety profile in terms of major bleeding.

With major bleeding, protamine sulfate can be used to reverse partially the anticoagulant effects of LMWH. Anti–factor Xa levels, however, are often not fully normalized [10]. LMWH also has a much longer half-life. In the setting of major bleeding, it takes longer for coagulation to return to normal with LMWH.

Other potential adverse events with the use of LMWH are thrombocytopenia and osteopenia. The risk of HIT with LMWH is discussed later. Although UFH can lead to osteopenia, LMWH has the advantage of reduced activation of osteoclasts, thereby causing less bone loss.

Indications

Of the three LMWHs available in the United States, enoxaparin has the most approved clinical indications, although interchange of agents is common. Enoxaparin is approved for prophylaxis of VTE in selected medical and surgical conditions. A multicenter randomized double-blind study examined rates of VTE in hospitalized elderly medical patients on enoxaparin compared with UFH. The results showed equal efficacy and safety profiles [30]. With LMWH's other benefits of a longer half-life, more predictable pharmacokinetics, decreased effects on platelets, and less activation of osteoclasts, LMWH is often preferred to UFH for VTE prophylaxis.

Enoxaparin is also indicated for treatment of DVT and PE. The movement of DVT treatment to the outpatient setting has revolutionized therapy for the thousands of patients with DVT each year. This is particularly true for the elderly who avoid hospitalization and the complications that often accompany their stay.

Due to recent studies demonstrating both safety and efficacy of enoxaparin in the setting of both ACS and ST-segment elevation myocardial infarction (STEMI), enoxaparin is approved for both of these indications. In a recent meta-analysis of 6 randomized controlled trials of nearly 22,000 patients comparing enoxaparin to UFH, there was a statistically significant difference in the combined endpoint of death or non-fatal myocardial infarction (MI) at 30 days, in favor of enoxaparin [31]. Furthermore, there was no significant difference in blood transfusions or major bleeding. A limitation of this large meta-analysis however, is that patients included in the study had variable rates of cardiac catheterization and use of glycoprotein IIB/IIIA inhibitors. Nonetheless, many practitioners prefer enoxaparin as the initial treatment for ACS given its safety, efficacy, and ease of administration.

Interventional cardiologists have also become more comfortable performing cardiac catheterizations in the setting of enoxaparin, as more safety data has emerged. Previously, invasive stenting was only performed using UFH, as it had a long track record and levels of anticoagulation could be rapidly assessed using bedside ACT assays. With more ACS patients initially treated in the emergency department with enoxaparin however, the question whether it was safe to undergo catheterization and possible stenting while on enoxaparin arose. The SYNERGY trial examined over 10,000 high risk ACS patients in whom an early invasive strategy had already been planned [32]. Patients were randomized to either UFH or enoxaparin and then brought to the catheterization laboratory. There was no difference in the primary efficacy endpoint of all cause death or non-fatal MI at 30 days. There was however a statistically significant increased risk of major bleeding in the enoxaparin arm, using the Thrombosis in Myocardial Infarction (TIMI) definition of major bleeding. Using the definition by the Global Use of Strategies to Open Occluded Coronary Arteries (GUSTO) investigators however, there was no statistically significant increase in major bleeding. Enoxaparin is now widely used in cardiac catheterization laboratories, particularly in ACS patients.

Tinzaparin has a more limited indication profile because it is currently only approved for the initial treatment of DVT and PE in the inpatient setting. Dalteparin has a wider spectrum of approved uses, with indications for DVT prophylaxis and treatment, and for ACS [9].

Pentasaccharides

Pharmacology and monitoring

Fondaparinux sodium is a further refinement of the heparin moiety that binds to antithrombin. The structure of fondaparinux is based on the pentasaccharide region of the heparin molecule specific for antithrombin binding. It is a synthesized molecule rather than being extracted from animal tissue. Fondaparinux selectively inhibits factor Xa by binding to antithrombin. This binding produces a conformational change in the structure of antithrombin, allowing it effectively to inhibit factor Xa [33,34]. Because fondaparinux lacks the longer saccharide chains that bind to thrombin, it has no ability to neutralize thrombin and is entirely specific for factor Xa.

Because of absence of binding to other plasma proteins, fondaparinux has nearly 100% bioavailability and predictable pharmacokinetics. Through the subcutaneous route, it reaches peak plasma level in 2 hours and has an elimination half-life of 17 hours. Clearance is by the kidneys [33]. As a result of the predictable effects of fondaparinux, it is not necessary to monitor its anticoagulant effect. Monitoring is possible however with an anti–factor Xa assay calibrated with fondaparinux [35].

Dosing

Because of the long half-life of fondaparinux, once-daily dosing is available for both treatment and prophylaxis of VTE. This is very attractive, especially for elderly patients in the outpatient setting where no monitoring is necessary. Dose ranging studies have been performed for both treatment and prophylaxis of VTE. For treatment, the suggested dose is 7.5 mg subcutaneous once daily [33]. When comparing the safety and efficacy of fondaparinux with enoxaparin in VTE prophylaxis, all doses of fondaparinux resulted in a lower incidence of VTE [36]. The recommended dose for VTE prophylaxis is 2.5 mg subcutaneous once daily.

Because of its renal excretion, reduced dosage is recommended for patients with moderate renal dysfunction, and contraindicated in those with a creatinine clearance of less than 30 mL/min [37]. Patients who are either underweight or morbidly obese also require alteration in dosage [9].

Adverse effects

Like other anticoagulants, bleeding is the most common complication of fondaparinux. To complicate matters, there is no drug that can reverse the anticoagulant effect of fondaparinux. In the setting of a major bleed, supportive measures and transfusions of fresh frozen plasma or factor concentrates, specifically recombinant factor VIIa, are the only tools available. In the Matisse-PE trial, rates of major bleeding were similar for both fondaparinux and UFH. The incidence was 1.3% in the fondaparinux group compared with 1.1% in the UFH arm [38].

Although thrombocytopenia has rarely been reported with fondaparinux use, the typical HIT and thrombosis syndrome does not occur [9].

Indications

Several recent trials have established the effectiveness of fondaparinux compared with enoxaparin for the prevention of VTE in orthopedic surgery. Two studies examined patients undergoing hip replacement surgery for rates of development of VTE by postoperative day 11. Patients were either administered fondaparinux or enoxaparin in daily subcutaneous doses. With no differences in major bleeding or death, the investigators found relative risk reductions between 26% and 56% for the development of VTE with the use of fondaparinux when compared with enoxaparin

[39,40]. Rates of VTE using fondaparinux also have been examined in hip fracture surgery. A randomized double-blind study of over 1700 patients was conducted where patients received either fondaparinux or enoxaparin for the prevention of VTE postoperatively by day 11. A relative risk reduction of 56.4% was found in favor of fondaparinux [41].

Fondaparinux has also been studied in knee replacement surgery. One trial of more than 1000 patients randomized to fondaparinux versus enoxaparin showed a greater than 50% relative risk reduction for total VTE in the fondaparinux group (12.5% versus 27.8%, $P < .001$), and an almost significant reduction in proximal DVT. Although the fondaparinux group had a higher frequency of major bleeding, there was no statistical difference when comparing the rate of death or re-operation because of bleeding [42].

Extended prophylaxis with fondaparinux was examined in the PENTHIFRA Plus study. The group found that extended prophylaxis for up to 31 days was associated with a VTE relative risk reduction of 96% ($P < .001$) when compared with no prophylaxis. There was also no increase in clinically relevant bleeding [43–45]. While fondaparinux is approved for surgical patients, it is important to note that it is not approved for prophylaxis of VTE in medical patients.

Fondaparinux has also been examined with respect to its efficacy in treatment for DVT and PE. In a double-blind study of 2205 patients with acute DVT randomized between fondaparinux and enoxaparin for the initial treatment, followed by 3 months of warfarin, there was no significant difference in recurrence of VTE (3.9% and 4.1%, respectively) or major bleeding (1.1% and 1.2%, respectively) [46].

A randomized open label noninferiority study involving 2213 patients with hemodynamically stable PE compared efficacy of fondaparinux with UFH. Recurrent DVT-PE occurred in 2.4% of patients treated with fondaparinux compared with 3.6% of patients treated with UFH. Rates of major bleeding were also similar, 1.3% for fondaparinux and 1.1% for UFH [38]. Fondaparinux is currently approved for the inpatient treatment of PE, and for both the inpatient and outpatient treatment of DVT.

Off label indications

While fondaparinux has only been approved for both prevention and treatment of VTE, there has been extensive research involving its use in ACS and cardiac catheterization patients. In the Oasis 5 trial, investigators randomized ACS patients to receive either enoxaparin or fondaparinux (2.5 mg dose) [47]. Groups had similar endpoints of death, MI, or refractory ischemia at 9 days, and the fondaparinux group had a trend toward reduced endpoints at 30 and 180 days. Major bleeding was significantly less with fondaparinux (2.2% versus 4.1%, $P < .001$). It is interesting to note that the dosage of fondaparinux for ACS is lower than that for VTE. The PENTUA study was a dose finding study for patients with ACS comparing doses of 2.5 mg, 4 mg, 8 mg, and 12 mg [48]. There was no difference in the primary composite endpoint of death, MI, or recurrent ischemia. Thus, the lower, 2.5 mg dose is the one most commonly used in ACS.

The Oasis 6 trial then randomized STEMI patients to receive fondaparinux versus placebo when no UFH was indicated or to fondaparinux versus UFH, when an anticoagulant was indicated [49]. Fondaparinux showed a reduction in the endpoint of death or reinfarction at 30 days, but only in patients not undergoing percutaneous coronary intervention (PCI). Since PCI is the preferred treatment strategy for patients with STEMI, it is unlikely that fondaparinux will be approved for use in this setting.

Fondaparinux has also been studied in the setting of elective and urgent PCI in the ASPIRE trial [50]. Investigators randomized 350 patients to either UFH, 2.5 mg of fondaparinux, or 5 mg of fondaparinux. Patients were also stratified to use of glycoprotein IIB/IIIA inhibitors. The groups had similar safety and efficacy, with a trend lower bleeding with the lower fondaparinux dose.

Heparin-induced thrombocytopenia

Pathophysiology and diagnosis

There are two forms of HIT: an early benign form that is non-immune mediated, and a second more dangerous immune-mediated form [20]. In the latter case, an IgG antibody–mediated activation of platelets occurs that can lead to severe thrombocytopenia and life-threatening thrombosis. Heparin binds to platelet factor 4, an endogenous platelet protein released from platelets, and in some cases induces an immune response to a newly formed epitope [51]. The IgG bound to the heparin–platelet factor 4 complex may then bind to Fc receptors on the platelet surface, and

by so doing activate platelets leading to the generation of prothrombotic platelet microparticles or to the aggregation of platelets [52]. In the process, thrombocytopenia occurs, and in 25% to 50% of patients a paradoxical thrombosis may occur in either the venous or arterial circulation.

For patients receiving heparin in treatment or prophylaxis doses, platelet monitoring is recommended every-other or every-third day for the first 7 to 14 days. The diagnosis of HIT should be suspected in any patients receiving heparin or having an exposure in the previous 3 months who develop a drop in platelets by greater than 50%, an absolute count of less than 150,000, or a new thrombotic event. Heparin-dependant IgG antibodies should be measured, if available, but a diagnosis of HIT is usually based on clinical criteria. These criteria include thrombocytopenia in the presence of heparin or its recent use and exclusion of other causes. There are no data to support the testing for HIT antibodies in the absence of any clinical evidence of HIT. The risk for development of HIT is greatest in post surgical patients, followed by medical patients, and least likely in the setting of pregnancy [53].

Heparin-induced thrombocytopenia with other anticoagulants

HIT can occur with LMWH, although much less frequently than with UFH [54]. In a study of 665 patients randomized to UFH or enoxaparin for prophylaxis of VTE after hip surgery, HIT occurred in 9 of 332 in the heparin group compared with 0 of 333 in the enoxaparin group ($P = .0018$). In addition, eight of the nine patients with HIT also had evidence of thrombosis [54].

Although patients exposed to fondaparinux may test positive for heparin-dependent IgG antibodies, there is no evidence that fondaparinux leads to immune-mediated HIT [55]. For patients with a history of HIT, fondaparinux is being studied as an acceptable alternative for VTE prophylaxis.

Treatment of heparin-induced thrombocytopenia

When HIT is diagnosed, it is important to stop heparin and to avoid the use of LMWH [53]. Because of the increased risk of thrombosis, however, continuation of an anticoagulant must be considered. The drugs currently approved for the treatment of HIT in the United States are direct thrombin inhibitors argatroban and lepirudin (Table 2). These drugs are to be used whether or not clinically evident thrombosis is present.

Table 2
Dosing guidelines for lepirudin and argatroban in heparin-induced thrombocytopenia

Medication	Dosing route	Dose	Adjustments	Monitoring
Lepirudin	IV	0.4 mg/kg bolus then 0.15 mg/kg/h	Adjustment for renal impairment	aPTT
Argatroban	IV	2 µg/kg/min	Adjustment for hepatic impairment	aPTT

Abbreviations: aPTT, activated partial thromboplastin time; IV, intravenous.

Lepirudin is a recombinant form of the naturally occurring substance hirudin. Patients treated with lepirudin can develop drug-specific antibodies that have an unpredictable effect on the anticoagulant activity. In 45% of patients, anticoagulant activity is enhanced, whereas in 6% the activity is suppressed [56]. Close monitoring of the aPTT is necessary to prevent both bleeding and thrombotic complications of treatment. In the combined analysis of the HAT 1, 2, and 3 studies, which looked at HIT patients treated with lepirudin against historical controls, patients receiving lepirudin had fewer thrombotic events, but an unchanged rate of death [57].

Argatroban has a rapid onset of action and reversibility. Unlike lepirudin, there is no antibody formation with argatroban, so its anticoagulant properties are more predictable. Monitoring is achieved with the aPTT in low doses and the ACT in higher doses [58,59]. Caution must be used, however, in the setting of hepatic dysfunction because argatroban is metabolized by the liver [60]. The recommended dose for patients with hepatic dysfunction is 0.5 mcg/kg/min [61]. Argatroban has been demonstrated to reduce new thrombosis and death, but only compared with historical controls [62,63].

Argatroban is approved for both HIT and as an adjunct for PCI in the United States for both patients with and without HIT. Bivalirudin has similar indications to argatroban, as an adjunct for PCI in patients at risk for HIT, with HIT, and the general population. It is not approved however for the treatment of HIT independent of PCI.

Summary

UFH, LMWH, and fondaparinux each have advantages and disadvantages in the treatment and prophylaxis of VTE in the elderly and in the setting of ACS (Table 3). UFH's nonspecific binding to other plasma proteins makes achieving a therapeutic level difficult, and bleeding a significant risk. LMWH is safe in the elderly, although it needs to be used cautiously in patients with creatinine clearance less than 30 mL/min or those weighing over 150 kg. The anti–factor Xa activity level may be used in these settings. Fondaparinux, the newest of the group, seems to be effective and safe in the elderly. It also has the advantage of not causing HIT.

HIT occurs in the setting of UFH or less likely LMWH use and is manifested by thrombocytopenia and/or thrombosis. Argatroban or lepirudin, direct thrombin inhibitors, are recommended to increase platelets and prevent thrombosis in these patients with HIT.

With the ever aging population, the future will demand a better understanding of medications used for conditions like VTE and ACS that increase in prevalence with increasing age. Anticoagulants need to be further examined in elderly patients, because they carry potentially fatal risks if underdosed or overdosed. Few trials include patients at extremes of age, and such issues as normal age-related decreases in renal function and different volumes of distribution have not been adequately addressed. More trials need to be conducted that include large numbers of patients

Table 3
Comparison of pharmacokinetics and other aspects of commonly used anticoagulants

Medication	Dosing route	Half life	Excretion	Monitoring	Adverse effects
Unfractionated heparin	IV or SQ	~1 hour	Metabolized by liver, excreted by kidneys	aPTT or ACT	Bleeding, HIT, osteopenia
Low-molecular-weight heparin	SQ	3–7 h	Metabolized by liver, excreted by kidneys	None or Anti-factor Xa activity	Bleeding, HIT (less than UFH)
Fondaparinux	SQ	~20 h	Renal	None	Bleeding

Abbreviations: ACT, activated clotting time; aPTT, activated partial thromboplastin time; HIT, heparin-induced thrombocytopenia; IV, intravenous; SQ, subcutaneous.

over the age of 65 so that anticoagulation may be better understood in this growing population.

References

[1] Berman AR, Arnsten JH. Diagnosis and treatment of pulmonary embolism in the elderly. Clin Geriatr Med 2003;19:157–75.

[2] Oger E. Incidence of venous thromboembolism: a community-based study in Western France. EPI-GETBP Study Group. Groupe d'Etude de la Thrombose de Bretagne Occidentale. Thromb Haemost 2000;83:657–60.

[3] Oger E, Bressollette L, Nonent M, et al. High prevalence of asymptomatic deep vein thrombosis on admission in a medical unit among elderly patients. Thromb Haemost 2002;88:592–7.

[4] Jacobs LG. Prophylactic anticoagulation for venous thromboembolic disease in geriatric patients. J Am Geriatr Soc 2003;51:1472–8.

[5] Kniffin WD Jr, Baron JA, Barrett J, et al. The epidemiology of diagnosed pulmonary embolism and deep venous thrombosis in the elderly. Arch Intern Med 1994;154:861–6.

[6] Leizorovicz A, Mismetti P. Preventing venous thromboembolism in medical patients. Circulation 2004;110(Suppl 1):IV13–9.

[7] Goldhaber SZ, Dunn K, MacDougall RC. New onset of venous thromboembolism among hospitalized patients at Brigham and Women's Hospital is caused more often by prophylaxis failure than by withholding treatment. Chest 2000;118:1680–4.

[8] Ansell J. Anticoagulation, acute and chronic: indications and methods. In: Alpert J, editor. Cardiology for the primary care physician. 3rd edition. Philadelphia: Current Medicine; 2001. p. 407–18.

[9] Hoppensteadt D, Walenga JM, Fareed J, et al. Heparin, low-molecular-weight heparins, and heparin pentasaccharide: basic and clinical differentiation. Hematol Oncol Clin North Am 2003;17:313–41.

[10] Hirsh J, Raschke R. Heparin and low-molecular-weight heparin: the Seventh ACCP Conference on Antithrombotic and Thrombolytic Therapy. Chest 2004;126(Suppl 3):188S–203S.

[11] Hirsh J. Heparin. N Engl J Med 1991;324:1565–74.

[12] Hirsh J, Warkentin TE, Shaughnessy SG, et al. Heparin and low-molecular-weight heparin: mechanisms of action, pharmacokinetics, dosing, monitoring, efficacy, and safety. Chest 2001;119(Suppl 1):64S–94S.

[13] Rich MW. The management of venous thromboembolic disease in older adults. J Gerontol A Biol Sci Med Sci 2004;59:34–41.

[14] Heit JA, Silverstein MD, Mohr DN, et al. The epidemiology of venous thromboembolism in the community. Thromb Haemost 2001;86:452–63.

[15] de Groot MR, Buller HR, ten Cate JW, et al. Use of a heparin nomogram for treatment of patients with venous thromboembolism in a community hospital. Thromb Haemost 1998;80:70–3.

[16] Bernardi E, Piccioli A, Oliboni G, et al. Nomograms for the administration of unfractionated heparin in the initial treatment of acute thromboembolism: an overview. Thromb Haemost 2000;84:22–6.

[17] Hylek EM, Regan S, Henault LE, et al. Challenges to the effective use of unfractionated heparin in the hospitalized management of acute thrombosis. Arch Intern Med 2003;163:621–7.

[18] Kitchen S. Problems in laboratory monitoring of heparin dosage. Br J Haematol 2000;111:397–406.

[19] Simko RJ, Tsung FF, Stanek EJ. Activated clotting time versus activated partial thromboplastin time for therapeutic monitoring of heparin. Ann Pharmacother 1995;29:1015–21.

[20] Hirsh J, Raschke R, Warkentin TE, et al. Heparin: mechanism of action, pharmacokinetics, dosing considerations, monitoring, efficacy, and safety. Chest 1995;108(Suppl 4):258S–75S.

[21] Sethi GK, Copeland JG, Goldman S, et al. Implications of preoperative administration of aspirin in patients undergoing coronary artery bypass grafting. Department of Veterans Affairs cooperative study on antiplatelet therapy. J Am Coll Cardiol 1990; 15:15–20.

[22] Campbell NR, Hull RD, Brant R, et al. Aging and heparin-related bleeding. Arch Intern Med 1996; 156:857–60.

[23] Levine MN, Raskob G, Beyth RJ, et al. Hemorrhagic complications of anticoagulant treatment: the Seventh ACCP Conference on Antithrombotic and Thrombolytic Therapy. Chest 2004;126(Suppl 3): 287S–310S.

[24] Weitz JI. Low-molecular-weight heparins. N Engl J Med 1997;337:688–98.

[25] Couturaud F, Julian JA, Kearon C. Low molecular weight heparin administered once versus twice daily in patients with venous thromboembolism: a meta-analysis. Thromb Haemost 2001;86:980–4.

[26] Siguret V, Pautas E, Gouin I. Low molecular weight heparin treatment in elderly subjects with or without renal insufficiency: new insights between June 2002 and March 2004. Curr Opin Pulm Med 2004;10: 366–70.

[27] Mismetti P, Laporte-Simitsidis S, Navarro C, et al. Aging and venous thromboembolism influence the pharmacodynamics of the anti-factor Xa and antithrombin activities of a low molecular weight heparin (nadroparin). Thromb Haemost 1998;79:1162–5.

[28] Di Minno G, Tufano A. Challenges in the prevention of venous thromboembolism in the elderly. J Thromb Haemost 2004;2:1292–8.

[29] Mismetti P, Laporte-Simitsidis S, Tardy B, et al. Prevention of venous thromboembolism in internal medicine with unfractionated or low-molecular-weight heparins: a meta-analysis of randomised clinical trials. Thromb Haemost 2000;83:14–9.

[30] Bergmann JF, Neuhart E. A multicenter randomized double-blind study of enoxaparin compared with unfractionated heparin in the prevention of

venous thromboembolic disease in elderly inpatients bedridden for an acute medical illness. The Enoxaparin in Medicine Study Group. Thromb Haemost 1996;76:529–34.

[31] Peterson JL, Mahaffey KW, Hasselblad v, et al. Efficacy and bleeding complications among patients randomized to enoxaparin or unfractionated heparin for antithrombin therapy in non-ST-segment elevation acute coronary syndrome. JAMA 2004; 292:89–96.

[32] Fergusen JJ, Califf RM, Antman EM, et al. Enoxaparin vs unfractionated heparin in high-risk patients with non-ST-segment elevation acute coronary syndromes managed with an early invasive strategy: primary results of the SYNERGY randomized trial. JAMA 2004;292:45–54.

[33] Samama MM, Gerotziafas GT. Evaluation of the pharmacological properties and clinical results of the synthetic pentasaccharide (fondaparinux). Thromb Res 2003;109:1–11.

[34] Turpie AG. Pentasaccharides. Semin Hematol 2002; 39:158–71.

[35] Paolucci F, Frasa H, Van Aarle F, et al. Two sensitive and rapid chromogenic assays of fondaparinux sodium (Arixtra) in human plasma and other biological matrices. Clin Lab 2003;49:451–60.

[36] Turpie AG, Gallus AS, Hoek JA. A synthetic pentasaccharide for the prevention of deep-vein thrombosis after total hip replacement. N Engl J Med 2001; 344:619–25.

[37] Bauer KA, Hawkins DW, Peters PC, et al. Fondaparinux, a synthetic pentasaccharide: the first in a new class of antithrombotic agents–the selective factor Xa inhibitors. Cardiovasc Drug Rev 2002; 20:37–52.

[38] Buller HR, Davidson BL, Decousus H, et al. Subcutaneous fondaparinux versus intravenous unfractionated heparin in the initial treatment of pulmonary embolism. N Engl J Med 2003;349: 1695–702.

[39] Lassen MR, Bauer KA, Eriksson BI, et al. Postoperative fondaparinux versus preoperative enoxaparin for prevention of venous thromboembolism in elective hip-replacement surgery: a randomised double-blind comparison. Lancet 2002;359:1715–20.

[40] Turpie AG, Bauer KA, Eriksson BI, et al. Postoperative fondaparinux versus postoperative enoxaparin for prevention of venous thromboembolism after elective hip-replacement surgery: a randomised double-blind trial. Lancet 2002;359:1721–6.

[41] Eriksson BI, Bauer KA, Lassen MR, et al. Fondaparinux compared with enoxaparin for the prevention of venous thromboembolism after hip-fracture surgery. N Engl J Med 2001;345:1298–304.

[42] Bauer KA, Eriksson BI, Lassen MR, et al. Fondaparinux compared with enoxaparin for the prevention of venous thromboembolism after elective major knee surgery. N Engl J Med 2001;345: 1305–10.

[43] Eriksson BI, Lassen MR. Duration of prophylaxis against venous thromboembolism with fondaparinux after hip fracture surgery: a multicenter, randomized, placebo-controlled, double blind study. Arch Intern Med 2003;163:1337–42.

[44] Turpie AG. Overview of the clinical results of pentasaccharide in major orthopedic surgery. Haematologica 2001;86(Suppl 2):59–62.

[45] Turpie AG, Bauer KA, Eriksson BI, et al. Fondaparinux vs enoxaparin for the prevention of venous thromboembolism in major orthopedic surgery: a meta-analysis of 4 randomized double blind studies. Arch Intern Med 2002;162:1833–40.

[46] Buller HR, Davidson BL, Decousus H, et al. Fondaparinux or enoxaparin for the initial treatment of symptomatic deep venous thrombosis: a randomized trial. Ann Intern Med 2004;140:867–73.

[47] Yusuf S, Mehta SR, Chrolavicius S, et al. Comparison of fondaparinux and enoxaparin in acute coronary syndromes. N Engl J Med 2006;354:1464–76.

[48] Simoons ML, Bobbink IW, Boland J, et al. A dose-finding study of fondaparinux in patients with non-ST-segment elevation acute coronary syndromes: the Pentasaccharide in Unstable Angina (PENTUA) Study. J Am Coll Cardiol 2004;43:2183–90.

[49] Yusuf S, Mehta SR, Chrolavicius S, et al. Effects of fondaparinux on mortality and reinfarction in patients with acute ST-segment elevation myocardial infarction: the OASIS-6 randomized trial. JAMA 2006;295:1519–30.

[50] Mehta SR, Steg PG, Granger CB, et al. Randomized, blinded trial comparing fondaparinux with unfractionated heparin in patients undergoing contemporary percutaneous coronary intervention. Circulation 2005;111:1390–7.

[51] Greinacher A. Antigen generation in heparin-associated thrombocytopenia: the non immunologic type and the immunologic type are closely linked in their pathogenesis. Semin Thromb Hemost 1995;21: 106–16.

[52] Warkentin TE, Kelton JG. A 14-year study of heparin-induced thrombocytopenia. Am J Med 1996;101: 502–7.

[53] Warkentin TE, Greinacher A. Heparin-induced thrombocytopenia: recognition, treatment, and prevention: the Seventh ACCP Conference on Antithrombotic and Thrombolytic Therapy. Chest 2004; 126(Suppl 3):311S–37S.

[54] Warkentin TE, Levine MN, Hirsh J, et al. Heparin-induced thrombocytopenia in patients treated with low-molecular-weight heparin or unfractionated heparin. N Engl J Med 1995;332:1330–5.

[55] Ahmad S, Jeske WP, Walenga JM, et al. Synthetic pentasaccharides do not cause platelet activation by antiheparin-platelet factor 4 antibodies. Clin Appl Thromb Hemost 1999;5:259–66.

[56] Eichler P, Friesen HJ, Lubenow N, et al. Antihirudin antibodies in patients with heparin-induced thrombocytopenia treated with lepirudin: incidence, effects

on aPTT, and clinical relevance. Blood 2000;96: 2373–8.

[57] Lubenow N, Eichler P, Lietz T, et al. Lepirudin in patients with heparin-induced thrombocytopenia-results of the third prospective study (HAT-3) and a combined analysis of HAT-1, HAT-2, and HAT-3. J Thromb Haemost 2005;3:2428–36.

[58] Walenga JM. An overview of the direct thrombin inhibitor argatroban. Pathophysiol Haemost Thromb 2002;32(Suppl 3):9–14.

[59] Walenga JM, Ahmad S, Hoppensteadt D, et al. Argatroban therapy does not generate antibodies that alter its anticoagulant activity in patients with heparin-induced thrombocytopenia. Thromb Res 2002;105:401–5.

[60] Swan SK, Hursting MJ. The pharmacokinetics and pharmacodynamics of argatroban: effects of age, gender, and hepatic or renal dysfunction. Pharmacotherapy 2000;20:318–29.

[61] Levine RL, Hursting MJ, McCollum D. Argatroban therapy in heparin-induced thrombocytopenia with hepatic dysfunction. Chest 2006;129:1167–75.

[62] Lewis BE, Wallis DE, Berkowitz SD, et al. Argatroban anticoagulant therapy in patients with heparin-induced thrombocytopenia. Circulation 2001;103: 1838–43.

[63] Lewis BE, Wallis DE, Leya F, et al. Argatroban anticoagulation in patients with heparin-induced thrombocytopenia. Arch Intern Med 2003;163: 1849–56.

ELSEVIER
SAUNDERS

CARDIOLOGY
CLINICS

Cardiol Clin 26 (2008) 157–167

Warfarin Pharmacology, Clinical Management, and Evaluation of Hemorrhagic Risk for the Elderly

Laurie G. Jacobs, MD

Albert Einstein College of Medicine and Montefiore Medical Center, 111 East 210 Street, Bronx, NY 10467, USA

More than sixty years ago it was observed that cattle, after consuming sweet clover hay, frequently died from hemorrhage. Bishydroxycoumarin, or dicoumarol, was identified as the causative agent, and this discovery ultimately led to the subsequent synthesis of warfarin. Warfarin, a vitamin K antagonist, is currently the most extensively used oral anticoagulant world-wide. It is prescribed for a variety of indications, including primary and secondary prevention of venous thromboembolism, prevention of systemic embolism and stroke in patients with prosthetic heart valves and atrial fibrillation (AF), primary prevention of myocardial infarction, and in the acute management of myocardial infarction for prevention of stroke, recurrent infarction, and death [1]. Warfarin has undergone extensive clinical study, and may be used for other conditions as well.

Despite wide usage and considerable accumulated data from clinical trials demonstrating efficacy for a variety of thrombotic and thromboembolic conditions, wafarin is underutilized because its management is complex for both patients and physicians. For example, pooled data from a number of clinical trials has demonstrated that warfarin provides a 64% relative risk reduction for stroke in patients with AF [2]. In addition, in a study undertaken in Britain, stroke prophylaxis with warfarin for patients with AF has been demonstrated to be cost-saving relative to the cost of a stroke, inclusive of drug costs, monitoring, transportation, work missed, nursing visits, and costs associated with complications (bleeding-related visits, hospital admissions and procedures)

[3], yet warfarin remains underused for thromboprophylaxis in patients with AF.

Warfarin use for stroke prevention for patients with AF increased from 28% during 1991 to 1992, to 41% in the United States during 1999 to 2000 [4]. The greatest increase occurred in patients aged 80 years and older. In a 2003 national study undertaken in Ireland, in patients aged 75 or more 26% were on warfarin, 50% on aspirin, and 3% on both [5]. Despite an increase in use, these statistics still reflect under-use in the elderly, who often sustain the greatest risk for thromboembolic events [6]. There are many reasons for this, including physicians' perception and estimation of the potential risks associated with warfarin use—specifically bleeding—as well as incidence of thromboembolic events and magnitude of benefit provided by warfarin therapy for a given indication [7]. Warfarin use is also limited by the difficulty in managing this medication. It has a narrow therapeutic window, wide variability in dose-response across individuals, a significant number of drug and dietary interactions, and requires close laboratory monitoring with frequent dose adjustment. Despite these limitations, warfarin can be managed with relative safety, even in an elderly population in which many of these issues play a role.

Pharmacology

Mechanism of action

Warfarin is an anticoagulant that acts by inhibiting the vitamin K-dependent coagulation factors II (prothrombin), VII, IX, and X. It also has activity against the regulatory anticoagulant proteins C, S, and Z, which provides the potential for warfarin to act as a procoagulant as well.

A version of this article originally appeared in *Clinics in Geriatric Medicine*, volume 22, issue 1.

E-mail address: lajacobs@montefiore.org

Warfarin inhibits the interconversion of vitamin K and its vitamin K 2,3 epoxide, which modulates the γ-carboxylation of glutamate residues on the N-terminal regions of the coagulation proteins.

The efficacy of warfarin is usually attributed to its anticoagulant effect through suppression of synthesis of the vitamin K-dependent coagulation factors (II, IV, IX, and X). Some research seems to suggest that the antithrombotic effect (rather than simply the anticoagulant effect) is more closely associated with the reduction in prothrombin (II) and factor X levels. Prothrombin decreases the ability to generate thrombin, the main modulator of clot formation. A reduction in thrombin levels, which is involved in the clot and bound to fibrin, is thought to reduce thrombogenicity in addition to an anticoagulant effect [1].

Pharmacokinetics and pharmacodynamics

Warfarin exists as a racemic mixture of R and S enantiomers, with the S enantiomer having about two to five times greater intrinsic activity, although it is more rapidly cleared. Warfarin is readily absorbed after oral administration, with peak concentration within 4 hours. Concern about alterations in absorption with different formulations of warfarin have generally been unfounded [8], although a study in one country where universal generic substitution was undertaken indicated that the generic warfarin may have somewhat reduced bioavailability, particularly in the lowest doses [9].

Approximately 99% of warfarin is bound to plasma proteins. Warfarin is almost entirely eliminated through stereoselective metabolism by hepatic microsomal enzymes cytochrome P450-2C9 (CYP2C9) [10,11], with an effective mean half-life of 40 hours [12]. There are several variants of the gene that encode the hepatic microsomal enzyme P450-2C9 found among different ethnic groups, which have been associated with an increase in adverse clinical outcomes [1]. In the future, identification of these mutations for clinical testing may enable more specific dosing recommendations when warfarin therapy is initiated. A mutation in the gene encoding the enzyme responsible for oxidizing the S-isomer is common, producing an increased response to warfarin, and thus reduced dose requirements. Hepatic dysfunction can increase the response through impaired synthesis of clotting factors as well as decreased metabolism of the drug. Warfarin resistance is a very rare condition in which alteration of the receptor is present. Patients with a low body weight [13,14], low serum albumin, significant congestive heart failure, liver disease, or other medications with interactions may require lower doses. Renal clearance does not play a significant role in the response to warfarin.

Although there are no alterations in the pharmacokinetics of warfarin with age, older adults appear to exhibit a greater pharmacodynamic response to warfarin. There is a greater increase in the prothrombin time (PT) and international normalized ratio (INR) in response to the same dose in an older adult. The etiology of this effect is unknown.

Interactions with pharmaceutic and herbal compounds

The dose-response to warfarin varies significantly between individuals because of intrinsic genetic factors, concurrent consumption of other drugs, dietary factors, and comorbid disease states, each of which can affect its metabolism. Drug interactions that alter the pharmacokinetics of warfarin may include alterations in absorption (eg, cholestyramine), which would decrease the anticoagulant effect. Many drug interactions with warfarin are caused by alterations in metabolism either by 2C9 enzyme induction [15], which increases warfarin clearance and thereby reducing antithrombotic activity (eg, phenytoin, rifampin) [16], or stereoselective and nonselective enzyme inhibition (eg, amiodarone, cimetidine, sulfamethoxazole, metronidazole) [17], which increase its antithrombotic effect (and the INR). Reduced plasma-binding because of the presence of excessively albumin-bound drugs, causing an increase in free drug and therefore an increase in antithrombotic activity, is much more uncommon. Stereoselective interactions that inhibit the metabolism of the S-enantiomer preferentially will have a greater impact on the INR than those interacting with the R-enantiomer; a drug such as amiodarone [18] has a very significant impact because of its interaction with both. In addition, amiodarone, for example, may exhibit its interaction with warfarin over an extended period of time, as it is loaded slowly.

Pharmacodynamic interactions may include synergism because of impaired hemostasis (eg, with use of aspirin as an antiplatelet agent), reduced clotting factor synthesis (liver disease), competitive antagonism (dietary vitamin K), and alterations in the vitamin K control loop and receptor, causing warfarin resistance, an uncommon condition. The use of analgesic medications with warfarin in elderly individuals often presents the potential for interactions. In addition to the synergism with salicylates and nonsteroidal anti-inflammatory (NSAIDS) medications causing bleeding because of their antiplatelet effect as well as their potential to cause gastric ulceration, doses of salicylates greater than 1.5 grams per day [19] may increase the activity of warfarin (and the INR) because of interference with the microsomal P450 system. Even low dose aspirin (75 mg–100 mg) administered concurrently with warfarin is associated with increased rates of bleeding [20,21]. Weekly doses of 2,275 mg to 4,579 mg of acetaminophen has been associated with an increase in the INR to 6 or greater in a cohort of anticoagulation clinic patients [22].

Information regarding interactions of warfarin with herbal medications is limited but growing [23]. An interaction with ginkgo attributed to an inhibition of CYP2C9 [16] was described in several studies; however, a controlled trial failed to demonstrate this interaction [24]. Hyperforin found in St. John's wort has been credited with causing induction of the CYP2C9 microsomal enzymes and reducing the anticoagulant effect of warfarin [25]. Ginseng has also been found to inhibit warfarin. It has been postulated that ginseng accelerates the clearance of warfarin [16], but gingenosides have also been reported to alter platelet aggregation in vitro and cause an increase in bleeding in surgical patients [26]. An interaction between dietary supplements of fish oils (2 grams per day or more) and warfarin, causing an increase in the INR, has been described in a study. This interaction is attributed to the eicosapentaneoic acid and docosahexanoic acid of the omega-3-polyunsaturated fatty acids [27]. A registry of anticoagulant interactions with supplements is available at http://www.clotcare.com.

A detailed listing of prescription drug interactions with warfarin can be found in the drug labeling, other references, or through the use of computerized drug interaction programs. Data regarding interactions with herbal preparations are more difficult to obtain. In addition, many of the studies investigating drug interactions with warfarin were undertaken at a time when inclusion of elderly subjects was not required by the United States Food and Drug Administration or internationally. In addition, such studies are often undertaken with one compound at a time. Elderly individuals taking multiple medications

may be subject to unanticipated interactions. Because of the numerous potential drug interactions and the variable nature of these interactions in terms of direction (increase or decrease the INR), intensity, and timing, it is essential to closely monitor the INR when adding or eliminating a drug from a patient's regimen when that patient is concurrently taking warfarin.

Interactions caused by vitamin K, diet, and concomitant disease

Vitamin K is a fat-soluble vitamin generally derived from phylloquinones in plant material that can alter warfarin's dose-response relationship significantly [28]. Patient education is essential to develop a diet with a relatively constant level of vitamin K and to identify foods rich in vitamin K. Dietary supplements (Table 1) and specialized vitamin and mineral supplements, such as Viactiv, a popular calcium supplement, may also contain vitamin K and be administered unknowingly to older adults receiving warfarin. Patients taking warfarin should be educated to examine nutritional labeling of foods and dietary supplements. Grapefruit juice, however, does not appear to alter the anticoagulant response to warfarin [29].

A variety of medications, foods, and comorbid diseases can interfere with absorption, as well as intestinal bacterial synthesis of vitamin K. Serious comorbid diseases leading to poor oral intake and malnutrition can cause an increase in the activity of warfarin because of a decline in vitamin K intake, stores, and hepatic synthesis of clotting factors. Broad-spectrum antibiotics can alter the production of vitamin K by gastrointestinal flora, particularly in patients with poor nutrition and limited stores. Chronic alcohol use can increase the clearance of warfarin [1], but the presence of concomitant liver disease can potentiate the action of warfarin. Significant wine use in patients taking warfarin apparently has little effect on the PT [30]. The metabolic rate has an impact upon warfarin metabolism as well; increased catabolism of coagulation factors occurs with fever, excess use of thyroxine, and hyperthyroidism.

Warfarin skin necrosis

Warfarin skin necrosis is the most serious adverse effect of warfarin outside of the risk of hemorrhage, and is induced by a transient hypercoagulable state. This is often associated with the administration of large loading doses of warfarin,

Table 1
Selected nutritional supplements and dietary vitamin K[1]

Product	Vitamin K (% daily needs)
Novartis Boost Drink	40
Novartis Boost/High Protein	40
Novartis Boost Breeze	0
Novartis Boost Plus	40
Novartis Boost Pudding	25
Equate	25
Equate; Plus	25
Ross Ensure; Plus	25
Ross Ensure; with calcium	35
Ross Ensure; with fiber	25
Ross Ensure	25
Ross Ensure High Protein	25
Ross Ensure Plus HN	25
Ross Ensure Powder	15
Ross Ensure Pudding	15
Ross AlitraQ	54 mg
Ross Enlive!	25
Ross Glucerna Meal Bars	28 mg
Ross Glucerna Shake	25
Ross Glucerna Snack Bars	15
Ross ProSure Shake	20 mg/8 fl oz
Ross NutriFocus	20 mg/8 fl oz
NESTLÉ Carnation Instant Breakfast Powder	24
NESTLÉ Carnation Instant Breakfast Ready-To-Drink	24
NESTLÉ Carnation Instant Breakfast for the Carb Conscious	24
NESTLÉ Carnation Instant Breakfast Lactose Free	11
NESTLÉ Carnation Instant Breakfast Lactose Free Plus	17
NESTLÉ Carnation Instant Breakfast Lactose Free VHC	35
NESTLÉ Carnation Instant Breakfast Juice Drink	5
Novartis Resource Standard	25
Novartis Resource Plus	25
Novartis Resource Fruit Beverage	15
Novartis Resource Arginaid EXTRA	20
Novartis Impact Recover	20
Novartis Novasource 2.0	25

Ensure, AlitraQ, Enlive!, Glucerna, Prosure and NutriFocus are registered trademarks of Ross Products, a division of Abbott Laboratories.

Boost, Resource, Resource Plus, Impact Recover, Arginaid and NovaSource are registered trademarks of the Novartis Company.

Equate is a registered trademark of the Solartek Dist. Company.

Carnation Instant Breakfast is a registered trademark of the Nestle Corporation.

Adapted from http://www.ptinr.com/data/templates/article.aspx?articleid=192&zoneid=1.

and may effect individuals with congenital or acquired protein C or S deficiency, acquired functional protein C deficiency, and factor V Leiden [31,32]. Affected individuals develop skin lesions within several days. They begin as an erythematous macule that, if untreated, progresses to an indurated lesion with purpuric regions, which ultimately becomes necrotic.

Clinical management

Optimal therapeutic range

The response to warfarin can be assessed through use of the PT. The PT increases, as compared with a control value, with a reduction in levels of factors II, VII, and X, each according to their half-life, because of warfarin suppression of new synthesis of the vitamin K-dependent factors. The PT test requires thromboplastin. Different thromboplastins vary in responsiveness, as quantified by their international sensitivity index (ISI). The INR is a standardized method of monitoring and reporting the response to warfarin. It is calculated from the PT, which has been calibrated for the ISI of the thromboplastin used. With administration of warfarin, the INR initially increases because of a reduction of factor VII, which has a 6-hour half-life, the shortest of the vitamin K-dependent coagulation factors. Despite the early change in INR, however, the suppression of factor VII levels confers a minor antithrombotic effect.

The optimal intensity of warfarin treatment for the major clinical indications, as designated by a range of values for the INR [1], has been determined by consensus, informed by clinical trials, case series, and other studies. These guidelines for the target INR reflect differences in the thrombogenic potential of various conditions, and therefore vary according to the indication. The upper limit of the therapeutic range for a given indication reflects data regarding bleeding risk along with thrombogenic potential. The lower limit of the recommended range is determined by efficacy of various intensities of the warfarin examined. When prescribing therapy for an individual patient, however, an individual assessment of bleeding risk and thrombogenic potential, based upon risk factors, is needed. The use of a lower target for the INR in older adults (ie, "low dose" warfarin) is controversial and may not be supported by current data for various indications [33,34].

Initiation of therapy

As the anticoagulant and antithrombotic effects of warfarin take several days to occur. Patients at immediate risk require concurrent treatment with other anticoagulants, such as heparin or low molecular weight heparins. Heparin is usually continued until the INR is the therapeutic range. Heparin at therapeutic levels has a minimal impact on the INR.

A number of investigators have sought to identify the ideal regimen for initiating warfarin therapy. Several studies undertaken in the hospital setting indicate that larger loading doses (20 mg) provide no advantage in achieving a therapeutic level in a timely fashion, often leading to a high INR, and have a greater potential to induce a transient hypercoagulable state by causing a sudden decrease in protein C during the first 36 hours of warfarin therapy. Furthermore, initiation with a 5-mg initial dose was found to be superior to 10 mg [35,36]. A study of subjects treated with warfarin after heart valve replacement, who were randomized to receive an initial dose of either 2.5 mg or 5 mg of warfarin, showed that the lower dose was more effective [37]. Conversely, in subjects with acute venous thrombosis in whom warfarin was initiated in the out-patient setting, initial administration of 10 mg of warfarin allowed a more rapid achievement of a therapeutic INR [38]. This sample, however, did not consist of exclusively elderly patients.

Subsequent dosing also requires careful selection of dose amounts. In a recent study of warfarin induction in elderly inpatients, most of whom had acute venous thromboembolic disease, a 4-mg dose was given for the first 3 days of treatment. The dosage was then adjusted according to the INR on day 3 through use of an algorithm, which predicted the maintenance dose with a low rate of overanticoagulation [39]. Several nomograms [35,36,40] have been used to assist dosing. Computer software programs [41–43] are also available to assist with determining initial and subsequent doses of warfarin. The time-in-therapeutic range (TTR) is comparable or somewhat superior to manual dosing by experienced medical staff at lower INR ranges (71% versus 68%) [44], but the major advantage was seen for higher doses, as clinicians may be over cautious dosing in this range. Computerized dose management has not been demonstrated to provide improved clinical care, but may assist in clinical settings in which access to medical staff

experienced with warfarin dose adjustment is limited. Some programs can establish dosing from induction of therapy, whereas others are only useful in maintenance dosing and require prior data.

Gage [45] has examined the use of nomograms and computer modeling for warfarin dosing. He suggests the following: a patient with a baseline INR of 1, who achieves an INR greater than 1.5 obtained 15 to 24 hours after the initial dose, will require a very low daily dosage of warfarin (eg, 1 mg). If the INR is 1.2 to 1.3, the patient will require a low daily dosage (2 mg–3 mg) and a second dose of 5 mg should be given. If the INR remains 1 to 1.1 after a second dose of 5 mg, a higher dose (eg, 7.5 mg) can be given.

Warfarin dosing varies with age and gender because of pharmacodynamic issues, dietary changes, polypharmacy, and clinical status. A recent study of warfarin maintenance dosing patterns in clinical practice indicated that the median dose for men with AF, aged 60 to 69, was 4.6, whereas for women it was 4. For men aged 70 to 79, the median dose was 4.3, versus 3.5 for women; and for men aged 80 to 89 it was 3.9, versus 3.2 for women. The median doses were slightly greater for patients receiving anticoagulation for venous thromboembolic disease, but demonstrated the same trend of decreased dose with age and female gender [46].

Each study has examined dosing regimens in different groups of patients according to age and pathology, and in different settings. It is clear, however, that a uniform dosing regimen will not fit all patients, and that lower initial and maintenance doses are required in the elderly because of the increased pharmacodynamic effect. In addition, consideration of the patient's body weight, serum albumin, significant comorbid diseases (particularly congestive heart failure or liver disease) and the use of medications with potential interactions, require adjustment of initial dosing regimens.

Monitoring of maintenance therapy

Warfarin is often initiated in the hospital setting, where it is often administered in the evening. The INR is obtained with morning laboratory testing, allowing time in the afternoon to obtain the results and determine the next dose for that evening. This may not allow for sufficient time for the warfarin effect to be demonstrated. Gage suggests that INR testing be done 15 hours or more following administration of the first dose

[45]. Warfarin should be administered in the afternoon if INR monitoring is done the following morning; if warfarin is administered in the evening, INR monitoring should occur the following afternoon. Many patients continue to dose warfarin in the evening following hospital discharge, believing there is a rationale for this timing. The relationship of timing of dosing and adherence to warfarin therapy has not been studied. Adherence with warfarin therapy has been significantly associated with older age and higher income [47].

The optimal frequency of INR testing to maintain patients within therapeutic range is not clear, and individual patients exhibit fluctuations of the INR with changes in diet, medications, clinical status, and medication adherence. At these times, more frequent testing is advisable. When warfarin therapy is initiated, INR monitoring is usually done every few days until a result within the optimal therapeutic range is achieved. The INR is then usually obtained weekly for 1 to 2 weeks or more, to verify dosing by stability of the INR within range. Commonly, testing is then obtained biweekly for 1 to 2 weeks. If the INR remains stable within the therapeutic range and all else remains constant, the duration between tests can be extended to no less often than monthly. Consensus guidelines recommend that the frequency of testing not exceed every 4 weeks [1], and some data suggest that the quality of management is improved if testing is more frequent.

The quality of anticoagulation management, meaning the proportion of time that patients are within the TTR, has been used as a tool to assess different models for monitoring warfarin with different testing frequencies. In addition to the intensity of therapy, the stability of therapy is also important, as the time during which the INR fluctuates above the therapeutic range presents periods of increased risk for hemorrhage. The elderly can be managed to achieve a similar TTR as patients of other ages. In a study of warfarin management by an anticoagulation clinic, the elderly patients had a similar TTR and rate of hemorrhage [48].

In addition, TTR and stability of INR values have been found to improve after the first 6 to 12 weeks of therapy. It is unclear if this reflects any physiologic change, or that individuals who are difficult to manage or experience hemorrhages early are eliminated from study, producing a "survivor bias." Nevertheless, in a meta-analysis of patients treated with warfarin with venous thromboembolism, the case-fatality rate for major bleeding was 13.4% across 33 trials, and 9.1% after 3 months of therapy. The rate of intracranial hemorrhage was 1.15 per 100 patient-years for all patients, and 0.65 per 100 patient-years after 3 months of therapy [49], demonstrating that the greater stability in INR achieved over time reduced the risk of hemorrhage from excessive anticoagulation.

Systems for monitoring maintenance therapy

Clinical systems for monitoring warfarin therapy include "usual care," in which the INR is obtained at physicians' offices, anticoagulation management services or clinics which obtain the INR and manage therapy, and home monitoring. Point-of-care monitoring systems in which the INR is determined from a fingerstick sample of blood can be employed at home, in the doctor's office, or in a clinic. The TTR across several studies of usual care in physicians' offices ranges from 34% to 64%, as compared with 61% to 92% for anticoagulation management services [1]. Although anticoagulation management systems appear to achieve a superior TTR, the frequency of testing was not comparable between studies, and often the patient samples studied were not randomized. Randomized controlled trials of warfarin have achieved TTR from 44% to 83%.

Point-of-care PT monitoring systems calculate a PT or INR from measured thromboplastin clotting times on fingerstick samples, and can be used within medical settings or for patient self-testing at home. Studies of point-of-care home monitoring demonstrate a TTR of 56% to 93%. Issues remain regarding calibration and the reproducibility of INR results on different systems [1]. One study compared the cost of care for INR testing by home health nurses caring for 35 homebound elderly patients, between obtaining the sample at the patient's home and transporting them to a central laboratory—including materials, procedures, transportation and labor—with a point-of-care PT monitoring system. The cost to obtain an INR test was $6.86 with the point-of-service model, versus $17.30, with close agreement between the two values for those results falling below an INR of 3.5, but with greater disparity for higher values [50].

Management of nontherapeutic INRs

Recommendations for management of patients in whom an INR result is above the therapeutic range are based upon clinical experience and consensus guidelines, as clinical trials have not been undertaken. Options for management include withholding further doses, administration of vitamin K, and the administration of coagulation factors. Decisions about management of a patient with an INR above the therapeutic range not only rests upon the value of the INR and the clinical status of the patient with regard to bleeding, but is also influenced by other factors. In patients with an INR greater than 6, in whom two doses of warfarin were withheld, the INR returned more slowly to baseline in patients of older age, those with a lower maintenance dose, and in those with decompensated congestive heart failure or cancer.

The current guidelines established by the Seventh American College of Chest Physicians Conference on Antithrombotic and Thrombolytic Therapy [1] recommend:

INR less than 5 and no significant bleeding: lower the dose or omit a dose, monitor more frequently, and resume therapy at a lower dose when the INR has fallen into the therapeutic range.

INR 5 to less than 9 without bleeding: omit the next one to two doses, monitor more frequently, and resume therapy at a lower dose; or, alternatively, omit a dose and administer vitamin K1 (1 mg–2.5 mg) orally, which should result in a reduction of the INR in 24 hours.

INR greater than 9 and no significant bleeding: hold warfarin and administer vitamin K1 (5 mg–10 mg) orally, which should result in a reduction of the INR in 12 to 24 hours; the INR can be monitored closely and additional vitamin K1 can be given as necessary. Warfarin can be resumed at a lower dose when the INR reaches therapeutic levels.

In patients with serious bleeding and elevated INRs: recommendations are to hold warfarin and give vitamin K1 (10 mg) by slow intravenous infusion supplemented with fresh frozen plasma, prothrombin complex concentrate, or recombinant factor VIIa, depending on the urgency of the situation.

With life-threatening bleeding and elevated INRs: warfarin should be held and prothrombin complex concentrate or recombinant factor VIIa, and vitamin K1 (10mg) by slow intravenous infusion should be given.

Oral vitamin K is preferred over subcutaneous or intravenous therapy, as it was found to lower the INR more rapidly in asymptomatic patients who have INR values above the therapeutic range while receiving warfarin [51]. Oral vitamin K, however, is most often available in the United States in 5-mg tablets, allowing dosing of 2.5 mg for low dose therapy rather than 1 mg. Nevertheless, a reduction in the INR occurs 6 to 12 hours following vitamin K administration. Prothrombin complex concentrate contains factors II, IX, and X, and low levels of factor VII. Fresh frozen plasma can be added as a source of factor VII. Both can more rapidly reduce the INR, although they require a significant infusion of fluid and products.

Hemorrhagic risk

Intracranial hemorrhage is the most feared site for hemorrhage associated with warfarin therapy, as patients rarely fully recover. The most common sites for bleeding in patients treated with anticoagulants are the gastrointestinal tract, genitourinary tract, and soft tissues [52–54]. In a meta-analysis of six clinical trials of anticoagulation for AF, major bleeding occurred in 2.2 patients per 100 patient-years, with hemorrhagic stroke in 0.5 patients per 100 patient-years, and lethal bleeding in 0.4 patients per 100 patient-years [55]. In the SPORTIF III and V trials in which warfarin was a comparator for prevention of stroke in patients with nonvalvular atrial fibrillation, the rate of intracranial hemorrhage, including both hemorrhagic strokes and subdural hematomas, was 0.4%, and the rate for major hemorrhage was 2.5% per year [56,57].

Rates of hemorrhage in clinical trials may not reflect that experienced in the community. In a prospective study of rates of hemorrhage in elderly patients in the community, the cumulative incidence of major hemorrhage for patient less than 80 years of age was 13.1 per 100 person-years, versus 4.7 for those aged 65 to 80 years [58]. In addition, both treatment-specific factors, which are potentially modifiable (the intensity, stability, and duration of coumadin use, as well as use of other medications increasing bleeding risk), as well as patient-specific risk factors (which are not usually modifiable) must be assessed when estimating the risk of hemorrhage in an individual patient.

Treatment characteristics and bleeding risk

It is clear from clinical trial data that the intensity of warfarin therapy is the most important risk factor for hemorrhage from any site, independent of the risk factor [59,60]. An INR greater than 4 confers a markedly increased risk for intracranial hemorrhage [61]. The rate of war-farin-associated major hemorrhage and intracra-nial hemorrhage among patients admitted to the Brigham and Women's hospital has increased from 20.2% and 1.9%, respectively, from the pe-riod 1995 to 1998, to 33.3% and 7.8% during the period 1998 to 2002 [62]. Excess anticoagula-tion contributed independently to the increase in morbidity and mortality [63]. The intensity of therapy is described by the recommended thera-peutic range; the recommended duration of ther-apy is determined by the indication, which is discussed in subsequent articles in this issue.

The use of concomitant medications that po-tentiate bleeding risk, such as aspirin, clopidogrel, and NSAIDs, further increases the risk for hemor-rhage while being treated with warfarin. These medications are commonly prescribed for elderly individuals because of the prevalence of cardiovas-cular disease and osteoarthritis in this population.

Patient characteristics and bleeding risk

Despite the fact that age is also associated with other independent risk factors for hemorrhage and with the use of medications, which may interact with warfarin or potentiate bleeding risk, it appears that age is an independent risk factor for major hemorrhage, although this re-mains controversial. In the Stroke Prevention in Atrial Fibrillation trial, the rate of major bleeding for subjects receiving warfarin was 2.3% per year; however, the rate for those under the age of 75 was 1.7% and for those above, 4.2% per year [64]. In addition to increasing the risk for nonspecific hemorrhage, it appears that age is a specific risk factor for intracranial hemorrhage, with a 40% in-crease per decade [61].

The risk for bleeding increases with the pres-ence of several comorbid conditions, habits, and medications. Patients with recent hemorrhage or a history of gastrointestinal hemorrhage, stroke, liver disease, and renal insufficiency are at increased risk. Uncontrolled hypertension and treated hypertension, stroke, and cancer have also been associated with an increased risk of hemorrhage for patients treated with warfarin.

A recent study reviewed the literature regard-ing gastrointestinal hemorrhage in patients treated with warfarin, and applied decision-ana-lytic modeling to define risk factors. It concluded that persons with spontaneous (ie, non-NSAID related) upper gastrointestinal tract bleeding which has resolved, and who have been evaluated

and treated for *Helicobacter pylori*, if appropriate, appear to have no increased risk of hemorrhage than persons without a history of upper gastroin-testinal hemorrhage [65].

Patients who fall have presented another group of patients in whom the risk of hemorrhage may be increased, particularly intracranial hemorrhage. Many physicians have been reluctant to prescribe anticoagulants for fallers. Man-Song-Hing and colleagues conducted a Markov decision analysis to evaluate the risk of falling and sustaining a sub-dural hematoma (SDH), versus the benefit of stroke prevention for older adults with AF treated with warfarin and average risks of stroke and falls [66]. After an extensive review of the literature, they began their analysis with the following assump-tions: 33% of community-dwelling elderly fall yearly and the rate of SDH in the elderly is 0.0004 per patient-year; thus, the relative risk of developing an SDH in persons who fall as com-pared with those who do not is 1.4. They concluded that for patients with an average risk of stroke (5% per year if untreated), the risk of SDH from falling is so small that the individual would need to fall 300 times a year for the risks of anticoagulant therapy to outweigh its benefits.

Assessment of bleeding risk

Prediction rules can assist in assessing bleeding risk. The modified Outpatient Bleeding Risk Index [67] assigns one point each for age greater than 65 years, history of gastrointestinal bleeding, history of stroke, and one or more specific comorbid condi-tion (recent myocardial infarction, hematocrit of less than 30%, renal insufficiency with a creatinine of greater than 1.5mg/dl, or diabetes mellitus). A low risk for major bleeding (0 points) using this instrument confers a 2% risk within 3 months and 3% for 12 months; an intermediate risk (1–2 points) confers a 5% 3-month risk and a 12% 12-month risk; and a high risk (3–4 points) confers a 23% risk for major bleeding within 3 months and a 48% risk within 12 months. Using the Outpatient Bleeding Risk Index to stratify patients for risk, Beyth and colleagues undertook a randomized study of usual care versus a multicomponent inter-vention to prevent major bleeding complications in older patients receiving warfarin for treatment of a thromboembolic disease. The intervention con-sisted of patient education about warfarin, training to increase patient participation, self-monitoring of the PT, and nomogram-based management of warfarin dosing. At 6 months, the TTR for the intervention group was 56% versus 32% in controls, major bleeding was 5.6% versus 12% in controls, and death and thromboembolic complications was similar between the two groups. Other risk assessment instruments may include and weigh risk factors for bleeding differently [68,69].

Summary

Elderly patients as a group may present more of a challenge in managing warfarin therapy because of alterations in pharmacokinetics from other medications, diet, and disease; pharmacodynamic changes; increased risk for hemorrhage; and difficulty in monitoring. The elderly, however, may derive the most benefit from warfarin therapy for certain indications, such as the prevention of stroke in atrial fibrillation or recurrent events following deep venous thrombosis, as their risk of thromboembolic disease is often significantly greater than that observed in other populations. With careful attention to these issues, warfarin can be managed as effectively as in other populations.

References

[1] Ansell J, Hirsch J, Poller L, et al. The pharmacology and management of the vitamin K antagonists. The Seventh ACCP Conference on Antithrombotic and Thrombolytic Therapy. Chest 2004;126:204S–33S.

[2] Hart RG, Pearce LA, Aguilar MI. Meta-analysis: antithrombotic therapy to prevent stroke in patients who have non-valvular atrial fibrillation. Ann Intern Med 2007;146:857–67.

[3] Abdelhafiz AH, Wheeldon NM. Use of resources and cost implications of stroke prophylaxis with warfarin for patients with nonvalvular atrial fibrillation. Am J Geriatr Phamacother 2003;1:53–60.

[4] Fang MC, Stafford RS, Urskin JN, et al. National trends in antiarrythmic and antithrombotic medication use in atrial fibrillation. Arch Intern Med 2004; 164:55–60.

[5] Mahmud A, Bennett K, Okechukwu I, et al. National underuse of antithrombotic therapy in chronic atrial fibrillation identified from digoxin prescribing. Br J Clin Pharmacol 2007;64(5):706–9.

[6] Schatz IJ, Masaki K, Yano K, et al. Cholesterol and all-cause mortality in elderly people from the Honolulu Heart Program: a cohort study. Lancet 2001;358:351–66.

[7] Gross CP, Vogel EW, Dhond AJ, et al. Factors influencing physicians' reported use of anticoagulation therapy in nonvalvular atrial fibrillation: a cross-sectional study. Clin Ther 2003;25:1750–64.

[8] Swenson CN, Fundak G. Observational cohort study of switching warfarin sodium products in a managed care organization. Am J Health Syst Pharm 2000;71:115–21.

[9] Halkin H, Shapiro J, Durnik D, et al. Increased warfarin doses and decreased international normalized ratio response after nationwide switching. Clin Pharmacol Ther 2003;74:215–21.

[10] Yamazaki H, Shimada T. Human liver cytochrome P450 enzymes involved in the 7-hydroxylation of R- and S-warfarin enantiomers. Biochem Pharmacol 1997;54:1195–203.

[11] Kaminsky LS, Shang S-Y. Human P450 metabolism of warfarin. Pharmacol Ther 1997;73:67–74.

[12] Coumadin tablets (Warfarin sodium tablets USP) package insert, Revised April, 1998.

[13] Dobrzanski S, Duncan SE, Harkiss A, et al. Age and weight as determinants of warfarin requirements. J Clin Hosp Pharm 1983;8:75–7.

[14] Routledge PA, chapman PH, Davies DM, et al. Factors affecting warfarin requirements. A prospective population study. Eur J Clin Pharmacol 1979; 15:319–22.

[15] Cropp JS, Bussey HI. A review of enzyme induction of warfarin metabolism with recommendations for patient management. Pharmacotherapy 1997;17: 917–28.

[16] Greenblatt DJ, von Moltke LL. Interaction of warfarin with drugs, natural substances, and foods. J Clin Pharmacol 2005;45:127–32.

[17] Breckenridge A, Orme M, Wesseling H, et al. Pharmacokinetics and pharmacodynamics of the enantiomers of warfarin in man. Clin Pharmacol Ther 1974;15:424–30.

[18] O'Reilly RA, Trager WF, Rettie AE, et al. Interaction of amiodarone with racemic warfarin and its separated enantiomorphs in humans. Clin Pharmacol Ther 1987;42:290–4.

[19] Rothschild BM. Commentary: hematological perturbations associated with salicylate. Clin Pharmacol Ther 1979;26:145–52.

[20] Turpie AGG, Gent M, Laupacis A, et al. Aspirin and warfarin after heart-valve replacement: a comparison of aspirin with placebo in patients treated with warfarin after heart-valve replacement. N Engl J Med 1993;329:524–9.

[21] The Medical Research Council's General Practice Research Framework. Thrombosis prevention trial: randomized trial of low-intensity oral anticoagulation with warfarin and low-dose aspirin in the primary prevention is ischaemic heart disease in men at increased risk. Lancet 1998;351:233–41.

[22] Hylek EM, Heiman H, Skates SJ, et al. Acetaminophen and other risk factors for excessive warfarin anticoagulation. J Am Med Assoc 1998;279:657–62.

[23] Wittkowsky AK. Dietary supplements, herbs and oral anticoagulants: the nature of the evidence. J Thromb Thrombolysis 2008;25:72–7.

[24] Engelsen J, Nielsen JD, Winther K. Effect of coenzyme Q10 an ginkgo biloba on warfarin dosage in stable, long-term warfarin treated outpatients: a randomized, double blind, placebo-crossover trial. Thromb Haemost 2008;25:2526–32.

[25] Ioannides C. Pharmacokinetic interactions between herbal remedies and medicinal drugs. Xenobiotica 2002;32:451–78.

[26] Ang-Lee MK, Moss J, Yuan CS. Herbal medicines and perioperative care. J Am Med Assoc 2001;286:208–16.

[27] Buchley MS, Goff AD, Knapp WE. Fish oil interaction with warfarin. Ann Pharmacother 2004;38:50–3.

[28] Franco V, Polanczyk CA, Clausell N. Role of vitamin K intake in chronic oral anticoagulation: prospective evidence from observational and randomized protocols. Am J Med 2004;116:711–3.

[29] Sullivan DM, Ford MA, Boyden TW. Grapefruit juice and the response to warfarin. Am J Health Syst Pharm 1998;55:1581–3.

[30] O'Reilly RA. Lack of effect of fortified wine ingested during fasting and anticoagulant therapy. Arch Intern Med 1981;141:458–9.

[31] Conway EM, Bauer KA, Barzegar S. Suppression of hemostatic system activation by oral anticoagulants in the blood of patient with thrombotic diatheses. J Clin Invest 1987;80:1535–44.

[32] McGehee WG, Klotz TA, Epstein DJ, et al. Coumarin necrosis associated with hereditary protein C deficiency. Ann Intern Med 1984;101:59–60.

[33] Hylek EM, Skates SJ, Sheehan MA, et al. An analysis of the lowest effective intensity of prophylactic anticoagulation for patients with nonrheumatic atrial fibrillation. N Engl J Med 1996;335:540–6.

[34] Hart RJ, Aguilar MI. Anticoagulation in atrial fibrillation: selected controversies including optimal anticoagulation intensity, treatment of intracerebral hemorrhage. J Thromb Thrombolysis September 29, 2007.

[35] Harrison L, Johnston M, Massicotte MP, et al. Comparison of 5-mg and 10-mg loading doses in initiation of warfarin therapy. Ann Intern Med 1997;126:133–6.

[36] Crowther MA, Ginsberg JB, Kearon C, et al. A randomized trial comparing 5 mg and 10 mg warfarin loading doses. Arch Intern Med 1999;159:46–8.

[37] Ageno W, Turpie AGG, Steidl L, et al. Comparison of a daily fixed 2.5 mg warfarin dose with a 5 mg, international ratio adjusted, warfarin dose initially following heart valve replacement. Am J Cardiol 2001;88(1):40–4.

[38] Kovacs MJ, Rodger M, Anderson DR, et al. Comparison of 10-mg and 5-mg warfarin initiation nomograms together with low-molecular-weight heparin for outpatient treatment of acute venous thromboembolism. A randomized double-blind, controlled trial. Ann Intern Med 2003;138:714–9.

[39] Siguret V, Gouin I, Debray M, et al. Initiation of warfarin therapy in elderly medical inpatients: a safe and accurate regimen. Am J Med 2004;118:137–42.

[40] Schulman S. Care of patients receiving long-term anticoagulant therapy. 2003;349:675–83 Appendix 1. Available at: www.nejm.org in supplementary material.

[41] White RH, Hong R, Venook AP, et al. Initiation of warfarin therapy: comparison of physician dosing with computer-predicted dosing. J Gen Intern Med. 1987;2:141–8.

[42] White RH, Mungall D. Outpatient management of warfarin therapy: comparison of computer-predicted dosage adjustment to skilled professional care. Ther Drug Monit 1991;13:46–50.

[43] Dawn AC. Integrated Induction Management System Available at: www.4s-dawn.com/dawnac.

[44] Manotti C, Moia M, Palareti G, et al. Effect of computer aided management on the quality of treatment in anticoagulated patients: a prospective, randomized, multicenter trial of APROAT. Haematologica 2001;86:1060–70.

[45] Gage BF, Finh SD, White RH. Warfarin therapy for an octogenarian who has atrial fibrillation. Ann Intern Med 2001;134:465–74.

[46] Garcia D, Regan S, Crowther M, et al. Warfarin maintenance dosing patterns in clinical practice. Implications for safer anticoagulation in the elderly population. Chest 2005;127(6):2049–56.

[47] Davis NJ, Billett HH, Cohen HW, et al. Impact of adherence knowledge, and quality of life on anticoagulation control. Ann Phamacother 2005;39:632–6.

[48] Copeland M, Walker ID, Tait RC. Oral anticoagulation and hemorrhagic complications in an elderly population with atrial fibrillation. Arch Intern Med 2001;161:2125–8.

[49] Linkins L-A, Choi PT, Douketis JD. Clinical impact of bleeding in patients taking oral anticoagulant therapy for venous thromboembolism. A meta-analysis. Ann Intern Med 2003;139:893–900.

[50] Cheung DS, Heizer D, Wilson J, et al. Cost-saving analysis of using a portable coagulometer for monitoring homebound elderly patients taking warfarin. Am J Geriatr Cardiol 2003;12(5):283–7.

[51] Crowther MA, Douketis JD, Schnurr T, et al. Oral vitamin K lowers the international normalized ratio more rapidly than subcutaneous vitamin K in the treatment of warfarin-associated coagulopathy: a randomized controlled trial. Ann Intern Med 2002;137:251–4.

[52] Landefeld CS, Beyth RJ. Anticoagulant-related bleeding: clinical epidemiology, prediction and prevention. Am J Med 1993;95:315–28.

[53] Fihn SD, McDonell M, Martin D, et al. Risk factors for complications of chronic anticoagulation. A multicenter study. Warfarin Optimized Outpatient Follow-up Study Group. Ann Intern Med 1993;118:511–20.

[54] Palareti G, Leali N, Coccheri S, et al. Bleeding complications of oral anticoagulant treatment: an inception-cohort, prospective collaborative study (ISCOAT). Lancet 1996;348:423–8.

[55] Van Walraven C, Hart RG, Singer DE, et al. Oral anticoagulants vs aspirin in nonvalvular atrial fibrillation. An individual patient meta-analysis. J Am Med Assoc 2002;288:2441–8.

[56] Olsson SB, Executive Steering Committee of the SPORTIF III Investigators. Stroke prevention with the oral direct thrombin inhibitor ximelagatran compared with warfarin in patients with non-valvular atrial fibrillation (SPORTIF III): randomised controlled trial. Lancet 2003;362:1691–8.

[57] SPORTIF Executive Steering Committee for the SPORTIF V Investigators. Ximelagatran versus warfarin for stroke prevention in patients with nonvalvular atrial fibrillation: a randomized trial. J Am Med Assoc 2005;293:690–8.

[58] Hylek E, Evans-Molina C, Shea C, et al. Major hemorrhage and tolerability of warfarin in the first year of therapy among elderly patients with atrial fibrillation. Circulation 2007;115:2689–96.

[59] Fihn SD, Callahan CM, Martin DC, et al. White RH for the National Consortium of Anticoagulation Clinics. The risk for and severity of bleeding complications in elderly patients treated with warfarin. Ann Intern Med 1996;124:970–9.

[60] Levine MN, Raskob G, Beyth RJ, et al. Hemorrhagic complications of anticoagulant treatment. The Seventh ACCP Conference on Antithrombotic and Thrombolytic Therapy. Chest 2004;126:287S–310S.

[61] Hylek EM, Singer DE. Risk factors for intracranial hemorrhage in outpatients taking warfarin. Ann Intern Med 1994;120:897–902.

[62] Kucher N, Castellanos LR, Quiroz R, et al. Time trends in warfarin-associated hemorrhage. Am J Cardiol 2004;94:403–6.

[63] Koo S, Kucher N, Nguyen PL, et al. The effect of excessive anticoagulation on mortality and morbidity in hospitalized patient with anticoagulant-related major hemorrhage. Arch Intern Med 2004;164: 1557–60.

[64] The Stroke Prevention in Atrial Fibrillation Investigators. Bleeding during antithrombotic therapy in patients with atrial fibrillation. Arch Intern Med 1996;156:409–16.

[65] Man-Son-Hing M, Laupacis A. Balancing the risks of stroke and upper gastrointestinal tract bleeding in older patients with atrial fibrillation. Arch Intern Med 2002;162:541–50.

[66] Man-Son-Hing M, Nichol G, Lau A, et al. Choosing antithrombotic therapy for elderly patient with atrial fibrillation who are at risk for falls. Arch Intern Med 1999;159:677–85.

[67] Beyth RJ, Quinn LM, Landefeld CS. Prospective evaluation of an index for predicting the risk of major bleeding in outpatients treated with warfarin. Am J Med 1998;105:91–9.

[68] Kakar P, Lane D, Lip GY. Bleeding risk stratification models in deciding on anticoagulation in patients with atrial fibrillation: a useful complement to stroke risk stratification schema. Chest 2006;130: 1296–9.

[69] Shireman TI, Mahnken JD, Howard PA, et al. Development of a contemporary bleeding risk model for elderly warfarin recipients. Chest 2006;130: 1390–6.

New Anticoagulant Agents: Direct Thrombin Inhibitors

Edith A. Nutescu, PharmD, FCCP*, Nancy L. Shapiro, PharmD,
Aimee Chevalier, PharmD

Department of Pharmacy Practice, Antithrombosis Center, University of Illinois at Chicago, College of Pharmacy and Medical Center, 833 South Wood Street, M/C 886, Room 164, Chicago, IL 60612, USA

Thrombin is the key effector enzyme responsible for the final step in thrombus formation. Because of the central role it plays in thrombus generation, propagation, and stabilization, effective inhibition of thrombin is crucial in the prevention and treatment of thrombotic disorders. Thrombin can be inhibited indirectly or directly. Traditional anticoagulants, such as heparin (unfractionated and fractionated) and vitamin K antagonists are indirect inhibitors of thrombin. Indirect thrombin inhibitors have comprised the most frequently used anticoagulants in clinical practice for the last five decades. Although effective if appropriately used, these traditional anticoagulant agents are also fraught with many limitations, such as unpredictable anticoagulant response, need for routine dose adjustments and anticoagulant monitoring, heparin-induced thrombocytopenia (HIT), genetic variations in response, binding to various proteins and cells, and lack of inhibition of clot bound thrombin [1]. In recent years, much emphasis has been placed on the development of direct thrombin inhibitors (DTI) and other novel classes of antithrombotic agents with more selective mechanisms of action that may offer benefits over traditional agents in the treatment and prevention of various thrombotic disorders. The DTIs exert their effect by interacting directly with the thrombin molecule without the need of a cofactor. These agents offer

many advantages over heparin including the inhibition of both circulating and clot-bound thrombin; a more predictable anticoagulant response because they do not bind to plasma proteins and are not neutralized by platelet factor 4; lack of required cofactors, such as antithrombin or heparin cofactor II; inhibiting thrombin-induced platelet aggregation; and absence of induction of immune-mediated thrombocytopenia. The DTIs have been studied for many indications, such as HIT, prophylaxis and treatment of venous thromboembolism (VTE), acute coronary syndromes with and without percutaneous transluminal coronary angioplasty, and nonvalvular atrial fibrillation (AF) [2]. The prototype of this class is hirudin, which was originally isolated from the salivary glands of the medicinal leech, *Hirudo medicinalis*. More recently, through recombinant DNA technology several synthetic analogues have also been produced. Currently, four parenteral agents (lepirudin, desirudin, bivalirudin, and argatroban) have been approved for use in the United States, and various oral compounds are in clinical development (Table 1).

Parenteral direct thrombin inhibitors

Hirudin

Hirudin was the first agent of the DTI class developed for clinical use. Hirudin is a 65–amino acid polypeptide (7000 d), originally produced from the salivary glands of the medicinal leech (*H medicinalis*) [3]. Hirudin itself is not commercially available; however, its discovery led to the development by recombinant technology of

A version of this article originally appeared in *Clinics in Geriatric Medicine*, volume 22, issue 1.

* Corresponding author.
E-mail address: enutescu@uic.edu (E.A. Nutescu).

Table 1
Pharmacologic and clinical properties of direct thrombin inhibitors

Properties	Lepirudin	Desirudin	Bivalirudin	Argatroban	Ximelagatran	Dabigatran
Route of administration	IV or SC (bid)	IV or SC (bid)	IV	IV	PO ximelagatran SC melagatran	PO (qd or bid)
Indication	Prophylaxis or treatment of thrombosis in patients with HIT	DVT prevention after THA (not available in the US)	Patients with UA undergoing PTCA; PCI with provisional use of GPI; Patients with or at risk of HIT/HITTS undergoing PCI	Prophylaxis or treatment of thrombosis in patients with HIT; patients at risk for HIT undergoing PCI	Investigated for VTE prevention and treatment and stroke prevention in AF; Approval denied by FDA in October, 2004	Investigational for VTE prevention and treatment and stroke prevention in AF
Binding to thrombin	Irreversible catalytic site and exosite-1	Irreversible catalytic site and exosite-1	Partially reversible catalytic site and exosite-1	Reversible catalytic site	Reversible catalytic site	Reversible catalytic site
Half-life in healthy subjects	1.3–2 h	2–3 h	25 min	40–50 min	3–5 h	14 h–17 h
Monitoring	aPTT (IV) SCr/CrCL	aPTT (IV) SCr/CrCL	aPTT/ACT SCr/CrCL	aPTT/ACT Liver function	* SCr/CrCL Liver function	* SCr/CrCL Effect on liver function unclear at this time
Clearance	Renal	Renal	Proteolytic and renal	Hepatic	Renal	Renal
Antibody development	Antihirudin antibodies in up to 60% of patients	Not reported	May cross-react with antihirudin antibodies	No	Unknown	Unknown
Effect on INR	Slight increase	Slight increase	Slight increase	Increase	Unpredictable and variable	Unpredictable and variable

Abbreviations: ACT, activated clotting time; AF, atrial fibrillation; aPTT, activated partial thromboplastin time; bid, twice daily; CrCL, creatine clearance; DVT, deep vein thrombosis; GPI, glycoprotein IIb-IIIa inhibitor; HIT, heparin-induced thrombocytopenia; HITTS, heparin-induced thrombocytopenia and thrombosis syndrome; IV, intravenous; PCI, percutaneous coronary intervention; PO, oral; PTCA, percutaneous transluminal coronary angioplasty; qd, daily; SC, subcutaneous; SCr, serum creatinine; THA, total hip arthroplasty; UA, unstable angina; VTE, venous thromboembolism.

* Routine monitoring of anticoagulant effect may not be necessary.

derivatives, namely lepirudin and desirudin. Lepirudin is available in the United States, whereas desirudin is available in Europe [4]. Hirudins are potent and specific thrombin inhibitors, forming a stoichiometric and very slowly reversible complex by binding to both the active site and exosite-1 of the thrombin molecule (Fig. 1). Because of this bivalent binding, hirudins are considered the most potent inhibitors of thrombin [3].

Lepirudin

Because of this strong, almost irreversible bond between lepirudin and thrombin, bleeding problems have been associated with its use. A meta-analysis of studies in patients with acute coronary syndrome showed hirudin to be associated with more bleeding than heparin (1.7% versus 1.3%; odds ratio 1.28; 95% confidence interval [CI], 1.06–1.55) [5]. Currently, there is no pharmacologic antidote available to reverse the effects of hirudin or its derivatives.

Lepirudin distributes to extracellular fluids and is characterized by an initial half-life of approximately 10 minutes after intravenous (IV) infusion. Elimination follows a first-order process and is characterized by a terminal half-life of 1.3 hours in young healthy volunteers. Metabolism occurs by release of amino acids by way of catabolic hydrolysis of the parent drug. Lepirudin is primarily eliminated renally as unchanged drug

(35%); dose adjustments are needed for patients with renal impairment. In patients with marked renal insufficiency (creatinine clearance <15 mL/min) and on hemodialysis, elimination half-lives are prolonged up to 2 days. The dose should be monitored and adjusted to an activated partial thromboplastin time (aPTT) ratio of 1.5 to 2.5 × baseline because the bleeding risk increases above this range with no increase in efficacy [2–4,6].

Lepirudin is indicated for anticoagulation in patients with HIT and associated thrombosis to prevent further thromboembolic complications. It is contraindicated in patients with known hypersensitivity to hirudins or to any of the components of lepirudin [6]. Efficacy of lepirudin for HIT has been documented through three prospective cohort trials using historical controls. In one trial, a significant reduction in the combined end point of mortality, amputation, and thromboembolism was achieved with lepirudin compared with control patients (10% versus 23% at day 7 and 25% versus 52% at day 35, $P = .014$) [7]. The second trial found a nonsignificant trend favoring lepirudin, but there were more frequent bleeds reported in the lepirudin group compared with controls (44.6% versus 27.2% at 35 days; RR 2.57; $P = .0001$, log-rank test) [8]. No difference was seen in bleeding events requiring transfusion, however, and there were no intracranial bleeds observed in the lepirudin group. In the third trial,

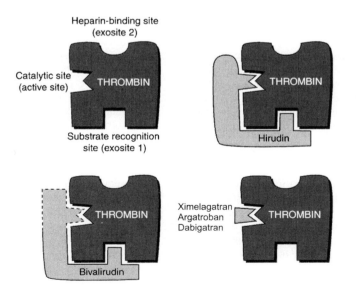

Fig. 1. Mechanism of action of direct thrombin inhibitors. (*Adapted from* Lefkovits J, Topol EJ. Direct thrombin inhibitors in cardiovascular medicine. Circulation 1994;90:1522–36; with permission.)

the combined endpoint occurred in 21% of patients, with major bleeding occurring in 19.5% of patients [9]. A combined analysis of all three HAT trials (HAT-1, HAT-2, HAT-3, n = 403 total) showed a combined endpoint occuring in 82 patients (20.3%), with 47 deaths (11.7%), 22 limb amputations (5.5%), 30 new thromboembolic complications (7.4%), and 71 (17.6%) major bleeds [9]. Compared to the controls, the combined endpoint after start of treatment was reduced (29.7% vs. 52.1%, p = 0.0473), primarily due to the reduction in new thromboses (11.9% vs. 32.1%, p = 0.0008). Mean lepirudin maintenance doses ranged from 0.07 to 0.11 mg/kg/hr. Major bleeding was more frequent in the lepirudin patients (29.4% vs. 9.1%, p = 0.0148). A retrospective observational analysis in 181 patients with confirmed HIT treated in routine practice used a mean lepirudin dose of 0.06 mg/kg/hr [10]. Thrombotic events occurred in 13.8% of patients and 20.4% of patients experienced major bleeding. Mean lepirudin dose was not a significant predictor of thrombosis. However, mean lepirudin dose greater than 0.07 mg/kg/hr, long duration of treatment, and moderate to severe renal impairment were significant positive factors for major bleeding. These authors suggested that the recommended lepirudin dose of 0.15 mg/kg/hr is too high, and the use of reduced doses may be safer with regard to bleeding without compromising efficacy. Other studies have reported that actual doses of lepirudin given in HIT patients were lower than those recommended [11–13].

Research is also being conducted on the use of lepirudin for other indications. In a meta-analysis of six trials with 28,545 total acute coronary syndrome patients, using various forms of hirudin, including lepirudin, significant reductions in the risk of death or myocardial infarction (MI) were reported compared with heparin-treated patients (odds ratio 0.81, 95% CI, 0.73–0.91) [5]. Lepirudin given at 1.25 mg/kg subcutaneously (SC) twice daily was identified in a small dose-ranging study of 121 patients as effective and safe for the treatment of proximal deep vein thrombosis (DVT), and caused fewer ventilation-perfusion abnormalities after 5 days of treatment compared with patients given IV heparin (P = .006). There was no difference between the groups in thrombus extension or regression, major bleeding complications, or serious adverse events [14]. Other potential uses include maintenance of graft patency in hemodialysis patients and percutaneous coronary intervention (PCI) [3,15].

Product information recommends that lepirudin is given as an initial IV bolus of 0.4 mg/kg, up to a maximum of 110 kg, given over 15 to 20 seconds, then a continuous IV infusion of 0.15 mg/kg/h [6]. However, due to concerns of potential anaphylaxis, a bolus dose is now only recommended when life-threatening thrombosis is present. Thus, patients with isolated HIT should be treated with an initial infusion of 0.1mg/kg/hour without a bolus [16]. The aPTT should be checked 4 hours after starting the infusion, and at least daily during treatment. If the aPTT is above the target range of 1.5 to 2.5, the infusion should be stopped for 2 hours, then restarted at an infusion rate reduced by 50%, with no additional IV bolus. The aPTT should be checked again in 4 hours. If the confirmed aPTT is below the target range, the infusion rate should be increased in steps of 20%, with a repeat aPTT determined 4 hours later. In general, the infusion rate of 0.2 mg/kg/h should not be exceeded without checking for coagulation abnormalities, which might be preventive of an appropriate aPTT response [6]. Because the agent is renally eliminated, dosage adjustments and careful monitoring are recommended in patients with renal impairment (Table 2). When converting patients from IV lepirudin to an oral anticoagulant, the lepirudin dose should be tapered to an aPTT ratio of slightly more than 1.5 before oral anticoagulation therapy (warfarin) is initiated. To avoid inducing a prothrombotic effect when initiating oral anticoagulation, parenteral anticoagulation should also be continued for 4 to 5 days to overlap with warfarin. Lepirudin should be discontinued when the international normalized ratio (INR) reaches the intended therapeutic range. Warfarin loading doses are not recommended, and warfarin should only be initiated once platelet counts have begun to normalize [3,6,15].

As with all anticoagulants, hemorrhage can occur at any site in patients taking lepirudin. For patients with increased risk of bleeding, careful assessment of risks and benefits is recommended. Concomitant use of lepirudin and thrombolytics can increase the risk for bleeding complications and enhance the effect of lepirudin on aPTT prolongation. Formation of antihirudin antibodies was observed in 40% to 60% of HIT patients treated with lepirudin. This may increase the anticoagulant effect of lepirudin possibly because of delayed renal elimination of active lepirudin-antihirudin complexes. Strict monitoring of aPTT is necessary during prolonged

Table 2
Dosing considerations for direct thrombin inhibitors in patients with renal and hepatic dysfunction

	Lepirudin	Desirudin	Bivalirudin	Argatroban	Ximelagatran	Dabigatran
Renal impairment	[a]Bolus: 0.2 mg/kg Infusion: CrCL 45–60: 0.075 mg/kg/h; CrCL 30–44: 0.045 mg/kg/h; CrCL 15–29: 0.0225 mg/kg/h; CrCL <15: avoid or stop infusion; HD: stop infusion & additional IV bolus doses of 0.1 mg/kg qod should be considered if the aPTT ratio falls below 1.5	CrCl 31–60: 5mg SC q12h; CrCL <30: 1.7 mg SC q12h	[b]Bolus: no dose adjustment; Infusion: CrCL <30: 1 mg/kg/h; HD:0.25 mg/kg/h	Dose adjustment not required per product information[c]	Dose adjustment required; degree of dose decrease not defined.	Dose adjustment required; degree of dose decrease not defined at this time.
Hepatic impairment	Dose adjustment not required	Dose adjustment not required	Dose adjustment not required	[d]Initiate at 0.5 µg/kg/min, then titrate to aPTT 1.5–3 × baseline	FDA approval denied due to liver toxicity	Unclear at this time

Abbreviations: aPTT, activated partial thromboplastin time; CrCL, creatinine clearance mL/min; HD, hemodialysis; SC, subcutaneous.

[a] Bolus dose should only be used when life-threatening thromboses is present; No bolus dose is recommended in patients with isolated HIT.
[b] In treatment of HIT, a lower dose of ~ 0.15 mg/kg/hr has been suggested without an initial bolus dose.
[c] Mean dose of 0.8 mcg/kg/min in patients with CrCL < 30mL/min has been recently reported.
[d] Limited experience suggests that even lower doses may be needed.

therapy. Because of coagulation defects secondary to reduced production of vitamin K–dependent clotting factors, serious liver injury, such as cirrhosis, may enhance the effects of lepirudin [2,3,6].

Desirudin

The technical difficulties of isolating sufficient quantities of hirudin also led to the development of desirudin. Desirudin (a recombinant hirudin) is currently approved in the United States for DVT prophylaxis in patients undergoing total hip replacement. Although approved for use, the agent is not currently marketed in the United States; however, it is available in Europe [4]. Desirudin has been compared with both unfractionated heparin (UFH) and low-molecular-weight heparin (LMWH) for DVT prevention in patients undergoing major orthopedic surgery. In one trial, 445 patients were randomized to desirudin, 15 mg SC twice daily, or UFH, 5000 units SC three times daily, for 8 to 11 days. The first doses of both agents were administered preoperatively. Desirudin was superior for prevention of total and proximal DVT. Confirmed DVT occurred in 7% versus 23% of patients in the desirudin and heparin groups, respectively ($P < .0001$), and proximal DVT in 3% versus 16% ($P < .0001$). There were no cases of pulmonary embolism (PE) during the period when the medications were given; however, in the 6-week follow-up period, four PEs were confirmed, all in patients who had received heparin. No significant differences in blood loss, transfusions, or bleeding complications were noted between the treatment groups [17]. The results of a large clinical trial of 2079 patients showed that desirudin, 15 mg SC twice daily administered 30 minutes before surgery, is more effective than enoxaparin, 40 mg SC once daily started the evening before surgery, in preventing total VTE in patients after total hip replacement (18.4 versus 25.5%, $P = .0001$, relative risk reduction 28%) and proximal DVT-PE (4.5% versus 17.5%; $P = .01$; relative risk reduction = 40%) and has a similar safety profile [18]. It has been suggested that the benefit from desirudin comes from a more efficient mode of action, and timing of the initial dose. Desirudin was also studied in PCI in the HELVETICA randomized double-blind study of patients undergoing angioplasty and in a subset of patients with acute coronary syndromes undergoing early PCI in the GUSTO-IIb trial [19,20]. Both studies demonstrated improved effectiveness of desirudin over heparin, particularly among high-risk patients.

Desirudin reaches maximum concentration after being administered by the SC route after 1 to 3 hours, has a terminal elimination half-life after SC dosing of approximately 2 hours, and 80% to 90% of the elimination is by renal clearance and metabolism. The total urinary excretion of unchanged drug amounts to 40% to 50% of the administered dose. The aPTT should be monitored with desirudin in patients with hepatic dysfunction or moderate renal impairment. In patients with moderate renal impairment (creatinine clearance 31–60 mL/min), mean area under the curve was increased threefold, and in severe renal failure (creatinine clearance <31 mL/min) mean area under the curve was increased ninefold compared with patients with normal renal function. Dose reductions are recommended for patients with renal impairment (see Table 2). Daily aPTT levels and daily serum creatinine levels should be monitored. Peak aPTT should not rise to greater than two times control. If the peak aPTT rises above this level, dose reductions are made accordingly, and if necessary, the dose should be held until the aPTT returns to less than two times control. No specific pharmacologic antidote for desirudin exists; however, the anticoagulant effect can be partially reversed by thrombin-rich plasma concentrates, whereas aPTT levels can be reduced by IV desmopressin, 0.3 μg/kg [2–4,15,21,22].

Bivalirudin

Bivalirudin is a specific and reversible DTI, consisting of a bivalent synthetic 20–amino acid polypeptide, which is approved by the Food and Drug Administration (FDA) for use in patients with unstable angina undergoing percutaneous transluminal coronary angioplasty, with provisional use of glycoprotein IIb-IIIa inhibitor (GPI) for use as an anticoagulant in patients undergoing PCI, and in patients with or at risk for HIT/HITTS undergoing PCI [23]. It directly inhibits thrombin by specifically binding to both the catalytic site and the anion-binding exosite of circulating and clot-bound thrombin. The binding of bivalirudin to thrombin is reversible because thrombin slowly cleaves the bivalirudin-Arg3-Pro4 bond, resulting in recovery of thrombin-active site functions [1–3,21]. This reversible binding to thrombin is a proposed mechanism for an improved safety profile of bivalirudin as compared with hirudin and heparin [1,24]. Similarly to the other DTIs, no pharmacologic antidote is currently available to reverse its effects. Bivalirudin is mostly cleared by proteolytic cleavage and by hepatic metabolism, with approximately 20% eliminated renally. Patients with moderate (creatinine clearance 30–60 mL/min) and severe (creatinine clearance 10–29 mL/min) renal impairment exhibit a 20% decrease in drug clearance [21,23]. In patients with renal impairment the bivalirudin infusion rate needs to be adjusted and monitoring of anticoagulation status performed (see Table 2) [21,23]. In patients who are hemodialysis dependent the clearance of bivalirudin is reduced by 80% and approximately 25% is removed by hemodialysis. The half-life of the drug in patients with normal renal function is approximately 25 minutes [21,23]. The activated clotting time can be used to monitor the anticoagulant effect of bivalirudin. Therapeutic activated clotting time levels are achieved within 5 minutes after initiating bivalirudin therapy, and activated clotting time levels return back to subtherapeutic levels within 1 hour of discontinuing the infusion [21,23].

Bivalirudin dosing based on manufacturer's recommendation is 0.75 mg/kg IV bolus, followed by an IV infusion at a rate of 1.75 mg/kg/h for the duration of the PCI procedure that can be maintained up to 4 hours. After the 4-hour initial infusion, the rate is decreased to 0.2 mg/kg/h and the infusion can be maintained for up to 20 hours if needed [23]. In contrast to patients undergoing PCI, in the treatment of patients with HIT no bolus dose and lower bivaliruin infusion doses have been evaluated: 0.15-0.2 mg/kg/hr [16].

Various studies have evaluated the use of bivalirudin in patients with acute coronary syndromes undergoing PCI. The Bivalirudin Angioplasty Study is the first such large clinical trial that compared bivalirudin with high-dose heparin in 4312 patients undergoing PCI for non–ST elevation acute coronary syndromes or postinfarction angina [25]. An intent-to-treat analysis comparing differences in rates of death, MI, or repeat revascularization at 7, 90, and 180 days after angioplasty was conducted. Compared with heparin, bivalirudin reduced the composite end point in patients undergoing PCI at 7 days (6.2% versus 7.9%, $P = .039$), a benefit that was sustained at 90 days (15.7% versus 18.5%, $P = .012$), but was no longer significant by 180 days (23% versus 24.7%, $P = .153$). Bleeding occurred in 3.5% of

the bivalirudin patients versus 9.3% in the heparin group by 7 days ($P < .001$). This trial showed that bivalirudin reduces ischemic complications and bleeding after angioplasty, and that further comparison trials with GPI and for coronary stenting were needed [25]. In the Comparison of Abciximab Complications with Hirulog for Ischemic Events Trial (CACHET), a pilot trial, 268 patients undergoing elective PCI were randomized to low-dose heparin plus abciximab; bivalirudin (1 mg/kg bolus, followed by 2.5 mg/kg/h for 4 hours) plus abciximab (FDA-approved dosing); or bivalirudin (0.5 or 0.75 mg/kg bolus followed by 1.75 mg/kg/h continued until the end of the procedure) with provisional abciximab [26]. Patients also received aspirin and clopidogrel. Provisional abciximab was used in 24% of the patients. No significant differences in efficacy or complications were observed, suggesting that bivalirudin with planned or provisional abciximab may be at least as safe and effective as heparin-abciximab during PCI [26].

The Randomized Evaluation in PCI Linking Angiomax to Reduced Clinical Events-1 (RE-PLACE-1) trial randomized 1056 patients undergoing elective or urgent revascularization in a large-scale pilot study to heparin (70 units/kg bolus) or bivalirudin (0.75 mg/kg bolus, 1.75 mg/kg/h infusion during the procedure) [27]. All patients received aspirin; pretreatment with clopidogrel was encouraged and occurred in 56% of patients, and GPI blockade was at the physician's discretion, occurring in 72% of cases. Stents were placed in 85% of patients. The activated clotting times were higher among patients randomized to bivalirudin than among those given heparin before device activation (median, 359 versus 293 seconds; $P < .001$). The composite efficacy end point of death, MI, or repeat revascularization before hospital discharge or within 48 hours occurred in 5.6% and 6.9% of patients in the bivalirudin and heparin groups, respectively ($P = .40$). Major bleeding occurred in 2.1% versus 2.7% of patients randomized to bivalirudin or heparin, respectively ($P = .52$) [27].

To determine whether bivalirudin with GPIs used in a provisional fashion if necessary during the procedure could provide protection from ischemic and bleeding complications of PCI comparable with the current efficacy standard of low-dose heparin plus routine GPI blockade, while offering a potential advantage with regard to cost, the authors conducted REPLACE-2. This was a randomized, double-blind, heparin-GPI controlled international trial in 6010 patients undergoing PCI [28]. Patients requiring reperfusion for acute MI were excluded. Patients were randomized to IV bivalirudin (0.75 mg/kg bolus plus 1.75 mg/kg/h infusion for the duration of the PCI) with provisional GPI (abciximab or eptifibatide, using FDA-approved dosing), or heparin and planned GPI. More than 85% of all patients received aspirin and a thienopyridine for at least 30 days after PCI. Provisional GPI was administered to 7.2% of patients in the bivalirudin group. At 30-day follow-up, the primary quadruple composite (death, MI, urgent repeat revascularization, or in-hospital major bleeding) occurred in 9.2% of patients in the bivalirudin group versus 10% in the UFH plus GPI group (odds ratio 0.92; 95% CI, 0.77–1.09; $P = .32$). The secondary triple composite end point (death, MI, urgent repeat revascularization) occurred in 7.6% of patients in the bivalirudin group compared with 7.1% of patients in the UFH plus GPI group (odds ratio 1.09; 95% CI, 0.90–1.32; $P = .40$). Both end points met formal statistical criteria for noninferiority to heparin plus planned GPI. Bivalirudin plus provisional GPI was associated with a significant 41% relative reduction in in-hospital bleeding (2.4% versus 4.1%; $P < .001$) [28]. In a subanalysis of patients with renal dysfunction (creatinine clearance <60 mL/min), bivalirudin provided suppression of ischemic events comparable with heparin and GPI inhibitors, regardless of renal function [29]. Fewer bleeding events were seen with bivalirudin irrespective of renal dysfunction. Both of these results are consistent with results of the overall trial. Long-term follow-up to REPLACE-2 showed that at 6 months there was no evidence that the 0.8% excess in non–Q-wave MI in the bivalirudin group translated into increases in mortality [30]. Nonsignificant trends toward lower 1-year mortality with bivalirudin were present in all patient subgroups analyzed. Long-term (1 year) follow-up with bivalirudin and provisional GPI is comparable with that of heparin and planned GPI. An economic evaluation of REPLACE-2 concluded that compared with heparin plus routine GPI use, bivalirudin plus provisional GPI use resulted in similar acute ischemic events and cost savings of $375 to $400 per patient depending on the analytic perspective [31]. In the Acute Catheterization and Urgent Intervention Triage Strategy (ACUITY) trial, 13,819 patients with acute coronary syndromes were randomized to one of three antithrombotic regimens:

unfractionated heparin or enoxaparin plus a glycoprotein IIb/IIIa inhibitor, bivalirudin plus a glycoprotein IIb/IIIa inhibitor, or bivalirudin alone [32]. Bivalirudin plus a glycoprotein IIb/IIIa inhibitor, as compared with heparin plus a glycoprotein IIb/IIIa inhibitor, was associated with noninferior 30-day rates of the composite ischemia end point (7.7% and 7.3%, respectively), major bleeding (5.3% and 5.7%), and the net clinical outcome end point (11.8% and 11.7%). Bivalirudin alone, as compared with heparin plus a glycoprotein IIb/IIIa inhibitor, was associated with a noninferior rate of the composite ischemia end point (7.8% and 7.3%, respectively; $P = 0.32$; relative risk, 1.08; 95% confidence interval [CI], 0.93 to 1.24) and significantly reduced rates of major bleeding (3.0% vs. 5.7%; $P < 0.001$; relative risk, 0.53; 95% CI, 0.43 to 0.65) and the net clinical outcome end point (10.1% vs. 11.7%; $P = 0.02$; relative risk, 0.86; 95% CI, 0.77 to 0.97).

Follow up results from the ACUITY trial measured composite ischemia (death, myocardial infarction, or unplanned revascularization for ischemia) at 1 year [33]. At 1 year, no statistically significant difference in rates of composite ischemia or mortality among patients with moderate- and high-risk ACS undergoing invasive treatment with the 3 therapies was found.

Additional studies have evaluated the use of bivalirudin in patients with acute ST elevation MI and patients with HIT. Bivalirudin was compared with heparin in 17,073 patients undergoing fibrinolysis with streptokinase for acute ST elevation MI [34]. Patients were given either an IV bolus and 48-hour infusion of bivalirudin or heparin together with a standard 1.5 million unit dose of streptokinase given directly after the antithrombotic bolus. The primary end point was 30-day mortality, which showed no difference; 10.8% of patients in the bivalirudin group and 10.9% in the heparin group had died ($P = .85$). There were significantly fewer reinfarctions within 96 hours in the bivalirudin group than in the heparin group (odds ratio 0.70; 95% CI, 0.56–0.87; $P = .001$). The rates of moderate and mild bleeding were significantly higher in the bivalirudin group than the heparin group (respectively 1.32, 95% CI, 1–1.74, $P = .05$; and 1.47, 95% CI, 1.34–1.62, $P < .0001$). No differences were found in rates of severe bleeding, intracerebral bleeding, and transfusions [34].

Various small trials and descriptive reports also support the use of bivalirudin in patients with HIT or history of HIT, [35–40]. In vitro studies showed no evidence of platelet aggregation response when bivalirudin was combined with sera from patients with history of HIT with or without thrombosis [17].

Argatroban

Argatroban is a small molecular weight (527 d) DTI that binds reversibly to the active site of thrombin. Like the other DTIs, it is a direct inhibitor of the thrombin molecule and does not require a cofactor (ie, antithrombin III). Argatroban exerts its antithrombotic activity by inhibition of thrombin-catalyzed or induced reactions, including fibrin formation; activation of coagulation factors V, VIII, and XIII; activation of protein C; and platelet aggregation [1–4,41]. It is selective for thrombin and has little effect on related serine proteases. Metabolism is hepatic by hydroxylation and aromatization. Metabolism by CYP3A4-5 to four known metabolites plays a minor role. Unchanged argatroban is the major plasma component. Plasma concentration of the M1 metabolite forms 0% to 20% of the parent drug and is threefold to fivefold weaker [15,22]. The elimination half-life is 39 to 51 minutes, but extends to approximately 181 minutes in hepatic impairment; the dose should be reduced when used in patients with hepatic dysfunction (see Table 2). Time to peak steady state for drug levels and anticoagulant activity is 1 to 3 hours. The aPTT and activated clotting time can be used to monitor the anticoagulant effect of argatroban. The agent is excreted primarily through biliary secretion, and no dose adjustment is required for renal impairment. The initial recommended dose for argatroban is 2 μg/kg/min given by IV infusion. However, recent reports indicate using doses of argatroban lower than 1.5 mcg/kg/min [16]. Dosing is usually titrated to maintain an aPTT of 1.5 to 3 times that of baseline (not to exceed 100 seconds); however, the maximum recommended dose is 10 μg/kg/min. In patients with hepatic impairment the dose is initiated at 0.5 μg/kg/min [41,42].

Argatroban does not interfere with heparin-induced antibodies, and it is FDA approved for the prophylaxis or treatment of thrombosis in patients with HIT and also as an anticoagulant in patients with HIT or at risk of HIT undergoing PCI [41]. In a prospective cohort study of 418 patients with HIT, argatroban was compared with 185 historical controls [44]. The primary end point was a composite of all-cause death, all-cause amputations, or new thrombosis in 37 days. In patients with isolated HIT, this end point was reduced with argatroban compared with control patients (28% versus 38.8%, $P = .04$). A nonsignificant trend toward a reduction in this end point was observed in patients with HIT-associated thrombosis (41.5% versus 56.5%, $P = .07$). Increased bleeding rates were not observed with argatroban. A second prospective cohort of similar design was performed in 160 HIT patients and 144 HIT–thrombosis syndrome patients treated with argatroban and 193 historical controls (147 with HIT, 46 with HIT–thrombosis syndrome) [45]. The same primary outcome measure was used for this trial and was reached more often in the HIT control group (25.6% versus 38.8%; $P = .014$). In the HIT–thrombosis syndrome group, significance was not reached (43.8% versus 56.5%; $P = .13$) for the primary outcome measurement. Significant between-group differences by time-to-event analysis of the composite end point favored argatroban treatment in HIT ($P = .010$) and HIT–thrombosis syndrome ($P = .014$). Argatroban therapy also significantly reduced new thrombosis and death caused by thrombosis ($P < .05$). Argatroban-treated patients achieved therapeutic aPTTs generally within 4 to 5 hours of starting therapy and, compared with control subjects, had a significantly more rapid rise in platelet counts ($P = .0001$). Bleeding events were similar between groups. The authors concluded from both trials that argatroban therapy compared with historical control improves outcomes, particularly new thrombosis and death caused by thrombosis, in patients with HIT without increasing bleeding risk. A retrospective analysis of acutely ill HIT patients identified 390 patients who received argatroban (mean dose 1.9 mcg/kg/min for a mean of 6 days) or historical control therapy (n = 98). The primary all-cause composite endpoint of death, amputation, or new thrombosis within 37 days occurred in 133 (34.1%) argatroban-treated patients and 38 (39.8%) controls (p = 0.41). Argatroban significantly reduced the primary thrombosis-related composite endpoint of death because of thrombosis, amputation secondary to ischemic complications of HIT, or new thrombosis (17.7% vs. 30.6%, p = 0.007), with similar rates of bleeding (7.7% vs. 8.2%, p = 0.84) [43].

Concomitant use of argatroban with warfarin can cause increased prolongation of the INR greater than that of warfarin alone and alternative guidelines for monitoring therapy should be followed. Loading doses of warfarin should not be used, but rather, it should be started at the expected daily dose. The INRs in patients on warfarin and argatroban can be predicted at doses between 1 and 2 μg/kg/min. At doses higher than 2 μg/kg/min, the INR for warfarin alone cannot reliably be predicted from the INR obtained for warfarin plus argatroban. Argatroban therapy can be stopped when the combined INR on warfarin and argatroban is >4. Repeat the INR measurement in 4 to 6 hours, and if the INR is below the therapeutic level, argatroban can be restarted. Repeat this procedure daily until the desired INR on warfarin alone is obtained. For patients receiving more than 2 μg/kg/min, it is recommended to reduce the dose of argatroban to 2 μg/kg/min, then measure the INR for argatroban and warfarin 4 to 6 hours after dose reduction [15,41,42]. In patients who are critically ill with normal hepatic function, excessive anticoagulation occurred with FDA-approved or lower starting doses of argatroban. Doses between 0.15 and 1.3 μg/kg/min were required to maintain aPTTs in the target range. Consider reducing the starting dose to 0.5 to 1 μg/kg/min in critically ill patients who may have impaired hepatic perfusion (ie, patients on vasopressors, having decreased cardiac output, having fluid overload). Patients with hepatic dysfunction may require more than 4 hours to achieve full reversal of argatroban's anticoagulant effect following treatment [41,42]. In critically ill patients with multiple organ dysfunction, a starting dose of 0.2 mcg/kg/min has been recommended by some [46].

Oral direct thrombin inhibitors

For the last five decades little progress has been made in the development of oral anticoagulants and the choices have been mainly limited to the vitamin K antagonists. "Sweet clover disease" first reported in the 1920s, a malady that consisted of cattle dying of hemorrhagic complications after the ingestion of spoiled sweet clover, eventually led to the discovery of coumarin derivatives in the early 1940s [47]. Since then, warfarin has basically remained the sole oral anticoagulant in North America and despite many efforts to develop alternative oral agents, to date none succeeded. Although an effective and widely used anticoagulant, warfarin has certain limitations including the need for frequent monitoring of anticoagulant effect by the INR, large interindividual dosing

differences based in part on P-450 CYP2C9 activity, a narrow therapeutic index, interactions with dietary vitamin K and a large number of other medications, the need for constant patient education, compliance, and frequent follow-up [48]. These limitations, make warfarin's use complex in the clinical setting, creating a burden for patients and health care providers alike. There is clearly a need for other oral anticoagulant agents that are less complex and easier for the clinician to administer and manage. Many novel oral antithrombotic agents are currently in development, with great potential to improve on the limitations of vitamin K antagonists. Several oral DTIs are being investigated [49]. Ximelagatran, the first agent in the oral DTI class to be investigated, never made it to the US market due to concerns around liver toxicity. Despite this, many lessons can be learned from the extensive clinical data published to date as the stage is being set for more novel compounds of the same class. Dabigatran is another promising oral DTI now in Phase III development.

Ximelagatran

Ximelagatran has been evaluated for thromboprophylaxis in patients undergoing major orthopedic surgery, stroke prevention in AF, and in the acute treatment and secondary prevention of VTE.

Chemistry, pharmacology, and pharmacokinetics

Ximelagatran is a prodrug that was specially designed to overcome the poor oral bioavailability of its active drug melagatran. Ximelagatran contains two protecting residues, a hydroxyl and ester group, creating a large increase in lipophilicity and permeability coefficient across epithelial cells, leading to an oral bioavailability of approximately 18% to 24% in humans with low interindividual variability in resultant melagatran plasma levels [50–53]. On absorption, ximelagatran is converted to melagatran by either reduction of the hydroxyamidine to ethylmelagatran followed by hydrolysis to melagatran, or hydrolysis first to hydroxylmelagatran followed by reduction to melagatran [50,53]. Melagatran does not undergo further metabolism, and is primarily excreted by the kidneys. Ximelagatran itself, and the hydroxylmelagatran, have minimal anticoagulant activity [50]. Melagatran is a small-molecule DTI, with a molecular weight of 429 d [51]. Melagatran's pharmacokinetic parameters after administration of oral ximelagatran have been measured using parenteral melagatran as a comparator. A first-order, linear one-compartment model has been described. A linear dose-proportional increase in area under the serum concentration curve observed suggests that bioavailability is independent of dose [50]. Ximelagatran is rapidly absorbed, with peak concentrations achieved approximately 1 hour after administration [52]. The mean bioavailability measured in young healthy males is approximately 20% [51]. After oral ximelagatran administration, the mean time to maximum melagatran plasma concentrations is 1.8 to 3.3 hours; volume of distribution 2 to 2.5 L/kg; plasma clearance 23 to 34 L/h (approximately 48 L/h if renally impaired); and elimination half-life between 2.6 and 4.8 hours (approximately 9 hours in renally impaired) [53]. Mild to moderate hepatic impairment has no apparent significant effect on the pharmacokinetics or pharmacodynamics of ximelagatran [54]. With the exception of individuals with significant renal impairment or very low body weights, dosing reduction is not needed in unique populations, such as obese patients (up to 141 kg); various major ethnic backgrounds; or advanced age (up to 77 years old) [55–58]. The therapeutic window of melagatran has been shown to be wider than that of warfarin in a rat model of arterial thrombosis [59]. Ximelagatran and melagatran are not metabolized by known hepatic microsomal enzymes and to date they seem to lack significant CYP450 drug and food interactions [60]. Ximelagatran's bioavailability is not affected if taken with concurrent food, if crushed and mixed in applesauce, or if dissolved in water and administered by a nasogastric tube [61]. Concurrent ethanol ingestion does not alter the pharmacodynamics or pharmacokinetics of ximelagatran [62]. As with any other anticoagulant, however, the concurrent use of ethanol can lead to impaired cognitive function creating an independent risk for bleeding complications. The apparent lack of drug-drug and drug-food interactions with ximelagatran could offer a major clinical and practical advantage over warfarin that is currently limited by a tremendous number of interactions.

Clinical efficacy

An extensive clinical trials program involving approximately 30,000 patients has been completed to test the effectiveness of ximelagatran for a variety of indications.

Orthopedic surgery

In patients undergoing major orthopedic surgery, such as total hip arthroplasty or total knee arthroplasty, current practice in North America is to use pneumatic compression stockings, warfarin, UFH, LMWH, fondaparinux, or some combination thereof for VTE prophylaxis. Several studies have compared the efficacy and safety of ximelagatran and melagatran with LMWH or warfarin for prophylaxis of VTE in patients undergoing total hip arthroplasty or total knee arthroplasty [63–69].

Melagatran-ximelagatran compared with low-molecular-weight heparin. The Melagatran as prophylaxis of THRombosis in Orthopedic surgery (METHRO II and METHRO III) trials and the EXpanded PRophylaxis Evaluation Surgery Study (EXPRESS) were primarily conducted in Europe in both hip and knee arthroplasty patients, and compared melagatran-ximelagatran with once-daily LMWH started preoperatively [63–65]. METHRO II was a phase II dose ranging study. All three studies administered 3 mg of SC melagatran at some point after surgery, followed by twice-daily dosing until initiation of oral ximelagatran was started (usually the morning after surgery) or when the patient could take oral medication. The LMWH comparator (enoxaparin, 40 mg, or dalteparin, 5000 units daily) was started the evening before surgery. One major methodologic difference between the three studies was the timing of the first SC melagatran dose. The VTE outcomes for the LWMH arms in the three trials were very similar, allowing for indirect comparison of the three different melagatran-ximelagatran treatment groups. In the METHRO II and EXPRESS trials where SC melagatran was initiated immediately after surgery, a significantly lower rate of PE, total and proximal DVT compared with LMWH was observed [63,65]. The melagatran-ximelagatran combination reduced proximal DVT and PE by greater than 40% in the knee patients and by 67% in the hip patients compared with LMWH. Drainage from the wound site was slightly higher in the ximelagatran arm, with bleeding requiring reoperation very low at less than 0.5% [65]. In the METHRO III trial, where SC melagatran was initiated 4 to 12 hours postoperatively, the only outcome reaching statistical significance was fewer total DVTs or PEs seen in the total hip replacement subgroup receiving enoxaparin ($P = .004$). A post hoc analysis of the METHRO III data showed a lower rate of total DVT-PE when melagatran was started at 4 to 8 hours (27%) versus 8 to 12 hours postoperatively (35.4%). This observation underscores the importance of the timing of initiation of anticoagulation therapy after total hip arthroplasty and total knee arthroplasty. The overall incidence of major bleeding for total hip arthroplasty and total knee arthroplasty combined was no different between agents [64]. Parenteral melagatran was not used in the studies predominantly enrolling patients in North America. Colwell and coworkers [66] observed no significant decreases in total DVT-PE or proximal DVT between enoxaparin, 30 mg SC twice daily, or ximelagatran, 24 mg given orally twice daily, both started the morning after surgery in patients undergoing total hip arthroplasty. Symptomatic DVT during treatment occurred in fewer patients receiving ximelagatran. As seen in the EXPRESS trial [65], postoperative wound drainage was slightly higher, but not statistically significant ($P = .372$) with the use of ximelagatran [66].

These four comparative trials of ximelagatran versus LMWH help underline the importance of the timing and the dose of the antithrombotic agent relative to surgery [63–66]. Oral ximelagatran in combination with SC melagatran given at the time of hip or knee surgery was more efficacious in two studies, but at the cost of slightly greater bleeding rates [63,65]. When SC melagatran was not administered immediately after surgery, bleeding rates were comparable with LMWH, but efficacy was relatively reduced [64,66].

Ximelagatran compared with warfarin. Three major trials are presently available comparing ximelagatran, 24 or 36 mg twice daily started the morning after surgery, with warfarin at an INR target of 2.5 (range 1.8–3) begun the evening of surgery in patients undergoing total knee arthroplasty [67–69]. The EXULT A trial [67] examined both 24- and 36-mg doses of ximelagatran, whereas Francis and coworkers [69] only evaluated the 24-mg twice-daily dose, and EXULT B the 36-mg twice-daily dose [68]. Although all the assessed thrombotic outcomes were less frequent in the ximelagatran arms, statistical significance was exhibited only in the ximelagatran 36-mg groups in regard to a lower incidence of total DVT-PE compared with the warfarin cohort (20.3% versus 27.6%, $P = .003$ in EXULT A; and 22.5% versus 31.9%, $P < .001$ in EXULT B) [67,68]. Major bleeding was not significantly different in any of the three total knee arthroplasty trials. No

difference in postoperative bleeding was observed between cohorts, and wound dehiscence occurred in only 3 of the 1526 patients receiving ximelagatran [67,68]. The degree of INR control differed between the three trials. In EXULT-A warfarin arm, 67% of the patients by day 3, and 75% of the patients by the day of venography (mean INR, 2.4), had an INR within 1.8 to 3 [67]. The results for EXULT B were similar to EXULT A [68], whereas achieving INR target goals in the first study by Francis and coworkers [69] was lower at 32% and 53%, respectively.

The magnitude of ximelagatran dose seems to be an important factor linked to efficacy of the drug in the three previously discussed trials. The 36-mg twice-daily dose used in the EXULT A and B trials seemed to confer greater efficacy without unduly increasing bleeding risk [67–69]. In EXULT-A, the 36-mg ximelagatran group had similar bleeding and proximal DVT-PE rates as the 24-mg dose group, but was significantly better than warfarin for total DVT-PE plus death (27.6% versus 20.3%, $P = .003$), whereas the 24-mg dose was not (27.6% versus 24.9%, $P = .28$) [67]. Based on these observations, the 36-mg dose of ximelagatran is most likely preferred in patients undergoing total knee arthroplasty.

Treatment of venous thrombosis

The current standard of treatment for VTE includes administration of either UFH or LMWH for a minimum of 5 days and continued until INR is >2 for 2 consecutive days. Warfarin is then continued for at least 3 to 6 months, or longer if indicated [70]. The role of ximelagatran in the treatment of VTE as a potential alternative to current anticoagulant therapies has also been investigated. The THRombin Inhibitor in Venous thrombo-Embolism (THRIVE) studies compared the treatment of ximelagatran with standard anticoagulation or placebo for the acute treatment of VTE and up to 6 months after the initial event (THRIVE Treatment), and for an additional 18 months after the initial 6 months of standard therapy (THRIVE III) [71,72].

The THRIVE treatment study evaluated the safety and efficacy of ximelagatran, 36 mg twice daily, in the treatment of acute DVT (of which 37% also had a PE) to at least 5 days of enoxaparin, 1 mg/kg SC twice daily, and warfarin adjusted to an INR of 2 to 3 over 6 months [71]. Ximelagatran was found to be noninferior to enoxaparin combined with warfarin in preventing recurrence of VTE after acute DVT with or without PE. Numerically, there was less major bleeding and all-cause mortality in the ximelagatran group compared with the enoxaparin-warfarin group; however, the difference was not statistically significant. Enrolled patients may have been at low risk for VTE as evidenced by the lower rate of recurrent VTE regardless of treatment assignment (1.5%–2.1%) compared with the typical expected rate of 3% to 6% using standard treatment with either UFH or LMWH. Nonetheless, the findings of this study raise the possibility of treating VTE in the near future with a single oral agent, potentially eliminating the need for the combination of heparin-warfarin anticoagulation.

The THRIVE III study compared a lower dose of ximelagatran (24 mg twice daily) with placebo for 18 months of extended anticoagulation for secondary VTE prevention after an initial standard 6 months of anticoagulation with warfarin [72]. The estimated cumulative rate for recurrent VTE was significantly greater in the placebo group, 12.6%, compared with the ximelagatran group at 2.8% ($P < .001$). The major and minor bleeding event rates were similar for treatment and placebo groups. Further reduction in events using the 36-mg dose (which has not been studied in secondary prevention of VTE) of ximelagatran may be possible and warrants further consideration. This trial demonstrates the benefit of long-term anticoagulation with low-dose ximelagatran for the prevention of recurrent VTE beyond 6 months of standard anticoagulant therapy.

Stroke prevention in atrial fibrillation

Patients with AF are at high risk of stroke and require anticoagulation therapy. The incidence of stroke is even higher in patients with additional risk factors, such as congestive heart failure and left ventricular failure, coronary artery disease, hypertension, advanced age, diabetes mellitus, history of a stroke, or transient ischemic attack [73]. Warfarin is the standard of therapy in high-risk AF patients because it has been shown to reduce the risk of stroke by approximately two thirds. Despite this, warfarin is underused and it is only prescribed in 47% to 59% of eligible patients [73]. The development of novel antithrombotic agents may allow for the removal of existing barriers that prevent patients with AF from receiving effective prophylactic therapy.

The Stroke Prevention by ORal Thrombin Inhibition in atrial Fibrillation (SPORTIF) studies compared ximelagatran with standard warfarin therapy for the prevention of stroke in patients with nonvalvular AF and at least one additional risk factor for stroke [74–76]. SPORTIF III, a large (N = 3467) phase III, randomized, open-label trial compared ximelagatran, 36 mg twice daily, with adjusted-dose warfarin (INR of 2–3). Patients from 23 countries were included in this study and followed for an average of 17 months (range, 12–26 months per patient) [74,75]. More than one additional stroke risk factor was present in 72% of patients. The primary end point of the study was to demonstrate that ximelagatran was noninferior compared with warfarin for the prevention of stroke and systemic embolic events. The intention to treat event rate was not significantly different between the two groups: 1.6% per year with ximelagatran, and 2.3% per year with warfarin. Total bleeding rate (major and minor) was significantly less for ximelagatran (25.5%) compared with warfarin (29.5%) ($P = .007$; 14% relative risk reduction). Hemorrhagic strokes occurred in four (0.2% per year) of the patients receiving ximelagatran and nine (0.4% per year) of the patients receiving warfarin. The intracranial bleeding rates were similar to those observed with warfarin (0.3%) in several recent AF trials. The secondary combined end point of death, stroke, or major bleed for the on-treatment analysis was significantly lower in the ximelagatran treatment group (4.6%) as compared with warfarin (6.1%) (25% relative risk reduction, $P = .022$). The quality of warfarin INR control was 66% of the time in the typical target range of 2–3 and 81% time in range of 1.8 to 3.2. This INR control is much higher than what is typically achieved in clinical practice. It is possible that a higher primary event rate for warfarin-treated patients would be expected in clinical practice where poor INR control is common [77].

SPORTIF V was another large, randomized trial designed similarly to SPORTIF III, but was double blinded and mainly conducted in North America. SPORTIF V also compared ximelagatran, 36 mg twice daily, with adjusted-dose warfarin to an INR of 2–3 [74,76]. In the patients enrolled, 75% had more than one stroke risk factor. The incidence of stroke and systemic embolism was 1.6% per year in the ximelagatran group versus 1.2% in the warfarin group ($P = .13$). The combined incidence of primary events, major bleeding, and death in SPORTIF V (on-treatment analysis) was 5.8% for ximelagatran and 6.3% for warfarin (relative risk reduction 7%, $P = .527$). Similar to the SPORTIFF III trial,

63% of patients were maintained with INR values between 2 and 3, and 83% between 1.8 and 3.2. This suggests that the warfarin arm received the best possible therapy for analysis, which might not occur in general clinical practice. The SPORTIF trials demonstrated that ximelagatran is equivalent to well-controlled warfarin for stroke prevention in patients with AF.

Safety considerations

One of the major safety concerns associated with ximelagatran use is the potential of developing drug-induced liver toxicity. An increase in liver function tests (specifically alanine aminotransferase increases of more than three times the upper limit of normal) with ximelagatran have been reported in several trials. In the THRIVE III extended prophylaxis trial [72], increased alanine aminotransferase greater than three times upper limit of normal was observed in 6% of patients (compared with 1% in the placebo), with an estimated cumulative incidence rate of 5.4% at 4 months and 6.4% at 18 months. The enzyme levels normalized over a similar time course whether the ximelagatran was continued or stopped. Enzyme levels normalized in all but four patients. No patients progressed to symptomatic hepatic dysfunction in this study. In the THRIVE Treatment study [71] the incidence of alanine aminotransferase elevation greater than three times upper limit of normal was 9.6% in the ximelagatran arm and 2% in the warfarin arm. Nine patients in this study on ximelagatran also had bilirubin elevations greater than two times normal. One of these patients developed a suspected drug-induced hepatitis without an alternative explanation, but did recover after ximelagatran discontinuation. Another patient with elevated bilirubin died of fulminant hepatitis B. In the SPORTIF III and V trials [75,76], the increase in alanine aminotransferase of more than three times upper limit of normal was seen in 6.1% and 6% of patients receiving ximelagatran versus 0.8% on warfarin ($P \leq .001$). The increase was most commonly seen in the first 2 to 6 months of therapy. In SPORTIF III [75], 55% of the ximelagatran patients with alanine aminotransferase greater than three times upper limit of normal continued treatment, for which 93% returned to normal. Of the 45% where treatment was stopped, 8% of patients did not completely normalize. In SPORTIF III [75] four patients developed jaundice. In SPORTIF V [76] 14 patients had an increase in total bilirubin greater than two times normal within

1 month of an alanine aminotransferase rise greater than three times normal, an indicator of a possible severe insult on the liver. A total of five of these cases did not have an alternative diagnosis and two of these five patients died. Based on the summary of these data, the FDA has estimated that the rate of severe liver injury caused by ximelagatran was 1 in 200 patients [78]. Some experts believe 10% of these individuals progress to liver failure, liver transplant, or death [79]. If 1 in 200 patients have a sever liver insult on ximelagatran and 10% of these lead to overt liver failure, it is estimated that 1 in 2000 patients treated with long-term ximelagatran progress to overt liver failure. In fact, three patients did die with circumstances the FDA believed could reasonably be related to ximelagatran use, which is consistent with the 1 in 2000 rate because this analysis had 6948 patients [78].

Another concerning finding from the pooled Exult A and B studies [67,68] were coronary artery disease–related adverse events. The number and percentage of patients with these events (MI or ischemia-angina) was 20 (0.75%) in the ximelagatran group and 5 (0.26%) in the warfarin group ($P = .028$). The number and percentage of patients with MI was 16 (0.6%) in the ximelagatran group and 4 (0.21%) in the warfarin group ($P = .04951$). Considering that no differences in important demographics were present in the groups and that ximelagatran is an antithrombin agent with potential for use in cardiology, these findings were also concerning and unexpected [78].

The combination of melagatran and ximelagatran for short-term VTE prophylaxis after total hip arthroplasty or total knee arthroplasty was approved in Europe in May 2004, however it was subsequently withdrawn from the market due to concerns of liver toxicity. In the United States, however, the approval status of the agent took a different turn. In October 2004, the FDA denied approval of ximelagatran for all indications submitted (prevention of VTE after total knee replacement surgery, the long-term prevention of VTE recurrence after standard therapy, and stroke prevention because of AF). This decision was mainly because of increased rates of coronary artery disease events in ximelagatran patients in some studies and the possibility of ximelagatran-induced hepatic failure when it is used for long-term therapy [78].

Ironically, ximelagatran was the first oral agent in the last 50 years to come close to overcoming the major clinical challenges presented by warfarin. However, these benefits of ximelagatran did not outweigh the risks when compared with traditional anticoagulant therapies.

Dabigatran

Dabigatran is another emerging low-molecular-weight oral DTI currently in clinical development. Because dabigatran has poor oral bioavailability, an orally active prodrug dabigatran etexilate has been developed to overcome this problem. Like melagatran, dabigatran is a specific, competitive, and reversible thrombin inhibitor. The bioavailability of dabigatran is 3.5% to 5%. The agent is renally excreted; dose decreases will be necessary in patients with renal insufficiency. The metabolism of dabigatran is independent of the CYP450 enzyme system. The elimination half-life is 14 to 17 hours, longer as compared with ximelagatran; once-daily administration may be an appropriate approach [80]. To date, two phase II dose-ranging studies and three Phase III clinical trials have been completed in patients undergoing orthopedic surgery [81–85]. A pooled analysis of major VTE and VTE-related mortality in patients undergoing elective knee and hip replacement surgery across more than 8,000 randomized patients that were included in the three phase 3 trials (RE-MODEL, RE-MOBILIZE, and RE-NOVATE) was conducted [86]. The pooled analysis concluded that dabigatran was non-inferior to enoxaparin in the prevention of major VTE and VTE-related mortality after both knee and hip replacement. Major VTE and VTE-related mortality occurred in 3.8% of the 150 mg dabigatran etexilate group and 3.0% of the 220 mg dabigatran etexilate group, versus 3.3% of the enoxaparin group. Major bleeding events were similar across all treatment groups (1.1%, 1.4% and 1.4% respectively). Additional phase III clinical trials are under way for various indications including VTE prevention and treatment, and stroke prevention in AF. Like ximelagatran, dabigatran can be administered in fixed doses without anticoagulation monitoring and it seems void of clinically significant food and drug interactions [80–82]. In the short-term orthopedic studies no liver enzyme elevation has been noted; however, its effect on liver function with longer administration ≥ 1 month is unknown at this time.

Summary

Decades of research have been devoted to developing effective, safe, and convenient anticoagulant agents. Although effective, traditional anticoagulants are complex to administer and are fraught with limitations, such as unpredictable anticoagulant effect, frequent monitoring, and dosing adjustments. In recent years, much emphasis has been placed on the development of DTIs that offer benefits over agents like heparin and warfarin including the inhibition of both circulating and clot-bound thrombin; a more predictable anticoagulant response because they do not bind to plasma proteins and are not neutralized by platelet factor 4; lack of required cofactors, such as antithrombin or heparin cofactor II; inhibiting thrombin-induced platelet aggregation; and absence of induction of immune-mediated thrombocytopenia. Various injectable DTIs are currently available and used for many indications, such as HIT, prophylaxis of VTE, and acute coronary syndromes with and without PCI. In addition, research is now focusing on oral DTIs that seem promising and offer various advantages, such as oral administration, predictable pharmacokinetics and pharmacodynamics, a broad therapeutic window, no routine monitoring, no significant drug interactions, and fixed-dose administration. The first oral DTI to make it to the United States market may revolutionize antithrombotic therapy, allowing for more convenient and less complex therapeutic options.

References

[1] Bates SM, Weitz JL. The mechanism of action of thrombin inhibitors. J Invasive Cardiol 2000; 12(Suppl F):27–32.

[2] Nutescu EA, Wittkowsky AK. Direct thrombin inhibitors for anticoagulation. Ann Pharmacother 2004;38:99–109.

[3] Weitz JI, Hirsh J, Samama MM. New anticoagulant drugs: the Seventh ACCP Conference on Antithrombotic and Thrombolytic Therapy. Chest 2004; 126:265–86.

[4] Nutescu EA, Shapiro NL, Chevalier A, et al. A pharmacologic overview of current and emerging anticoagulants. Cleve Clin J Med 2005;72(Suppl 1):S2–6.

[5] Direct Thrombin Inhibitor Trialists' Collaborative Group. Direct thrombin inhibitors in acute coronary syndromes: principal results of a meta-analysis based on individual patients' data. Lancet 2002; 359:294–302.

[6] Berlex Laboratories. Product information: refludan (Lepirudin) rDNA. Available at: www.refludan.com. Accessed July 5, 2005.

[7] Greinacher A, Volpel H, Janssens U, et al. Recombinant hirudin (lepirudin) provides safe and effective anticoagulation in patients with heparin-induced

thrombocytopenia: a prospective study. Circulation 1999;99:73–80.

[8] Greinacher A, Janssens U, Berg G, et al. Lepirudin (recombinant hirudin) for parenteral anticoagulation in patients with heparin-induced thrombocytopenia. Heparin-Associated Thrombocytopenia Study (HAT) investigators. Circulation 1999;100:587–93.

[9] Lubenow N, Eichler P, Lietz T, et al. for the HIT Investigators Group. Lepirudin in patients with heparin-induced thrombocytopenia—results of the third prospective study (HAT-3) and a combined analysis of HAT-1, HAT-2, and HAT-3. J Thromb Haemost 2005;3:2428–36.

[10] Tardy B, Lecompte T, Boelhen F, et al. Predictive factors for thrombosis and major bleeding in an observational study in 181 patients with heparin-induced thrombocytopenia treated with lepirudin. Blood 2006;108:1492–6.

[11] McDaniel M, Soff G. Decreasing adverse drug events associated with lepirudin and argatroban for the treatment of heparin-induced thrombocytopenia [abstract]. Blood 2004;104:495.

[12] Hacquard M, Maistre E, Lecompte T. Lepirudin: is the approved dosing schedule too high? J Thromb Haemost 2005;3:2593–6.

[13] Kiser TH, Jung R, Maclaren R, et al. Evaluation of diagnostic tests and argatroban or lepirudin therapy in patients with suspected heparininduced thrombocytopenia. Pharmacotherapy 2005;25:1736–45.

[14] Schiele F, Lindgaerde F, Eriksson H, et al. Subcutaneous recombinant hirudin (HBW 023) versus intravenous sodium heparin in treatment of established acute deep vein thrombosis of the legs: a multicentre prospective dose-ranging randomized trial. International Multicentre Hirudin Study Group. Thromb Haemost 1997;77:834–8.

[15] Frenkel EP, Shen YM, Haley BB. The direct thrombin inhibitors: their role and use for rational anticoagulation. Hematol Oncol Clin North Am 2005;19:119–45.

[16] Dager WE, Dougherty JA, Nguyen PH. Heparin-induced thrombocytopenia: Treatment options and special considerations. Pharmacotherapy 2007;27(4):564–87.

[17] Eriksson BI, Ekman S, Lindbratt S, et al. Prevention of thromboembolism with use of recombinant hirudin: results of a double-blind, multicenter trial comparing the efficacy of desirudin (Revasc) with that of unfractionated heparin in patients having a total hip replacement. J Bone Joint Surg Am 1997;79:326–33.

[18] Erikkson BI, Wille-Jorgensen P, Kalebo P, et al. A comparison of recombinant hirudin with a low-molecular-weight heparin to prevent thromboembolic complications after total hip replacement. N Engl J Med 1997;337:1329–35.

[19] Serruys PW, Herrman JP, Simon R, et al. A comparison of hirudin with heparin in the prevention of restenosis after coronary angioplasty. The Helvetica Investigators. N Engl J Med 1995;333:757–63.

[20] The GUSTO-IIb Investigators. A comparison of recombinant hirudin with heparin for the treatment of acute coronary syndromes. The Global Use of Strategies to Open Occluded Coronary Arteries (GUSTO)-IIb Investigators. N Engl J Med 1996;335:775–82.

[21] Warkentin TE. Bivalent direct thrombin inhibitors: hirudin and bivalirudin. Best Pract Res Clin Haematol 2004;17:105–25.

[22] Monreal M, Costa J, Salva P. Pharmacological properties of hirudin and its derivatives. Drug Ther (NY) 1996;8:171–82.

[23] The Medicines Company. Product information: angiomax (Bivalirudin). Available at: www.angiomax.com. Accessed July 5, 2005.

[24] Lui HK. Dosage, pharmacological effects and clinical outcomes for bivalirudin in percutaneous coronary intervention. J Invasive Cardiol 2000;12(Suppl F):41–52.

[25] Bittl JA, Chaitman BR, Feit F, et al. Bivalirudin versus heparin during coronary angioplasty for unstable or postinfarction angina: final report reanalysis of the Bivalirudin Angioplasty Study. Am Heart J 2001;142:952–9.

[26] Lincoff AM, Kleiman NS, Kottke-Marchant K, et al. Bivalirudin with planned or provisional abciximab versus low-dose heparin and abciximab during percutaneous coronary revascularization: results of the Comparison of Abciximab Complications with Hirulog for Ischemic Events Trial (CACHET). Am Heart J 2002;143:847–53.

[27] Lincoff AM, Bittl JA, Kleiman NS, et al. Comparison of bivalirudin versus heparin during percutaneous coronary intervention. The Randomized Evaluation of PCI Linking Angiomax to Reduced Clinical Events (REPLACE)–1 Trial. Am J Cardiol 2004;93:1092–6.

[28] Lincoff AM, Bittl JA, Harrington RA, et al. Bivalirudin and provisional glycoprotein IIb/IIIa blockade compared with heparin and planned glycoprotein IIb/IIIa blockade during percutaneous coronary intervention. REPLACE-2 randomized trial. JAMA 2003;289:853–63.

[29] Chew DP, Lincoff AM, Gurm H, et al. Bivalirudin versus heparin and glycoprotein IIb/IIIa inhibition among patients with renal impairment undergoing percutaneous coronary intervention: a subanalysis of the REPLACE-2 trial. Am J Cardiol 2005;95:581–5.

[30] Lincoff AM, Kleiman NS, Kereiakes DJ, et al. Long-term efficacy of bivalirudin and provisional glycoprotein IIb/IIIa blockade vs heparin and planned glycoprotein IIb/IIIa blockade during percutaneous coronary revascularization. REPLACE-2 randomized trial. JAMA 2004;292:696–703.

[31] Cohen DJ, Lincoff AM, Lavelle TA, et al. Economic evaluation of bivalirudin with provisional glycoprotein IIB/IIIA inhibition versus heparin with routine glycoprotein IIB/IIIA inhibition for percutaneous coronary intervention: results from the REPLACE-2 trial. J Am Coll Cardiol 2004;44:1792–800.

[32] Stone GW, McLaurin BT, Cox DA, et al. Bivalirudin for patients with acute coronary syndromes. N Engl J Med 2006;355:2203–16.

[33] Stone GW, Ware JH, Bertrand ME, et al. Antithrombotic strategies in patients with acute coronary syndromes undergoing early invasive management: one-year results from the ACUITY trial. JAMA 2007;298(21):2497–506.

[34] White H. Thrombin-specific anticoagulation with bivalirudin versus heparin in patients receiving fibrinolytic therapy for acute myocardial infarction: the HERO-2 randomised trial. Lancet 2001;358:1855–63.

[35] Mahaffey KW, Lewis BE, Wildermann NM, et al. The anticoagulant therapy with bivalirudin to assist in the performance of percutaneous coronary intervention in patients with heparin-induced thrombocytopenia (ATBAT) study: main results. J Invasive Cardiol 2003;15:611–6.

[36] Francis JL, Drexler A, Gwyn G, et al. Successful use of bivalirudin in the treatment of patients suspected, or at risk for, heparin-induced thrombocytopenia. Blood 2004;104:4077.

[37] Koster A, Dyke CM, Aldea G, et al. Bivalirudin during cardiopulmonary bypass in patients with previous or acute heparin-induced thrombocytopenia and heparin antibodies: results of the CHOOSE-ON trial. Ann Thorac Surg 2007;83:572–7.

[38] Mann MJ, Tseng E, Ratcliffe M, et al. Use of bivalirudin, a direct thrombin inhibitor, and its reversal with modified ultrafiltration during heart transplantation in a patient with heparin-induced thrombocytopenia. J Heart Lung Transplant 2005;24:222–5.

[39] Clayton SB, Ascell JR, Crumbley AJ, et al. Cardiopulmonary bypass with bivalirudin in type II heparin-induced thrombocytopenia. Ann Thorac Surg 2004;78:2167–9.

[40] Gordon G, Rastegar H, Schumann R, et al. Successful use of bivalirudin for cardiopulmonary bypass in a patient with heparin-induced thrombocytopenia. J Cardiothorac Vasc Anesth 2003;17:632–5.

[41] Glaxo Smith Kline. Product information: argatroban. Available at: www.argatroban.com. Accessed July 5, 2005.

[42] LaMonte MP, Brown PM, Hursting MJ. Alternative parenteral anticoagulation with argatroban, a direct thrombin inhibitor. Expert Rev Cardiovasc Ther 2005;3:31–41.

[43] Gray A, Wallis DE, Hurstin MJ, et al. Argatroban therapy for heparin-induced thrombocytopenia in acutely ill patients. Clin Appl Thromb Hemost 2007;13:353–61.

[44] Lewis BE, Wallis DE, Leya F, et al. Argatroban anticoagulation in patients with heparin-induced thrombocytopenia. Arch Intern Med 2003;163:1849–56.

[45] Lewis BE, Wallis DE, Berkowitz SD, et al, ARG-911 Study Investigators. Argatroban anticoagulant therapy in patients with heparin-induced thrombocytopenia. Circulation 2001;103:1838–43.

[46] Beinderlinden M, Treschan TA, Gorlinger K, et al. Argatroban anticoagulation in critically ill patients. Ann Pharmacother 2007;41:749–54.

[47] Nutescu EA, Bauman JL. Shifting paradigms in oral anticoagulation management. J Cardiovasc Pharmacol Ther 2004;3:149–50.

[48] Ansell J, Hirsh J, Poller L, et al. The pharmacology and management of the vitamin K antagonists: the Seventh ACCP Conference on Antithrombotic and Thrombolytic Therapy. Chest 2004;126:204S–33S.

[49] Nutescu EA, Helgason CM, Briller J, et al. New blood thinner offers first potential alternative in 50 years: ximelagatran. J Cardiovasc Nurs 2004;19:374–83.

[50] Eriksson UG, Bredberg U, Hoffman KJ, et al. Absorption, distribution, metabolism, and excretion of ximelagatran, an oral direct thrombin inhibitor, in rats, dogs, and humans. Drug Metab Dispos 2003;31:294–305.

[51] Eriksson UG, Bredberg U, Gislen K, et al. Pharmacokinetics and pharmacodynamics of ximelagatran, a novel oral direct thrombin inhibitor, in young healthy male subjects. Eur J Clin Pharmacol 2003;59:35–43.

[52] Wolzt M, Wollbratt M, Svensson M, et al. Consistent pharmacokinetics of the oral direct thrombin inhibitor ximelagatran in patients with nonvalvular atrial fibrillation and in healthy subjects. Eur J Clin Pharmacol 2003;59:537–43.

[53] Gustafsson D, Elg M. The pharmacodynamics and pharmacokinetics of the oral direct thrombin inhibitor ximelagatran and its active metabolite melagatran: a mini-review. Thromb Res 2003;109:S9–15.

[54] Wahlander K, Eriksson-Lepkowska M, Frison L, et al. No influence of mild-to-moderate hepatic impairment on the pharmacokinetics and pharmacodynamics of ximelagatran, an oral direct thrombin inhibitor. Clin Pharmacokinet 2003;42:755–64.

[55] Sarich TC, Teng R, Peters GR, et al. No influence of obesity on the pharmacokinetics and pharmacodynamics of melagatran, the active form of the oral direct thrombin inhibitor ximelagatran. Clin Pharmacokinet 2003;42:485–92.

[56] Eriksson UG, Johansson S, Attman PO, et al. Influence of severe renal impairment on the pharmacokinetics and pharmacodynamics of oral ximelagatran and subcutaneous melagatran. Clin Pharmacokinet 2003;42:743–53.

[57] Johansson LC, Frison L, Logren U, et al. Influence of age on the pharmacokinetics and pharmacodynamics of ximelagatran, an oral direct thrombin inhibitor. Clin Pharmacokinet 2003;42:381–92.

[58] Johansson LC, Andersson M, Fager G, et al. No influence of ethnic origin on the pharmacokinetics and pharmacodynamics of melagatran following oral administration of ximelagatran, a novel oral direct thrombin inhibitor, to healthy male volunteers. Clin Pharmacokinet 2003;42:475–84.

[59] Elg M, Gustafsson D, Carlsson S. Antithrombotic effects and bleeding time of thrombin inhibitors and warfarin in the rat. Thromb Res 1999;94:187–97.

[60] Bredberg E, Andersson TB, Frison L, et al. Ximelagatran, an oral direct thrombin inhibitor, has a low potential for cytochrome P450-mediated drug-drug interactions. Clin Pharmacokinet 2003;42:765–77.

[61] Schutzer KM, Wall U, Lonnerstedt C, et al. Bioequivalence of ximelagatran, an oral direct thrombin inhibitor, as whole or crushed tablets or dissolved formulation. Curr Med Res Opin 2004;20:325–31.

[62] Sarich TC, Johansson S, Schutzer KM, et al. The pharmacokinetics and pharmacodynamics of ximelagatran, an oral direct thrombin inhibitor, are unaffected by a single dose of alcohol. J Clin Pharmacol 2004;44:388–93.

[63] Eriksson BI, Bergqvist D, Kalebo P, et al. Ximelagatran and melagatran compared with dalteparin for prevention of venous thromboembolism after total hip or knee replacement: the METHRO II randomized trial. Lancet 2002;360:1441–7.

[64] Eriksson BI, Agnelli G, Cohen AT, et al. Direct thrombin inhibitor melagatran followed by oral ximelagatran in comparison with enoxaprin for prevention of venous thromboembolism after total hip or knee replacement: the METHRO III study. Thromb Haemost 2003;89:288–96.

[65] Eriksson BI, Agnelli G, Cohen AT, et al. The direct thrombin inhibitor melagatran followed by oral ximelagatran compared with enoxaparin for the prevention of venous thromboembolism after total hip or knee replacement: the EXPRESS study. J Thromb Haemost 2003;1:2490–6.

[66] Colwell CW, Berkowitz SD, Davidson BL, et al. Comparison of ximelagatran, an oral direct thrombin inhibitor, with enoxaparin for the prevention of venous thromboembolism following total hip replacement: a randomized, double-blind study. J Thromb Haemost 2003;1:2119–30.

[67] Francis CW, Berkowitz SD, Comp PC, et al. Comparison of ximelagatran with warfarin for the prevention of venous thromboembolism after total knee replacement. N Engl J Med 2003;349:1703–12.

[68] Colwell CW, Berkowitz SD, Comp PC, et al. Randomized, double-blind comparison of ximelagatran, an oral direct thrombin inhibitor, and warfarin to prevent venous thromboembolism (VTE) after total knee replacement (TKR). Blood 2003;102 (11 part 1):14a.

[69] Francis CW, Davidson BL, Berkowitz SD, et al. Ximelagatran versus warfarin for the prevention of venous thromboembolism after total knee arthroplasty: a randomized, double-blinded trial. Ann Intern Med 2002;137:648–55.

[70] Buller HR, Agnelli G, Hull RD, et al. Antithrombotic therapy for venous thromboembolic disease: the Seventh ACCP Conference on Antithrombotic and Thrombolytic Therapy. Chest 2004;126:401S–28S.

[71] Fiessinger JN, Huisman MV, Davidson BL, et al. Ximelagatran vs low-molecular-weight heparin and warfarin for the treatment of deep vein thrombosis. JAMA 2005;293:681–9.

[72] Schulman S, Wahlander K, Lundstrom T, et al. Secondary prevention of venous thromboembolism with the oral direct thrombin inhibitor ximelagatran. N Engl J Med 2003;349:1713–21.

[73] Singer DE, Albers GW, Dalen JE, et al. Antithrombotic therapy in atrial fibrillation: the Seventh ACCP Conference on Antithrombotic and Thrombolytic Therapy. Chest 2004;126:429S–56S.

[74] Halperin JL. Ximelagatran compared with warfarin for prevention of thromboembolism in patients with nonvalvular atrial fibrillation: rationale, objectives, and design of a pair of clinical studies and baseline patient characteristics (SPORTIF III and V). Am Heart J 2003;146:431–8.

[75] Olsson SB. Stroke prevention with the oral direct thrombin inhibitor ximelagatran compared with warfarin in patients with non-valvular atrial fibrillation (SPORTIF III): randomized controlled trial. Lancet 2003;362:1691–8.

[76] SPORTIF Executive Steering Committee for the SPORTIF V Investigators. Ximelagatran vs warfarin for stroke prevention in patients with nonvalvular atrial fibrillation. JAMA 2005;293:690–8.

[77] Samsa GP, Matchar DB, Goldstein LB, et al. Quality of anticoagulation management among patients with atrial fibrillation: results of a review of medical records from 2 communities. Arch Intern Med 2000; 160:967–73.

[78] He R. Integrated executive summary for FDA review for NDA 21–686 Exanta (ximelagatran). Food and Drug Administration. Available at: http://www.fda.gov/ohrms/dockets/ac/04/briefing/2004-4069B1_03_FDA-Backgrounder-Execsummaryredacted.pdf. Accessed July 5, 2005.

[79] Zimmerman HJ. Drug-induce liver disease. In: Hepatotoxicity: the adverse effects of drugs and other chemicals on the liver. New York: Appleton-Century-Crofts; 1978.

[80] Stangier J, Erikkson BI, Dahl OE, et al. Pharmacokinetic profile of the oral direct thrombin inhibitor dabigatran etexilate in healthy volunteers and patients undergoing total hip replacement. J Clin Pharmacol 2005;45:555–63.

[81] Erikkson BI, Dahl OE, Ahnfelt L, et al. Dose escalating safety study of a new oral direct thrombin inhibitor, dabigatran etexilate, in patients undergoing total hip replacement: BISTRO I. J Thromb Haemost 2004;2:1573–80.

[82] Erikkson BI, Dahl OE, Buller HR, et al. A new oral direct thrombin inhibitor, dabigatran etexilate, compared with enoxaparin for prevention of thromboembolic events following total hip or knee replacement: the BISTRO II randomized trial. J Thromb Haemost 2005;3:103–11.

[83] Dahl OE, Rosencher N, Kurth AA, et al. RE-NOVATE Study Group. Dabigatran etexilate vs. enoxaparin for prevention of venous thromboembolism after total hip replacement: a randomised, double-blind, non-inferiority trial. Lancet 2007; 370(9591):949–56.

[84] Friedman RJ, Caprini JA, Comp PC et al. Dabigatran etexilate versus enoxaparin in preventing venous thromboembolism following total knee arthroplasty. Abstract presented at Congress of the International Society on Thrombosis and Haemostasis in Geneva, Switzerland, July 2007.

[85] Eriksson BI, Dahl OE, Rosencher N, et al. RE-MODEL Study Group. Oral dabigatran etexilate vs. subcutaneous enoxaparin for the prevention of venous thromboembolism after total knee replacement: the RE-MODEL randomized trial. J Thromb Haemost 2007;5(11):2178–85.

[86] Caprini JA, Hwang E, Hantel S et al. The oral direct thrombin inhibitor dabigatran etexilate is effective and safe for prevention of major venous thromboembolism following orthopaedic surgery. Abstract presented at Congress of the International Society on Thrombosis and Haemostasis in Geneva, Switzerland, July 2007.

ELSEVIER
SAUNDERS

Cardiol Clin 26 (2008) 189–201

CARDIOLOGY
CLINICS

Antiplatelet Agents and Arterial Thrombosis

Henny H. Billett, MD

*Albert Einstein College of Medicine, Thrombosis Prevention and Treatment Program, Department of Medicine,
Division of Hematology, Montefiore Medical Center, Bronx, NY 10467, USA*

There is an increase in arterial thrombotic events in the elderly. Elderly patients are more likely to have associated diseases such as diabetes, hypertension and hypercholesterolemia and when age is confounded by these other predisposing factors, the risk of an arterial ischemic event increases disproportionately, with data suggesting that the increased cardiovascular risk can be five times greater for those over 70 years of age compared with those under the age of 55 [1,2]. Antithrombotic therapy for geriatric patients is underused, even when one adjusts for potential drug contraindications [3]. This article focuses on the action of the currently available antiplatelet agents (aspirin, clopidogrel, and glycoprotein IIb/IIIa [GPIIb/IIIa] receptor antagonists) and assesses their effects in different disease states, with special attention to data that examine the geriatric population.

Although plasma anticoagulants have become the mainstay of venous thrombosis treatment, platelet-dependent arterial thromboses require a different therapeutic approach. Rupture of an atherosclerotic plaque in the high flow state of the arterial system mandates a rapid platelet reaction. To respond, platelets go through a complex series of responses: initiation, extension (recruitment), and perpetuation. These changes require the up-regulation or exposure of a multiplicity of receptors by a dizzying array of agonists, supported by a myriad of cytokines and aided by numerous secreted granular contents, all interacting with diverse ligands in the subendothelium and a wealth of interacting plasma factors. It

should come as no surprise then, despite making large strides in antithrombotic medical therapy within ever-bigger cardiovascular studies, abrogating the platelet response still eludes us.

Normal platelet physiology

The platelet has several transmembrane glycoproteins that serve as signal receptors. Glycoproteins IIb and IIIa are members of the integrin superfamily that are located on the platelet membrane. When activated, they join together to form the heterodimer GPIIb-IIIa. This heterodimer exposes a receptor for binding arginine-glycine-aspartic acid amino acid sequences, most notably the arginine-glycine-aspartic acid sequence of fibrinogen. There are approximately 50 to 80,000 copies of GPIIb-IIIa on the cell membrane. Fibrinogen bound to GPIIb-IIIa receptors on one platelet can crosslink other fibrinogen monomers attached to other platelet GPIIb-IIIa receptors, and a platelet-fibrinogen matrix forms.

On initial platelet activation, phospholipases split off the arachidonic acid moiety of another cell membrane phospholipid, phosphatidylinositol. The prostaglandin synthase cyclooxygenase I (COX-1) uses this arachidonic acid to form intermediate prostaglandins (PGG_2 and PGH_2). In the platelet, thromboxane synthase further transforms these intermediate prostaglandins to thromboxane A_2. Thromboxane A_2 increases platelet aggregation by increasing receptor-fibrinogen binding. In addition, thromboxane A_2 facilitates aggregation by inhibiting cAMP, opposes the actions of prostacyclin PGI_2, and causes vascular constriction. Anything that disturbs or inhibits COX-1 and the resultant pathway leads

A version of this article originally appeared in *Clinics in Geriatric Medicine*, volume 22, issue 1.

E-mail address: hbillett@montefiore.org

to decreased thromboxane A_2 formation and a disturbance in platelet function. The final common pathway then allows for clot formation, because the next step of platelet activation flips the phosphatidyl serine (PS) from the inner leaflet of the platelet membrane bilayer to the outer leaflet, exposing PS on the cell surface and activating the coagulation cascade.

Overview of antiplatelet agents and their mechanisms of action

Aspirin

Although a relatively weak antagonist of platelet action, aspirin's popularity arises from its low cost, physician and patient familiarity with the drug, lack of major adverse effects, and widespread availability. Derived from the white willow tree Saliz Alba, acetylsalicylic acid has been used pharmacologically as an antipyretic since the mid 1800s [4], but it was in the 1940s that the hemorrhagic effect of aspirin was noted. Twenty years later, it was recognized that the effect was platelet mediated; another 20 years ensued until the antiplatelet effect was noted to be prostaglandin mediated. Aspirin has a rapid onset of action, approximately 30 minutes, and exerts its effects by acetylating the serine 529 site of platelet COX-1 activity of prostaglandin H synthase [5]. COX-1 is present in small amounts in most tissues but is seen in increased amounts in platelets, stomach, and kidneys. Inhibition of COX-1 activity in the platelet interferes with thromboxane A_2 formation and renders the prostaglandin biosynthetic pathway incapable of increasing aggregation. This process occurs in mature megakaryocytes as well as platelets. Because of the anucleate platelet's inability to make new enzyme and the exquisite sensitivity of the platelet's prostanoid system to aspirin, the effect persists for the life of the platelet; the restoration of normal aggregation on cessation of aspirin therapy is caused by young newly released nonacetylated platelets replacing the aspirin-treated ones.

Aspirin also acetylates the COX activity of another prostaglandin synthase, COX-2, although at a different serine site (Ser 516). COX-2 is an inducible enzyme, responsive to inflammatory stimuli in monocytes, macrophages, fibroblasts, synovial cells, and vascular endothelial cells, and is constitutively expressed in others. The effect of aspirin on COX-1 activity is 50- to 100-fold greater than its effect on COX-2.

The platelet has minimal COX-2 activity in a resting state, but inducible COX-2 activity in megakaryocytes can be expressed in inflammatory states. COX-2 inhibition requires more frequent and higher aspirin dosing. Because both COX-1 and COX-2 are involved in the inflammatory response, however, the additional antithrombotic effect of aspirin may exist by way of downregulation of this COX-2 response, as demonstrated by its tight association with C-reactive protein. Since dosing is more important for COX-2, the lack of association of an antithrombotic effect with dosing, indicates that COX-2 inhibition probably does not play a major role in the effect of aspirin [5]. There is also some evidence that aspirin has a direct effect on thrombin generation and can antagonize the effects of vitamin K, but these effects do not seem to be of major significance in aspirin's pharmacologic profile.

Primary prevention

The Physicians Health Study [6] examined the effect of aspirin for primary prevention of cardiovascular events in over 22,000 patients over 5 years. They noted a 44% relative reduction in the risk of myocardial infarction associated with aspirin use. A smaller study, the British Male Doctors' Trial comprising 5139 men, showed only a 10% nonsignificant benefit in treated patients [7]. Three subsequent trials, the thrombosis prevention trial [8], the hypertension optimal treatment study [9], and the primary prevention project [10], agreed with the Physicians Health Study data, which demonstrated good primary prevention with aspirin use eliciting risk reduction in triple end points for most patients. The thrombosis prevention trial studied 5500 men treated with warfarin and aspirin and demonstrated an absolute risk reduction in cardiovascular risk with aspirin of 2.3 events per 1000 person-years. The hypertension optimal treatment study examined 18,800 patients and found that aspirin reduced major cardiovascular events by 15% ($P = .03$) and all myocardial infarction by 36% ($P = .002$), but had no effect on stroke. The primary prevention project study consisted of 4495 patients with one risk factor of whom 1031 had diabetes. The primary prevention project trial was stopped prematurely after subjects without diabetes were found to have a relative risk reduction in each of the triple end points, with a marked decrease in cardiovascular events (RRR 0.69). Interestingly, patients with diabetes had a nonsignificant increase in cardiovascular deaths

(RRR 1.23, 0.69–2.19). Using a meta-analysis based on these five trials, in 2002 the US Preventive Services Task Force recommended aspirin for the primary prevention of cardiovascular events [11].

When one examines these data for effects seen in the elderly, it is slightly less clear. The Physicians Health Study demonstrated that relative risk for first myocardial infarction was at least as significant for those 70 to 84 years old (RRR 0.49) as it was for those 60 to 69 years of age (RRR 0.46) [12]. In the hypertension optimal treatment study, patients over the age of 65 had a similar drug effect to that seen in younger patients [13]. However, in the thrombosis prevention trial where the maximum age of enrollment was 69 years of age, men above 65 did not demonstrate a benefit from aspirin. These data were further reviewed in a meta-analysis of the randomized participants, which demonstrated a 32% relative risk reduction for aspirin with a first myocardial infarction, and a 15% relative risk reduction for all vascular events [14,15].

Secondary prevention

In one of the first large-scale aspirin trials, the ISIS-2 trial, aspirin given within 24 hours of the onset of symptoms of an acute myocardial infarction, and continued for at least 5 weeks, resulted in a decrease in death, reinfarction, and ischemic stroke [16]. The 35-day mortality among patients with suspected myocardial infarction was 13.2% for those who did not receive streptokinase or aspirin, approximately 10.5% for those given one or the other, and only 8% for those receiving both agents [16]. This large beneficial effect of aspirin following myocardial infarction led to other secondary prevention trials. The International Stroke Trial and the Chinese Acute Stroke Trials [17,18] also demonstrated that the early use of aspirin after an event led to a significant decrease in subsequent vascular end points. Although the decrease was somewhat less in the stroke trials than those seen in coronary events, they were still highly significant.

Current recommendations for the use of aspirin in secondary prevention are based on several hundred trials, many of which included thousands of patients. An attempt to perform a major meta-analysis was painstakingly done by the Antithrombotic Trialists' collaboration. They examined 287 studies involving 13,000 high-risk patients, comparing cardiovascular outcome for patients on antiplatelet therapy versus placebo and further studied 77,000 patients on different antiplatelet regimens [19]. In this meta-analysis, patients with dementia were excluded but there were no exclusions or separate analysis based on age. Antiplatelet therapy was determined to be effective in reducing adverse cardiovascular events (nonfatal myocardial infarction, nonfatal stroke, or vascular death in high-risk patients), reducing the incidence of nonfatal myocardial infarction by one third, nonfatal stroke by one quarter, and vascular mortality by one sixth. Patients with prior myocardial infarction or cerebrovascular accident who were on aspirin for 2 years had an absolute risk reduction of 36 per 1000 events. Patients with acute myocardial infarction treated with aspirin for 1 month had a 38 per 1000 event reduction, and patients with acute strokes had an absolute risk reduction of 9 per 1000 if treated for 3 weeks with acetylsalicylic acid. Patients with peripheral arterial disease, atrial fibrillation, and stable angina each had a significantly decreased risk of an adverse outcome [19]. Aspirin reduced the relative risk of nonfatal strokes in patients with pre-existing disease by approximately 25% [19]. The decrease in fatal strokes (16%) was less than that for nonfatal, because of an increase in the relative incidence of hemorrhagic cerebrovascular accident. Importantly, there was no evidence of increased mortality from other causes. Indeed, there was a significant decrease in all cause mortality ($P < .0001$) and a decrease in nonvascular deaths, although the nonvascular deaths (caused by cancer and so forth) were not differentiated [19]. Recent data suggest that dual therapy, by adding a thienopyridine, may not enhance the effect of aspirin and may increase the adverse effects [20].

Aspirin versus warfarin or low-molecular-weight heparin in secondary prevention

Many studies have demonstrated the superiority of vitamin K antagonists and other venous anticoagulants in the prevention of embolic stroke for patients with atrial fibrillation. Data regarding the superiority, however, of either aspirin or vitamin K antagonists for ischemic, nonembolic strokes were less clear. The WARSS study compared aspirin with low- or medium-intensity dose warfarin (international normalized ratio 1.4–2.8). This study demonstrated conclusively that aspirin was the better choice for the prevention of recurrence of ischemic stroke [21]. A recent study that examined patients with transient ischemic attacks or stokes associated with a 55% to 99% intracranial artery stenosis randomized 569 patients to warfarin or high-dose aspirin (1300 mg/d) before the study was stopped because of concerns over the warfarin arm. After a mean follow-up of 1.8 years, they demonstrated a significant decrease in mortality in the aspirin group (4.3% versus 9.7%, hazard ratio 0.46) and a significantly lower incidence of major hemorrhage [22]. This group was not further separated by age.

Percutaneous coronary intervention

Because of the very high rate of thrombosis following percutaneous coronary intervention (PCI) and stenting, aspirin has been recommended for all patients within all age groups who undergo PCI [23]. Even with aspirin, however, the rate of rethrombosis is high and a plan of combination drug therapy is recommended. This is reviewed in the followings sections on thienopyridines.

Nonvalvular atrial fibrillation and venous thromboembolism: other indications for aspirin therapy?

The Stroke Prevention in Atrial Fibrillation study demonstrated that the effect of aspirin in atrial fibrillation, although smaller than that of vitamin K antagonists, reduced the risk of stroke by 24% over placebo. This implies that aspirin has a minor role to play in this disease. Following this trial, aspirin has become accepted therapy for use in patients at low risk for embolization [24]. Because age >75 years is considered a high risk, aspirin has a more limited use in the elderly but should be considered as an alternative when there are contraindications to vitamin K antagonists, or in those younger than 75. Similarly, although aspirin was found to significantly decrease deaths from pulmonary embolism in the PEP trial [25], the reduction was much smaller than that achieved by vitamin K antagonists, such as warfarin. A study using aspirin as primary prophylaxis for VTE in women did not demonstrate an advantageous effect [26]. The American College of Chest Physicians has not recommended aspirin therapy [27]. Whether aspirin therapy is at all useful for those intolerant of vitamin K antagonists or whether there is a different risk-benefit ratio for the elderly was not addressed by these guidelines.

Gender

The highest incidence of heart disease in women occurs about 12 to 15 years later than in men but heart disease is still the most common cause of death in women. Early studies of primary prevention focused solely on men and it was unclear whether the results could be extrapolated to women [6,7,12,]. Evidence-based guidelines analyzing gender are emerging for aspirin use for primary prevention for women [28]. More definitive data have emerged from the Women's Health Study [29]. This study looked at almost 40,000 women, 45 years of age or older, who randomly received either 100 mg of aspirin or placebo and monitored them for 10 years [29]. In the younger group, there was only a 9% relative reduction in the risk of first major cardiovascular event after 10 years (8.2–10.9); this difference was not statistically significant. Only stroke, when evaluated separately, had a significant 17% relative risk reduction ($P < .009$). When women over 65 were considered separately (N = 4097), however, there was a consistent benefit with regards to myocardial infarction ($P < .04$), ischemic stroke ($P < .05$), and major cardiovascular event ($P < .008$). Interestingly, the authors found no effect of menopausal status or the use of hormone replacement therapy on these data, but they did note a statistically significant increase in gastrointestinal hemorrhage requiring transfusion with aspirin use.

Side effects

The major side effect of aspirin is bleeding. An analysis by a group from Harvard found that aspirin complications occur in 1 out of 15 individuals and that, starting at age 50 years, the complication rate of aspirin was 6.8% and the mortality rate was 0.18% over a lifetime of aspirin therapy [30]. There is some evidence that gastrointestinal bleeding may be dose-related and may be partially alleviated with enteric-coated tablets. In some studies, lower dosages caused less gastrointestinal irritation and less bleeding, especially when used in combination with other antiplatelet agents [31,32]. The huge meta-analysis performed by the Antithrombotic Trialists' Group failed to identify an association of dosage with bleeding, however, noting that the absolute increase in major bleeding caused by aspirin was only 0.5 [19]. Bleeding risk in this meta-analysis was not stratified according to age. In a study done by Petty and coworkers [33], they noted that although the mean age of all patients who received aspirin was 73.9 years, the mean age of the patients who experienced complications was 79.7 years, suggesting that the sensitivity to aspirin increases with age. This increased sensitivity seen in the elderly, however, may be balanced (confounded?) by an increased incidence of "aspirin resistance."

Aspirin areas of concern: dose, tolerance, "resistance"

One of the worrisome issues associated with aspirin therapy, and an area of recent intense investigation, is identification of the correct dose. There are conflicting desires and worries. The bioavailability of aspirin is approximately 50%, which is decreased by enteric coating, but these tablets do seem to be associated with fewer gastrointestinal effects. Similarly, sustained-release tablets are available but do not seem to offer any advantage with regard to gastrointestinal adverse effects [5]. There is also some evidence that salicylate metabolism is different in the elderly and in women [34,35] and there are a few studies that have demonstrated that higher doses may actually be less beneficial [36]. The AMIS trial randomized patients to receive 1000 mg of aspirin versus placebo and found that mortality was not decreased in the treated group [37]. Other studies have also noted that there was an increased cardiovascular risk for patients on higher-dose aspirin [38]. This decrease in effect seen in the AMIS study with larger doses of aspirin is balanced by evidence from other studies that those on aspirin have an improved response and that at least a proportion of the nonresponders to aspirin increase their response with an increased dose. In one study by Syrbe and coworkers [39], 40% of all patients could be therapeutic, as demonstrated by decreased aggregation in platelet aggregation studies, with 30 mg/d, 50% required 100, and 10% required doses of > 300 mg/d. Most studies have used doses between 50 and 160 mg of aspirin and these dosages seem to be at least as effective as others, but the idea of tailoring dose to response had acquired several enthusiastic supporters [5,19].

There are data to indicate that patients with cardiovascular disease may become tolerant to the effects of aspirin. Pulcinelli and coworkers [40] tested 150 patients before and after 2, 6, 12, and 24 months of treatment with aspirin for their response to ADP and collagen-induced platelet aggregation. Initially, there was significant inhibition of platelet aggregation, but with time, this returned to normal in many patients, such that at 24 months, collagen-induced platelet aggregation was at baseline for 42% of the sampled population. This was not replicated when they tested ADP-induced aggregation response to the thienopyridine, ticlopidine. Aspirin tolerance has also been shown in another study on patients with stroke [41]. Helgason and coworkers [41] studied 306 patients treated with aspirin with prior stroke.

At initiation 228 of 306 patients showed immediate inhibition of platelet aggregation, whereas 78 demonstrated partial inhibition. Of these, 119 patients with immediate and complete inhibition underwent repeat testing. Thirty-nine of these patients (32.7%) had regained some aggregatory capability, again suggesting a tolerance or a reduced sensitivity to aspirin with time. These data may have special relevance for the elderly because they are more likely to be on medications for a longer period of time by virtue of their longevity and disease duration.

Recurrent thrombotic episodes occur despite aspirin, with a rate from 2% to 6% per year [42]. Although drug failure rates have been accepted for other medications, much effort has gone into examining the causes for aspirin failure. Adherence is a major issue because it has been demonstrated that 20% of patients may not be taking their medications [43]. In addition to these common causes, investigations have focused on a phenomenon now known as "aspirin resistance" [44]. This term has been defined as failing to obtain the expected aspirin-induced abnormalities as demonstrated by classical platelet aggregation studies; failure to prolong the closure time with the Platelet Function Analyzer (Dade Behring Inc., Deerfield, Illinois) [45], the clot time in the Verify Now Platelet Function Analyzer (Accumetrics, Inc., San Diego, California); failure to have the necessary decrease in thromboxane B_2 levels (the end product of thromboxane A_2, a platelet-specific prostaglandin); or other similar studies. The concordance of these tests is poor; patients may have one or several of these characteristics and it is not clear how the degree of aspirin resistance relates to any one test. What we have previously called resistance is probably best described now as a failure to suppress platelet aggregation despite aspirin therapy, thus allowing for other factors, even non-platelet factors to play a role in the lack of suppression of platelet activity. Whatever the cause, there are growing data that suggest that this aspirin resistance plays a role in cardiovascular mortality [46]. The prevalence of patients with aspirin resistance varies wildly from 5% to 75% across studies but most put the figure at approximately 15% [47]. Detecting aspirin resistance may be very important clinically, either because it may serve as a risk factor initially or as evidence of a need for alterations in therapy. Grotemeyer and coworkers [48] performed one of the earliest studies in 1993 in which they demonstrated that patients who were unresponsive to aspirin (fully a third of this population) were nine times more likely to have a vascular event than those who demonstrated sensitivity to acetylsalicylic acid. Grundman and coworkers [49] also looked at aspirin nonresponder status in patients with recurrent cerebrovascular accidents and noted that those patients also had a poorer prognosis. Gum and coworkers [50] followed patients prospectively and found that those who were aspirin resistant by aggregometry were at increased risk of myocardial infarction, stroke, or death when compared with patients who were sensitive to aspirin (24% versus 10%). Evidence from the Heart Outcomes Prevention Evaluation trial, in which 499 patients were compared with age and gender matched controls, showed that those patients who took aspirin but did not decrease their levels of thromboxane B_2 (a measure of aspirin resistance) were at higher risk for cardiovascular events [51,52]. Studies have demonstrated that patients with resistance to aspirin were more likely to be female, smokers, and older [53]. Even when age is controlled for, however, patients who are aspirin resistant were more likely to have a higher rate of cardiovascular events. The geriatric patient, who is more likely to be aspirin resistant, may not be getting the full value of aspirin therapy and may need additional medical treatment.

Several attempts have been made to explain aspirin resistance. Mutations in COX-1 have been documented by single nucleotide polymorphisms analyses (SNP) [54] and these may be responsible for different acetylation capabilities. Increased available thromboxane A_2 is another explanation. There may be a release of thromboxane A_2 from COX-2 of young platelets, monocytes, and macrophages. The inducible COX-2 in periods of stress has been postulated to increase the rate of low-dose aspirin resistance in patients who have recently undergone coronary artery bypass grafting (a period of increased COX-2 levels and of increased platelet turnover) [55]. Other possibilities are drug interference, particularly by nonsteroidal anti-inflammatory drugs. In a study performed in 2001, Catella-Lawson and coworkers [56] demonstrated that one dose of ibuprofen taken before aspirin could block the normal COX-1 activity in platelets, presumably by interfering with the docking site of the drug before acetylation. In this study, there was no effect of the COX-2 inhibitor, rofecoxib. Later studies have demonstrated, however, that there may be inhibition of aspirin benefits by the group of nonsteroidal anti-inflammatory drugs [57]. A study by Levesque and

coworkers [58] on elderly adults demonstrated that there was a 1.24 increased risk of acute myocardial infarction with high doses of rofecoxib and that this increase could be offset by aspirin if low-dose, but not high-dose, rofecoxib was used. These recent data on rofecoxib have caused the drug to be withdrawn and have cast suspicion on other COX-2 inhibitors and the entire class of nonsteroidal anti-inflammatory drugs with regard to increased cardiovascular complications [59].

Additional medications, such as the thienopyridines, may be primarily useful for the patients who are aspirin resistant and an argument can be made that little is added when thienopyridines are used with aspirin-sensitive patients. Data from Chen and colleagues [60], however, suggest that these two drugs work independently when they studied aspirin resistance in patients scheduled for PCI who were given aspirin and clopidogrel (a thienopyridine) and noted that aspirin-resistant patients were more likely to have elevated cardiac enzyme levels postprocedure (51.7% versus 24.6%) whether or not they were on clopidogrel. More studies are needed to investigate aspirin resistance and the mechanism of action, the sensitive population, and the potential remedies for this phenomenon. In addition, studies looking at aspirin in combination with other drugs, particularly clopidogrel, are important because there is evidence that clopidogrel resistance may also play an important role in treatment failures.

Clopidogrel

Clopidogrel is a member of the thienopyridine family, of which ticlopidine was the first agent to be used in cardiovascular disease [61]. These are potent platelet inhibitors and they work by irreversibly inhibiting the low-affinity ADP receptor, P_2Y_{12}, on the platelet membrane. The thienopyridines are rapidly absorbed and metabolized by hepatic cytochrome P-450 enzymes, CYP3A4 and CYP3A5. Inhibition of ADP-induced platelet aggregation can be seen within 2 hours after high-dose clopidogrel and, like aspirin, the effect remains for the life of the platelet. If daily doses of 75 mg/d are used, steady-state levels can be reached within 3 to 5 days [62]. For maximum effect, patients may be given a clopidogrel load (300–600 mg) and then the standard 75 mg/d. This results in ADP-induced platelet aggregation inhibition within 4 to 6 hours. Like aspirin, platelet aggregation studies return to normal within

1 week of stopping therapy as a result of the influx of new untreated platelets [63]. Clopidogrel is well absorbed in the elderly and has a comparable pharmacokinetic profile to that of younger patients.

Ticlopidine is an older thienopyridine that has been virtually abandoned because of the frequency of two major side effects: neutropenia (1%–2.4%) and thrombotic thrombocytopenia purpura (1 in 3000). Ticlopidine also requires twice daily dosing and costs more when the daily dose is considered. There is disagreement about whether there is any increased incidence of thrombotic thrombocytopenia purpura with clopidogrel use but, if there is an increased incidence, it is minimal compared with the benefit conferred [64]. Clopidogrel does not cause a significant neutropenia. When compared head-to-head with ticlopidine in the Classics stenting trial, it seemed to be more effective with fewer major adverse cardiovascular events [65]. AZD6140 and prasugrel, are new adenosine diphosphate receptor antagonists which may hold promise in acute coronary syndromes in preliminary trials [66,67].

One of the first trials to compare clopidogrel with aspirin was the CAPRIE study, which was performed in >19,000 patients over a period of up to 3 years. The study population consisted of patients with a recent cerebrovascular accident, myocardial infarction, or symptomatic peripheral arterial disease. When clopidogrel was compared with aspirin with regard to stroke, myocardial infarction, peripheral arterial disease, and overall event rate, there was a slight improvement in a composite cardiovascular triple end point, with clopidogrel having a relative risk reduction of 8.7% at the end of a mean of 2 years of study (5.32% versus 5.83%). The most significant reduction was in peripheral arterial disease, with a more modest benefit provided over acetylsalicylic acid when used in ischemic events [68]. The bleeding incidence in the CAPRIE study was approximately 9%, equivalent to aspirin. In its meta-analysis, the Antithrombotic Trialists' collaboration included only this study of clopidogrel and noted that clopidogrel reduced serious vascular events by 10% [19].

Because of the prevalence of aspirin use and its demonstrated efficacy, trials that studied clopidogrel used it in combination with aspirin. Since clopidogrel was found to be superior to aspirin in the CAPRIE study, the MATCH study was designed to assess whether the addition of aspirin to clopidogrel provides greater benefit as compared

with clopidogrel alone for the prevention of vascular events with potentially higher bleeding risk [69]. This study was a randomized, double-blind, placebo-controlled trial comparing clopidogrel with either placebo or aspirin (75 mg/d) in almost 7600 high-risk patients with recent ischemic stroke or transient ischemic attack and at least one additional vascular risk factor. The primary end point was a composite of ischemic stroke, myocardial infarction, vascular death, or rehospitalization for acute ischemia or worsening of peripheral arterial disease. At the end of 18 months, a small risk reduction in the dual-agent therapy group was noted (15.7% versus 16.7%; absolute risk reduction 1%), but this was more than compensated for by an increase in major bleeds (2.6% versus 1.3%; absolute risk increase 1.3%). No difference in mortality was noted.

When patients with an acute myocardial infarction were randomly allocated in the Clopidogrel and Aspirin: Determination of the Effects on Thrombogenicity trial to either aspirin (75 mg) or clopidogrel (75 mg), there was no significant clinical difference in adverse events or mortality [70]. In addition, this group measured some laboratory determinants known to be associated with increased thrombogenicity and demonstrated that both groups had similarly decreased fibrinogen, D dimer, von Willebrand's factor, factor VIII, and C-reactive protein levels at 1 and 6 months.

The CURE [71] trial also examined the effect of clopidogrel (with loading) versus placebo when added to aspirin. In this study of 12,562 patients who presented within 24 hours of symptoms, there was a 20% relative risk reduction in composite triple end point (nonfatal myocardial infarction, death, or stroke) with an 11.4% incidence in the aspirin and placebo groups versus 9.3% in the aspirin and clopidogrel group. As expected, there was significantly more bleeding (3.7% versus 2.7%) and a trend that was not statistically significant in major hemorrhage. Although the hemorrhagic component of this trial was aspirin dose-dependent, the efficacy was not.

Recently Sabatine and coworkers [72] reported on a group of almost 3500 patients under the age of 75 who had a myocardial infarction with ST segment elevation and who were receiving fibrinolytic agents, aspirin, and heparin. These patients were given either additional clopidogrel (loading dose of 300 mg, then 75 mg/d) or placebo. Efficacy was determined on the basis of blood flow and need for revascularization, death, or recurrent myocardial infarction. The triple end point occurred in 21.7% of placebo-treated and 15% of clopidogrel-treated patients, with a large relative reduction (36%) in favor of clopidogrel. Rates of major bleeding and intracranial hemorrhage were the same. No differences in rates of hemorrhage because of age in those under 75 were noted. Of note is that this study involved a relatively older population who received triple therapy and had improved outcomes without significant detriment in terms of major hemorrhage.

PCI has been a thorny issue. Many of the initial studies using dual-agent therapy were performed in studies investigating efficacy in PCI. Because of the high rate of rethrombosis in PCI, many of the initial investigations centered on PCI thrombosis risk reduction, a clinical setting in which ticlopidine had already proved to be useful. The CLASSICS trial demonstrated that clopidogrel was a better agent when used with aspirin for PCI therapy. It has become clear that clopidogrel timing may be important. When clopidogrel is given with a loading dose before stenting, the effects are improved, as compared with clopidogrel administered at the time of the procedure. When both aspirin and clopidogrel are continued beyond the PCI period of re-endoethelialization (typically 2–4 weeks) and extended to 9 to 12 months, these beneficial effects are further increased with a decrease in major adverse cardiovascular events [73,74].

Because of the CAPRIE data, clopidogrel has become accepted as optimal therapy for peripheral arterial disease. Other studies looking at the effect of clopidogrel for primary prevention are in progress. No data are currently available regarding very long-term therapy with clopidogrel, but it is clear that this drug is effective in the short and intermediate time frame [75].

Clopidogrel resistance

Despite aspirin and clopidogrel therapy, there is a high rate of rethrombosis after coronary events or after stenting. This has led the way for investigators to postulate that, in addition to an aspirin-resistance group, there may be a group with clopidogrel resistance [76]. Lack of inhibition of the ADP response has been demonstrated in some patients; part of the difficulty in assessing clopidogrel resistance is the lack of good measurement guidelines and the fact that most of these studies are confounded by aspirin ingestion. There is some suggestion that clopidogrel may have some

effect on the time lag of the Platelet Function Analyzer-100, but most studies have focused on flow cytometry outcomes, such as P-selectin exposure [77]. Studies looking at vasodilator-stimulated phosphoprotein (VASP) expression following the low-affinity ADP P_2Y_{12} blockade by clopidogrel have noted that as much as 30% of the treated population did not have the expected abnormal responses [78]. The causes for this clopidogrel resistance, aside from the medication adherence issues, are being investigated. There are known differences in ADP P_2Y_{12} receptor polymorphisms, differences in metabolism by the liver cytochrome P-450 isoenzymes, differences in the bioavailability of the active metabolite, and potential drug-drug interactions (especially with some of the statins that use similar cytochrome P-450 isozymes). Interestingly, recent studies demonstrate that the clinical outcome of these drug-induced clopidogrel resistant patients is not impacted by these statins [79] These are being studied as potential explanations for this phenomenon.

Dipyridamole

There are conflicting data on the role of dipyridamole in combination with aspirin in acute stroke. The European Stroke Prevention Study noted that the positive effect that they found was more profound in those younger than 70 years [80]. Although there are some data demonstrating increased efficacy of aspirin when dipyridamole is used in combination in older patients [81], most studies do not show a benefit, leaving little indication for use of dipyridamole in stroke [19].

Glycoprotein IIb-IIIa antagonists

The first GPIIb-IIIa inhibitor and still the most beneficial is abciximab, a human-murine Fab chimeric antibody fragment to the GPIIb-IIIa binding site. Abciximab is a large protein with a rapid and prolonged response, causing the bleeding time not to normalize until a full 12 hours after injection. Typically given as a bolus injection along with heparin and aspirin in patients with acute cardiovascular syndromes and before PCI, abciximab was demonstrated to deliver a 60% relative risk reduction in triple end points in the Epilog [82] and Epistent [83] trials with a long-term decrease in mortality. Abciximab has the capability to cross-react with other integrins, notably Mac-1 (alpha$_m$beta$_2$, CD11b/CD18), a leukocyte integrin, and vitronectin, an endothelial integrin. There is some suggestion that the increased effect of this drug over other GPIIb-IIIa antagonists stems from its ability to inhibit leukocyte adhesion by its anti–Mac-1 properties or endothelial adhesion by its antivitronectin properties. To date, abciximab is the only GPIIb-IIIa to demonstrate a prolonged survival benefit after PCI [84].

Major bleeding in the GPIIb-IIIa cardiovascular trials has been typically defined as any intracranial bleeding or a decrease in hemoglobin of ≥ 3 g/dL or in hematocrit of $\geq 15\%$ [85]. Although the rate of bleeding in the original trials was high (10.5% in the EPIC [86]), this has decreased as familiarity with its use has increased. In addition, it was recognized that the heparin dose could have been a factor and that bleeding at the vascular access site could be decreased with earlier sheath removal. With abciximab in particular, there were other issues. Because abciximab is a chimeric Fab, there is a tendency to cause human antichimeric antibodies, which limit repeated use but do not seem to interfere with function of the initial bolus medication. More importantly, there is a high incidence of thrombocytopenia with abciximab. Studies have demonstrated that a low platelet count occurs in approximately 5% of all patients but most of these (4%) are found to be spurious thrombocytopenia because of platelet clumping [87]. In the remainder, a true thrombocytopenia can develop, which can be rapid and severe, and result in profound bleeding. Although uncommon, it is more often seen in the elderly and those with lower baseline platelet counts. Treatment is rapid transfusion of platelets, which decreases individual receptor occupancy on the platelet membrane surface, restoring both platelet count and platelet function. Desmopressin has also been shown to be useful to help normalize the bleeding time [88].

Attempts to replicate abciximab have led to drugs like eptifibatide. Eptifibatide is a disintegrin derived from the southeastern pygmy rattlesnake. It is a small molecule that has an amino acid sequence specific for fibrinogen and has no vitronectin or Mac-1 effect. It is rapidly bound and rapidly reversed, with a normalization of the bleeding time within 1 to 4 hours. The effects of eptifibatide have been more modest and have been most impressive in those with milder disease, as noted in the PURSUIT trial, with approximately 11% relative risk reduction over placebo in patients with unstable angina [89]. As with abciximab, some studies examining the incidence of bleeding with eptifibatide have noted that older age increased

the bleeding risk [90], although a recent analysis did not find age to be a contributing factor [91].

Tirofiban is a small nonpeptide compound, stereochemically designed to interact with the arginine-glycine-aspartic acid fibrinogen receptor with similar attributes to eptifibatide in its reversibility, half-life, and bleeding time normalization. Results of tirofiban for patients with unstable angina in the PRISM studies have been mixed [92].

GPIIb-IIIa inhibitors improve patency and reduce reinfarction risk, with an increase in major bleeding. Intracranial hemorrhage was particularly increased in patients over 75 years of age [93], although a recent meta-analysis of six trials demonstrated that the elderly, while having the largest increase in bleeding with IIb/IIIa receptor blockers, also had the best outcomes in terms of reduction in non-fatal myocardial infarctions and overall mortality [94]. Nevertheless, the Antithrombotic Trialists' Group has recommended aspirin with the short-term addition of an intravenous GPIIb-IIIa antagonist for patients at risk for an immediate coronary event, noting a decrease in 20 events per 1000 in these patients. Attempts at manufacturing an effective oral GPIIb-IIIa antagonist that has long-term benefits have not yet met with success. Whether this is because of the presence of other effective medications, such that any additional benefit is lost, is not clear.

Summary

It seems justified and reasonable to prescribe low-dose aspirin for all geriatric patients, and for patients with peripheral arterial disease, clopidogrel for primary prevention. There is, at present, no place for the addition of dipyridamole or oral GPIIb-IIIa antagonists. GPIIb-IIIa antagonists may be indicated in acute events, requiring intervention. Whether patients should be screened for aspirin tolerance or resistance is not clear, but it may be prudent to place patients who fail therapy on a second antiplatelet agent, such as clopidogrel. There is no evidence to suggest that the increase in bleeding that may occur in the elderly should suggest that therapy be withheld and, indeed, there is some evidence that the elderly may derive a relatively increased benefit from the use of these antiplatelet agents.

References

[1] Sanmuganathan PS, Ghahramani P, Jackson PR. Aspirin for primary prevention of coronary heart

disease: safety and absolute benefit related to coronary risk derived from meta analysis of randomized trials. Heart 2001;85:265–71.

[2] Borgard V, Cambou JP, Lezorovcz A, et al. Comparison of cardiovascular risk factors and drug use in 14,544 French patients with a history of myocardial infarction, ischemic stroke and/or peripheral arterial disease. Eur J Cardiovasc Prev Rehab 2004;11: 394–402.

[3] Tran CT, Laupacis A, Mamdani MM, et al. Effect of age on the use of evidence based therapies for acute myocardial infarction. Am Heart J 2004;148: 834–41.

[4] Roth GJ, Calverley DC. Aspirin, platelets and thrombosis: theory and practice. Blood 1994;83: 885–98.

[5] Patrono C, Coller B, Fitzgerald GA, et al. Platelet active drugs: the relationships among dose, effectiveness and side effects. In: Hirsch J, Guyatt G, Albers G, et al, editors. The Seventh ACCP Conference on Antithrombotic and Thrombolytic Therapy: evidence-based guidelines. Chest 2004; 126:234S–64S.

[6] Steering Committee of the Physicians' Health Study Research Group. Final report on the aspirin component of the ongoing Physicians' Health Study. N Engl J Med 1989;321:129–35.

[7] Peto R, Gray R, Collins R, et al. Randomised trial of prophylactic daily aspirin in British male doctors. BMJ 1988;296:313–6.

[8] Thrombosis Prevention Trial. Randomized trial of low intensity oral anticoagulation with warfarin and low dose aspirin in the primary prevention of ischemic heart disease in men at increased risk. MRC General Practice Research Framework. Lancet 1998;351:233–41.

[9] Hansson L, Zanchett A, Carruthers SG, et al. Effect of intensive blood pressure lowering and low dose aspirin in patients with hypertension: principal results of the Hypertension Optimal Treatment randomized trial. HOT study group. Lancet 1998;351: 1755–62.

[10] Sacco M, Pellegrini F, Roncaglioni MC, et al. PPP Collaborative Group Primary prevention of cardiovascular events with low-dose aspirin and vitamin E in type 2 diabetic patients: results of the Primary Prevention Project (PPP) trial. Diabetes Care 2003;26: 3264–72.

[11] US Preventive Services Task force. Aspirin for the primary prevention of cardiovascular events: recommendation and rationale. Ann Intern Med 2002;136: 157–60.

[12] Eidelman RS, Hebert PR, Weisman SM, et al. An update on aspirin in the primary prevention of cardiovascular disease. Arch Intern Med 2003;163: 2006–10.

[13] Kjeldsen SE, Kolloch RE, Mallion LG, et al. Influence of gender and age on preventing cardiovascular disease by antihypertensive treatments and acetylsalicylic acid. The HOT Study. J Hypertens 2000;18:629–42.

[14] Cannon CP. Elderly patients with acute coronary syndromes; higher risk and greater benefit from antiplatelet therapy and/or interventional therapies. Am J Geriatr Cardiol 2003;12:259–62.

[15] Dornbrook-Lavender KA, Pieper JA, Roth MT. Primary prevention of coronary heart disease in the elderly. Ann Pharmacother 2003;37:1654–63.

[16] ISIS-2 (Second International Study of Infarct Survival) Collaborative Group. Randomized trial of intravenous streptokinase, oral aspirin, both or neither among 17,187 cases of suspected acute myocardial infarction: ISIS-2. Lancet 1988;2:349–80.

[17] Stroke Trial Collaborative Group. The International Stroke Trial: a randomized trial of aspirin, subcutaneous heparin, both or neither among 19,435 patients with acute ischemic stroke. Lancet 1997;349:1569–81.

[18] Chinese Acute Stroke Trial Collaborative Group. Randomized placebo controlled trial of early aspirin use in 20,000 patients with acute ischemic stroke. Lancet 1997;349:1641–9.

[19] Antithrombotic Trialists' Collaboration. Collaborative meta-analysis of randomized trials of antiplatelet therapy for prevention of death, myocardial infarction, and stroke in high risk patients. BMJ 2002;324:71–86.

[20] Bhatt DL, Fox KA, Hacke W, et al. Clopidogrel and aspirin versus aspirin alone for the prevention of atherothrombotic events. N Engl J Med 2006;354: 1706–17.

[21] Mohr J, Thompson JLP, Lazar RM, et al, for the Warfarin-Aspirin Recurrent Stroke Study Group. A comparison of warfarin and aspirin for the prevention of recurrent ischemic stroke. N Engl J Med 2001;345:1444–51.

[22] Chimowitz MI, Lynn MJ, Holett-Smith H, et al. Warfarin aspirin symptomatic intracranial disease trial investigators: comparison of warfarin and aspirin for symptomatic intracranial arterial stenosis. N Engl J Med 2005;352:1305–16.

[23] Lange RA, Hillis LD. Antiplatelet therapy for ischemic heart disease. N Engl J Med 2004;350: 277–80.

[24] Gage BF, van Walraven C, Pearce L, et al. Selecting patients with atrial fibrillation for anticoagulation: stroke risk stratification in patients taking aspirin. Circulation 2004;110:2287–92.

[25] Pulmonary Embolism Prevention Trial Collaborative Group. Prevention of pulmonary embolism and deep vein thrombosis with low dose aspirin. Lancet 2000;355:1295–302.

[26] Glynn RJ, Ridker PM, Goldhaber SZ, et al. Effect of low-dose aspirin on the occurrence of venous thromboembolism: a randomized trial. Ann Intern Med 2007;147:525–33.

[27] Geerts WH, Pineo GF, Heit JA, et al. Prevention of venous thromboembolism. In: Hirsch J, Guyatt G,

Albers G, et al, editors. The seventh ACCP conference on Antithrombotic and thrombolytic therapy: evidence-based guidelines. Chest 2004;126: 338S–400S.

[28] Mosca L, Appel LJ, Benjamin EJ, et al. Evidence based guidelines for cardiovascular disease prevention in women. Circulation 2004;109:672–93.

[29] Ridker PM, Cook NR, Lee IM, et al. A randomized trial of low dose ASA in the primary prevention of cardiovascular disease in women. N Engl J Med 2005;352:1293–304.

[30] Hur C, Simon LS, Gazelle GS. Analysis of aspirin associated risks in healthy individuals. Ann Pharmacother 2005;39:51–7.

[31] Peters RJG, Mehta RS, Fox KA. Effects of aspirin dose when used alone or in combination with clopidogrel in patients with acute coronary syndromes. Circulation 2003;108:1682–7.

[32] Dutch TIA, Trial study group. A comparison of two doses of aspirin in patients after a transient ischemic attack or minor ischemic stroke. N Engl J Med 1991; 325:1261–6.

[33] Petty GW, Brown RD, Whisnant JP, et al. Frequency of major complications of aspirin, warfarin and intravenous heparin for secondary stroke prevention. Ann Intern Med 1999;130:14–22.

[34] Montgomery PR, Berger LG, Mitenko PA, et al. Salicylate metabolism: effects of age and sex in adults. Clin Pharmacother 1986;39:571–6.

[35] Kjeldsen SE, Kolloch RE, Leonetti G, et al. Influence of gender and age on preventing cardiovascular disease by antihypertensive treatment and acetylsalicylic acid. The HOT study. J Hypertens 2000;18: 629–42.

[36] Taylor DV, Barnet HJM, Haynes RB, et al. low dose and high dose ASA for patients undergoing carotid endarterectomy: a randomized controlled trial. Lancet 1999;353:2179–84.

[37] Campbell CL, Steinhubl SR. Variability in response to aspirin: do we understand the clinical relevance. J Thromb Haemost 2005;3:665–9.

[38] Santopinto J, Garfinkel EP, Torres V, et al. Prior aspirin users with acute non-ST elevation coronary syndromes are at increased risk of cardiac events and benefit from enoxaparin. Am Heart J 2001; 141:566–72.

[39] Syrebe G, Redlich H, Weidlich B, et al. Individual dosing of aspirin prophylaxis by controlling platelet aggregation. Clin Appl Thromb Hemost 2001;7:209–13.

[40] Pulcinelli FM, Pignatelli P, Celestini A, et al. Inhibition of platelet aggregation by aspirin progressively decreases in long term treated patients. J Am Coll Cardiol 2004;43:979–84.

[41] Helgason CM, Bolin KM, Hoff JA, et al. Development of aspirin resistance in persons with previous ischemic stroke. Stroke 1994;25:2331–6.

[42] Sanderson S, Emery J, Baglin T, et al. Narrative review: aspirin resistance and its clinical implications. Ann Intern Med 2005;142:370–80.

[43] Waeber B, Leontetti G, Kolloch R, et al. Compliance with aspirin or placebo in the hypertension optimal treatment study. J Hypertens 1999;17:1041–5.

[44] Patrono C. Aspirin resistance: definition, mechanisms and clinical read-outs. J Thromb Haemost 2003;1:1710–3.

[45] Homoncik M, Jilma B, Hergovich N, et al. Monitoring of aspirin pharmacodynamics with the PFA-100. Thromb Haemost 2000;83:316–21.

[46] Krasopoulos G, Brister SJ, Beattie WS et al. Aspirin "resistance" and risk of cardiovascular morbidity: systematic review and meta-analysis. BMJ 2008; epub 17 Jan 2008.

[47] Bhatt DL. Aspirin resistance: more than just a laboratory curiosity. J Am Coll Cardiol 2004;43: 1127–9.

[48] Grotemeyer KH, Scharafinski HW, Husstedt IW. Two year follow up of aspirin responders and aspirin non-responders: a pilot study including 180 poststroke patients. Thromb Res 1993;71:397–403.

[49] Grundman K, Jasconek K, Kleine B, et al. Aspirin nonresponder status in patients with recurrent cerebral ischemic attacks. J Neurol 2003;250:63–6.

[50] Gum PA, Kottke-Marchant K, Welsh PA, et al. A prospective, blinded determination of the natural history of aspirin resistance among stable patients with cardiovascular disease. J Am Coll Cardiol 2003;41:961–5.

[51] Eikelboom JW, Hanky GJ. Aspirin resistance: a new independent predictor of vascular events. J Am Coll Cardiol 2003;1:2048–50.

[52] Eikelboom JW, Hirsh J, Weitz JI, et al. Aspirin-resistant thromboxane biosynthesis and the risk of myocardial infarction, stroke, or cardiovascular death in patients at high risk for cardiovascular events. Circulation 2002;105:1650–5.

[53] Gum PA, Kottke-Marchant K, Poggio ED, et al. Profile and prevalence of aspirin resistance in patients with cardiovascular disease. Am J Cardiol 2001;88:230–5.

[54] Halushka MK, Halushka PV. Why are some individuals resistant to the cardioprotective effects of aspirin? Could it be thromboxane A2? Circulation 2002;105:1620–2.

[55] Zimmermann N, Wenk A, Kim U, et al. Functional and biochemical evaluation of platelet aspirin resistance after coronary artery bypass surgery. Circulation 2003;108:542–7.

[56] Catella-Lawson F, Reilly MP, Kapoor SC, et al. Cyclooxygenase inhibitors and the antiplatelet effects of aspirin. N Engl J Med 2001;345:1809–17.

[57] Kurth T, Glynn RJ, Walker AM, et al. Inhibition of clinical benefits of aspirin on first myocardial infarction by nonsteroidal anti-inflammatory drugs. Circulation 2003;108:1191–5.

[58] Levesque LE, Brophy JM, Zhang B. The risk for myocardial infarction with cyclooxygenase –2 inhibitors: a population of elderly adults. Ann Intern Med 2005;142:481–9.

[59] Bresalier RS, Sandler RS, Quan H, et al, Adenomatous Polyp Prevention on Vioxx (APPROVE) Trial Investigators. Cardiovascular events associated with rofecoxib in a colorectal adenoma chemoprevention trial. N Engl J Med 2005;352:1092–102.

[60] Chen WH, Lee PY, Ng W, et al. Aspirin resistance is associated with a high incidence of myonecrosis after non-urgent percutaneous intervention despite clopidogrel treatment. J Am Coll Cardiol 2004;43:1122–6.

[61] Cattaneo M, Akkawat B, Lecchi A, et al. Ticlopidine selectively inhibits human platelet responses to adenosine diphosphate. Thromb Haemost 1991;66:694–9.

[62] Helft G, Osende JL, Worthley SG, et al. Acute antithrombotic effect of a front loaded regimen of clopidogrel in patients with atherosclerosis on aspirin. Arterioscler Thromb Vasc Biol 2000;20:2316–21.

[63] Weber AA, Braun M, Hohlfeld T, et al. Recovery of platelet function after discontinuation of clopidogrel treatment in healthy volunteers. Br J Clin Pharmacol 2001;52:333–6.

[64] Bennett CL, Connors JM, Carwile JM, et al. TTP associated with clopidogrel. N Engl J Med 2000;342:1773–7.

[65] Bertrand ME, Rupprecht HJ, Urban P, et al. Double blind study of the safety of clopidogrel with and without a loading dose in combination with aspirin compared with ticlopidine in combination with aspirin after coronary stenting. The clopidogrel aspirin stent international cooperative study CLASSICS. Circulation 2000;102:624–9.

[66] Storey RF, Husted S, Harrington RA J, et al. Inhibition of platelet aggregation by AZD6140, a reversible oral P2Y12 receptor antagonist, compared with clopidogrel in patients with acute coronary syndromes. Am Coll Cardiol 2007;50:1852–6.

[67] Wiviott SD, Braunwald E, McCabe CH et al. Prasugrel versus clopidogrel in patients with acute coronary syndromes. N Engl J Med 2007;357:2001–15.

[68] CAPRIE Steering Committee. A randomized, blinded trial of clopidogrel v. aspirin in patients at risk of ischemic events. Lancet 1996;348:1329–39.

[69] Diener HC, Bogousslavsky J, Brass LM, et al, MATCH investigators. Aspirin and clopidogrel compared with clopidogrel alone after recent ischaemic stroke or transient ischaemic attack in high-risk patients (MATCH): randomised, double-blind, placebo-controlled trial. Lancet 2004;364:331–7.

[70] Woodward M, Lower GDO, Francis MA, et al. A randomized comparison of the effects of aspirin and clopidogrel on thrombotic risk factors and C-reactive protein following MI: the CADET Trial. J Thromb Haemost 2004;2:1934–40.

[71] The Clopidogrel in Unstable Angina to Prevent Recurrent Ischemic Events Trial Investigators. Effects of clopidogrel in addition to aspirin in patients with non-ST segment elevation acute coronary syndromes. N Engl J Med 2001;345:494–502.

[72] Sabatine MS, Cannon CP, Gibson CM, et al. Clarity –TIMI. N Engl J Med 2005;352:1179–89.

[73] Steinhubl SR, Berger PB, Mann JT III, et al, The Clopidogrel for the Reduction of Events During Observation (CREDO) Investigators. Early and sustained dual oral antiplatelet therapy following percutaneous coronary intervention: a randomized controlled trial. JAMA 2002;288:2411–20.

[74] Mehta SR, Yusuf S, Peters RJ, et al, The Clopidogrel in Unstable angina to prevent Recurrent Events (CURE) Trial Investigators. Effects of pretreatment with clopidogrel and aspirin followed by long-term therapy in patients undergoing percutaneous coronary intervention: the PCI-CURE study. Lancet 2001;358:527–33.

[75] Gurbel PA, Bliden KP, Hiatt BL, et al. Clopidogrel for coronary stenting. Circulation 2003;107:2908–13.

[76] Matetzky S, Shenkman B, Guetta V, et al. Clopidogrel resistance is associated with increased risk of recurrent atherothrombotic events in patients with acute myocardial infarction. Circulation 2004;109:3171–5.

[77] Raman S, Jilma B. Time lag in platelet function inhibition by clopidogrel in stroke patients as measured by PFA-100. J Thromb Haemost 2004;2:2278–9.

[78] Aleil B, Ravanat C, Cazenave JP, et al. Flow cytometric analysis of intraplatelet VASP phosphorylation for the detection of clopidogrel resistance in patients with ischemic cardiovascular diseases. J Thromb Haemost 2005;3:85–92.

[79] Wenaweser P, Windecker S, Billinger M, et al. Effect of atorvastatin and pravastatin on platelet inhibition by aspirin and clopidogrel treatment in patients with coronary stent thrombosis. Am J Cardiol 2007;99:353–6.

[80] Sacco RL, Sivenius J, Diener HC. Efficacy of aspirin plus extended release dipyridamole in preventing recurrent stroke in high risk populations. Arch Neurol 2005;62:403–8.

[81] ESPS-2 group. European Stroke Prevention Study. 2. Efficacy and safety data. J Neurol Sci 1997;15S:S1–77.

[82] The EPILOG Investigators. Platelet GPIIb IIIa receptor blockade and low dose heparin during percutaneous coronary revascularization. N Engl J Med 1997;36:956–61.

[83] The EPISTENT Investigators. Randomised placebo-controlled and balloon-angioplasty-controlled trial to assess safety of coronary stenting with use of platelet glycoprotein-IIb/IIIa blockade. Evaluation of Platelet IIb/IIIa Inhibitor for Stenting. Lancet 1998;352:87–92.

[84] Kereiakes DJ, Runyon JP, Broderick TM, et al. IIb's are not IIb's. Am J Cardiol 2000;85:23C–31C.

[85] Blankenship JC. Bleeding complications of glycoprotein IIb-IIIa receptor inhibitors. Am Heart J 1999;138:S287–96.

[86] The EPIC Investigators. Use of monoclonal antibody directed against the platelet GPIIb IIIa

receptor in high risk coronary angioplasty. N Engl J Med 1994;330:956–61.

[87] Sane DC, Damaraju LV, Topol E, et al. Occurrence and clinical significance of pseudothrombocytopenia during abciximab therapy. J Am Coll Cardiol 2001;36:75–83.

[88] Reiter RA, Mayr F, Blazicek H. Desmopressin antagonizes the in-vitro platelet dysfunction induced by GPIIb IIIa inhibitors and aspirin. Blood 2003; 102:4594–9.

[89] Ronner E, Boersma E, Akkerhuis KM, et al. Patients with acute coronary syndromes without persistent ST elevation undergoing percutaneous coronary intervention benefit most from early intervention with protection by a glycoprotein IIb/IIIa receptor blocker. Eur Heart J 2002;23: 239–46.

[90] Mandak JS, Blankenship JC, Garndner LH, et al. Modifiable risk factors for vascular access site complications of angioplasty with glycoprotein IIb/IIIa

receptor inhibition in the impact II trial. J Am Coll Cardiol 1998;31:18–24.

[91] Brouse SD, Wiesehan VG. Evaluation of bleeding complications associated with GPIIb IIIa inhibitors. Ann Pharmacother 2004;38:1783–8.

[92] The Platelet Receptor Inhibition in Ischemic Syndrome Management (PRISM) Study Investigators. A comparison of aspirin plus tirofiban with aspirin plus heparin for unstable angina. N Engl J Med 1998;339:1498–505.

[93] Topol EJ, Gusto V Investigators. Reperfusion therapy for acute myocardial infarction with fibrinolytic therapy or combination reduced fibrinolytic therapy and platelet GPIIb IIIa inhibition. The GUSTO V randomized trial. Lancet 2001;357:1905–14.

[94] Hernandez AV, Westerhout CM, Steyerberg EW, et al. Effects of platelet glycoprotein IIb/IIIa receptor blockers in non-ST segment elevation acute coronary syndromes: benefit and harm in different age subgroups. Heart 2007;93:450–5.

CARDIOLOGY
CLINICS

Cardiol Clin 26 (2008) 203–219

ELSEVIER
SAUNDERS

Pathophysiology of Venous Thrombosis and the Diagnosis of Deep Vein Thrombosis–Pulmonary Embolism in the Elderly

Geno J. Merli, MD

Jefferson Center for Vascular Diseases, Jefferson Medical College, Thomas Jefferson University Hospital, 833 Chestnut Street, Suite 702, Philadelphia, PA 19107, USA

Venous thromboembolism (VTE) comprises deep vein thrombosis (DVT) and pulmonary embolism (PE) both of which account for >250,000 hospitalizations annually in the United States [1,2]. The most serious complication of DVT is PE which accounts for approximately 200,000 deaths per year and 10% of hospital deaths [1,2]. Other serious sequela of DVT is the development of postphlebitic syndrome which occurs in 20% to 50% of patients with lower extremities thrombotic events [3]. Studies have documented those susceptible groups which include elderly hospitalized patients or those that have had recent surgery, active cancer, or previous history of VTE have a high incidence of developing VTE [4,5].

The annual incidence of clinically recognized VTE increases with age in both men and women as documented by Anderson and colleagues [1] with a gradual rise beginning at age 45 followed by a sharp upswing after age 65. A similar pattern of age and VTE was demonstrated by Silverstein and colleagues [6] except that the incidence was higher in men than women. More importantly age specific survival rates in the first 2.5 years after hospitalization for VTE is highest for those less than 40 years and lowest for patients older than 70 years [1]. The purpose of this chapter is to review the pathophysiology of venous thrombosis, thrombophilia as it relates to the development of

thrombotic events, and the approach to confirming the diagnosis of VTE.

Pathophysiology of venous thrombosis

More than 150 years ago, our current understanding of the pathogenesis of venous thromboembolism was first outlined by Virchow. He proposed the triad of stasis, vascular injury, and hypercoagulability as the mechanism for the development of thrombosis [7]. Over the past 130 years, the roles of stasis and vascular injury in the pathogenesis of thrombosis have been extensively studied and led to the development of effective prophylaxis regimens to prevent these complications (Table 1).

Venous stasis

Venous return from the legs is enhanced by contraction of the calf muscles, which propels blood upward from the extremities and venous valves, which prevent blood from pooling in the lower extremities. Venous stasis may contribute to thrombogenesis by allowing stagnation of the blood with associated local hypoxia, which stimulates endothelial cell release of an activator of Factor X [8]. Venous stasis in the elderly can be produced by immobility (hospitalization, surgery, stroke), increased venous pressure (varicose veins, venous insufficiency from postthrombotic syndrome), and medical conditions which increase blood viscosity. Immobility causes pooling of blood in the intramuscular branches of the calf. This predisposes the patient to the development of thrombi which propagates into the deep venous

A version of this article originally appeared in *Clinics in Geriatric Medicine*, volume 22, issue 1.

E-mail address: geno.merli@jefferson.edu

Table 1
Virchow's triad: thrombosis risk in the elderly patient

1. Stasis	Immobilization
	Limb paralysis (stroke, plaster cast, spinal cord injury)
	Heart Failure
	Varicose Vein/Chronic Venous Insufficiency
2. Intimal Injury	Direct vessel Injury
	• Surgery
	• Central Venous Catheter
	• Trauma
	Indirect vessel injury
	• Chemotherapy
	• Vasculitis
	• Sepsis
	• Hyperhomocyteinemia
	• Sepsis
3. Hypercoagulability	Hereditary
	• Factor V Leiden
	• Prothrombin Gene Mutation
	• Antithrombin III Deficiency
	• Protein C
	• Proetin S
	Acquired
	• Malignancy
	• Hormone Replacement Therapy
	• Anticardiolipin Antibodies
	• Nephrotic Syndrome
	• Increased levels of clotting factors VIII

system of the extremity. Immobility has been studied extensively in populations such as spinal cord injury, stroke, orthopaedic surgery, and the hospitalized medically-ill patient. In each case immobility was an independent risk factor contributing to development of lower extremity DVT. Increased venous pressure contributes to stasis by reducing venous return as a result of varicosed veins or damaged valves which increase venous retrograde pressure. This latter complication causes increased retrograde pressure in the venous system and stasis of blood. Diseases that affect blood viscosity such as polycythemia, hypergammaglobulinemia, dysproteinemias, or cryoglobulinemia are sometimes manifested in an elderly population and contribute to stasis with resultant thrombois in the lower extremities.

Vascular injury

Although the normal endothelium is non-thrombogenic, damage or injury to the endothelium can trigger the activation of platelets and coagulation. This process leads to the expression of tissue factor, either directly by endothelial cells or by monocytes that are attracted to the site of damage. This process also leads to platelet adhesion and aggregation.

The vascular endothelium can be damaged by direct trauma, exposure to endotoxin, inflammatory cytokines such as interleukin-1 (IL-1) and tumor necrosis factor (TNF), thrombin, or low oxygen tension [9]. Injured endothelial cells synthesize tissue factor and PAI-1 and internalize thrombomodulin, all of which promote thrombogenesis [10]. Damaged endothelial cells also produce less t-PA, the principal activator of fibrinolysis which further tips the balance toward thrombosis. Common examples of direct venous injury in an elderly population include patients undergoing hip or knee surgery, prostatectomy, hysterectomy, or an extremity fracture. In addition this damaged endothelium is also exposed to thrombin and inflammatory mediators which contribute to thrombosis at the sites of injury.

Hypercoagulablility

Normally activated clotting factors are diluted in the flowing blood and are neutralized by inhibitors on the surface of endothelial cells or by circulating antiproteinases [11] Activated clotting factors that escape regulation, as a result of either reduced levels of inhibitors or sudden generation of overwhelming amounts of these factors, trigger the coagulation system, thereby leading to fibrin formation. A balancing mechanism immediately comes into play in an attempt to reduce the likelihood of thrombus formation. If thrombus forms, the fibrinolytic system is immediately activated as a result of the release of t-PA and urokinase from monocytes and leukocytes, which are attracted to the thrombus by released fibrinopeptides and platelet products [12].

Coagulation may be activated by contact of factor XII with collagen on exposed subendothelium of damaged vessels or by contact with prosthetic surfaces. Coagulation is further augmented by activated platelets. Coagulation also may be initiated by the exposure of blood to tissue factor made available locally as a result of vascular wall damage by activation of endothelial cells by cytokines, and by activated monocytes that migrate to areas of vascular injury [13,14]. Factor X can be activated directly by extracts of malignant cells that contain a cysteine protease which may be one of the mechanisms by which thrombosis is induced in patients with malignant disease [15]. A factor elaborated by hypoxic endothelial cells also can directly activate factor X potentially leading to thrombosis in patients with severe venous stasis, in which stagnant hypoxia occurs in the valve cusps [8].

The elderly population has a number of clinical risk factors that predispose patients to venous thromboembolism by activating blood coagulation including malignancy, joint replacement surgeries, trauma, systemic infections, and decreased mobility [8].

Thrombophilia

Up to 30% of patients with VTE have an inherited tendency for thrombophilia, which compares to approximately less than 10% of the general population [16]. Inherited thrombophilia frequently have their first presentation as a consequence of a temporal risk factor such as surgery, oral contraception, or estrogen replacement therapy use. Clues to an underlying genetic risk factor among patients with VTE include a thrombotic event under the age of 50 years, family history, recurrent thrombosis with or without anticoagulation, idiopathic thrombosis, thrombosis in unusual locations, or extensive thrombosis. The above issue of age often leads clinicians to discount the need to evaluate geriatric patients for hereditary thrombophilic states. Physicians should continue to evaluate the entirety of the clinical presentation of the patient and order appropriate testing to asses the etiology for the acute thrombotic event.

The most common forms of inherited thrombophilias are listed in the Table 2 [17]. Heterozygosity for the Factor V Leiden mutation is the most prevalent, occurring in 18% of Caucasians presenting with VTE [18]. This mutation is autosomal dominant and results in Factor V being resistant to inhibition by activated protein C an endogenous anticoagulant. The Factor V Leiden mutation accounts for approximately 40% of idiopathic thromboses. The Prothrombin Gene mutation 20,210 is seen in 7% of patients with VTE and is the result of an increase prothrombin levels caused by an inefficient F2 S' cleavage signal resulting in a gain of function mutation due to messenger RNA accumulation and an increase in prothrombin synthesis [19–21]. Both the Factor V Leiden and Prothrombin Gene mutation are uncommon in the African and Asian populations (see Table 2). High levels of homocyteine are associated with both venous and arterial thrombosis [22,23]. The mechanism by which hyperhomocyteinemia predisposes to thrombosis is unclear; however, potential mechanisms include endothelial activation, proliferation of smooth-muscle cells, changes in endothelial nitric oxide production or changes in enodtheilial sterol metabolism [24,25]. Hyperhomocysteinemia can be congenital

Table 2
Common inherited thrombophilic disorders

Disorder	Prevalence normals	Frequency Pts with VTE	Relative risk first VTE
Factor V Leiden (Heterozygous)		18.8%	7
Caucasians	4.8%	–	–
Hispanic American	2.21%	–	–
African American	1.23%	–	–
Native American	1.25%	–	–
Asian American	0.45%	–	–
African or Asian	0.05%	–	–
Factor V Leiden (Homozygous)	0.02%	–	80
Prothrombin Mutation (G20210A)		7.1%	2.8
Caucasian	2.7%	–	–
African or Asian	0.06%	–	–
Antithrombin III	0.02%	1.9%	20
Protein C	0.2–0.4%	3.7%	6.5
Protein S	0.003%	2.3%	5
Hyperhomocysteinemia (>18.5 umol/L)	5%–7%	10%	2.95

Data from Perry SL, Ortel TL. Clinical and laboratory evaluation of thrombophilia. Clin Chest Med 2003;24:153–70.

or acquired. Acquired forms are found in patients with dietary deficiencies of folate, vitamin B12, or vitamin B6. The most common hereditary hyper-homocysteinemia is associated with the methyle-netetrahydrafolate reductase (MTHFR) gene [26]. The homozygous state is asscociated with increased homocysteine levels. The relationship between this mutation and thrombosis, even in homozygous patients with increase homocysteine levels is controversial [27].

Screening for thrombophilia may benefit patients with clues to inherited hypercoagulability and VTE by allowing for family testing and counseling, safety during prophylactic anticoagulation in high risk settings as well as extended anticoagulation in special clinical scenarios and in situations where thrombotic risk is increased with drugs such as estrogen replacement, tamoxifen, and raloxifen. These potential benefits must be weighed against the test costs and the lack of definitive data to guide the optimal duration of anticoagulation therapy. Focusing genetic testing on patients with the highest suspicion of inherited thrombophilia may be the most cost-effective approach. Testing for the Factor V Leiden and Prothrombin Gene Mutation 20,210 can be performed at the time of presentation with acute thrombosis. Proteins C, S, and antithrombin levels (although rare as a cause of first time VTE in the elderly) should not be measured duration the acute thrombosis phase, since the levels are affected by the acute thrombotic process and the anticoagulants being used. Evaluation of these levels can be deferred until 2 to 4 weeks after the discontinuation of anticoagulation.

Diagnosis of deep vein thrombosis and pulmonary embolism

History and physical examination

Traditionally the history and physical examination of a patient suspected of having DVT included a detail history, careful inspection of the extremity for temperature and redness, measurement of leg circumference, elicitation of Homan's sign (calf pain with dorsiflexion of the foot). Three well designed trials evaluated the frequency of DVT symptoms and signs in patients with suspected thrombosis and confirmed their lack of sensitivity and specificity (Table 3) [28–30]. This sole use of clinical finding is artificial since clinicians couple the medical and surgical history, concomitant medical problems, medications, and risk factors (age, obesity, immobility etc) to decide on further testing to confirm DVT.

Wells and colleagues [31,32] developed the first clinical model for the diagnosis of patients presenting with suspected DVT. This model includes a thorough clinical examination and the identification of risk factors that predispose patients to having increased risk for thrombosis. In accordance with this model, patients are first divided into 3 risk categories (low, moderate, and high) and are further assessed through the use of D-dimer and ultrasonography (Fig. 1) and (Table 4). Clincial

Table 3
Frequency of symptoms and signs in patients with suspected DVT

Sign & symptoms	O'Donnell et al. [28]		Haeger et al. [29]		Molly et al. [30]	
	DVT+	DVT−	DVT+	DVT−	DVT+	DVT−
Pain	78%	75%	90%	97%	48%	23%
Tenderness	76%	89%	84%	74%	43%	35%
Edema	78%	67%	42%	32%	43%	26%
Homan's Sign	56%	61%	33%	21%	11%	11%
Swelling	85%	56%	.....	.....	41%	39%
Erythema	24%	38%	.....	.....	.....	.....

The DVT diagnosis was confirmed by venography.
DVT + indicates those with DVT.
DVT − indicates those without DVT.
O'Donnell et al. and Molloy et al. trials were Grade A studies since they were an independent blind comparisons of signs or symptoms with a criteria standard of diagnosis among a large number of consecutive patients suspected of having the target condition.
Haeger et al. was a Grade B study since it had the same criteria as above but a smaller number of patient.
..... = data not applicable.
Data from references [28–30].

practice guidelines for the diagnosis of DVT from the American Thoracic Society concur with this strategy, recommending the use of venography as a follow up to inconclusive compression ultrasound results, and the use of serial ultrasound or impedance plethysmography in patients with normal compression ultrasound results.

Pulmonary embolism has a wide spectrum of clinical presentation, from subtle clinical signs to hemodynamic instability resulting in death within an hour of acute onset. In most cases, PE goes undetected and is a 'silent' killer identified only at autopsy. An analysis of 200 autopsied cases showing massive or submassive PE performed between 1989 and 1995 revealed that in 78% of cases, major PE had not been diagnosed by physicians [33]. The most common signs and symptoms associated with PE are listed in Tables 5 and 6 [34]. For patients presenting with PE, shortness of breath, with or without leg pain, may be the first symptom, however there are a number of specific criteria that allow for a more accurate diagnosis. Similar to the clinical model for diagnosis of DVT, Wells and colleagues also defined a clinical algorithm for the diagnosis of PE, which when used in conjunction with D-dimer testing, safely reduces the need for expensive imaging diagnostics (Fig. 2) and (Table 7)

[35,36]. This model for assessment of PE uses a point system for calculating the low, moderate, or high pretest probability of PE. Points are assigned based on clinical symptoms of DVT, including heart rate of >100 beats per minute, immobilization for >3 days or recent surgery in the past 4 weeks, a clinical history of VTE, hemoptysis, malignancy, or the clinician determination that PE is as likely or more likely than another diagnosis. PE patient history and physical examination findings reported in the Prospective Investigation of Pulmonary Embolism Diagnosis trial illustrate the difficulty in quickly identifying or ruling out a diagnosis of PE. In PIOPED, the most common past and current physical findings included dyspnea, pleuritic chest pain, cough, tachycardia, and tachypnea [37]. These symptoms also can be indicative of heart failure, interstitial lung disease, or pneumonia. For this reason it is especially important to conduct thorough examination and risk stratification when examining patients for potential VTE.

Because of the lack of sensitivity and specificity associated with these findings, clinicians cannot unequivocally rely on them solely for diagnosing PE. Instead, clinical prediction rules have been developed that assess the pretest probability of pulmonary embolism. These scoring systems have

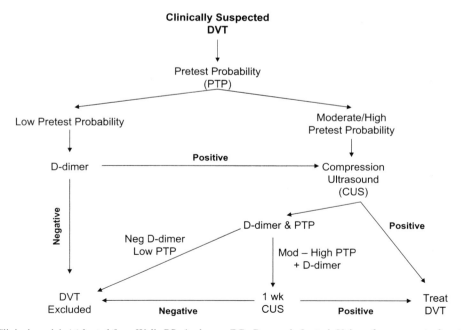

Fig. 1. Clinical model. (*Adapted from* Wells PS, Anderson DR, Bormanis J, et al. Value of assessment of pretest probability of DVT in clinical management. Lancet 1997;300:795–8; with permission).

Table 4
Pretest probability for DVT

Clinical characteristics	Score
1. Active cancer (treatment ongoing within previous 6 months or palliative)	1
2. Paralysis, paresis, or recent plaster immobilization of the lower extremities	1
3. Recently bedridden >3 days or major surgery within 12 weeks requiring general or regional anesthesia	1
4. Localized tenderness along the distribution of deep venous system	1
5. Entire swollen leg	1
6. Calf swelling 3 cm larger than asymptomatic side (measured 10 cm below tibial tuberosity)	1
7. Pitting edema confined to the symptomatic leg	1
8. Collateral superficial veins (non-varicose)	1
9. Alternative diagnosis at least as likely as deep vein thrombosis	−2

Scoring.
>3 points = High Probability.
1–2 points = Moderate Probability.
0 = Low Probability.
Adapted from Wells PS, Anderson DR, Bormanis J, et al. Value of assessment of pretest probability of DVT in clinical management. Lancet 1997;300:795–8; with permission.

been shown to be as accurate as experienced physicians using clinical gestalt assessment for pulmonary embolism [38]. These prediction rules allow clinicians to pursue further testing to prove or disprove the diagnosis.

Diagnostic testing for deep vein thrombosis and pulmonary embolism

Diagnostic evaluation of suspected VTE includes a clear correlation between clinical probability, test selection, and test interpretation. However, a variety of diagnostic approaches are feasible, and the availability and familiarity with particular technolgy may influence the choice of approach. Additionally, the sensitivity of certain diagonostic tests is affected by the location of the thrombus.

Diagnostic testing for deep vein thrombosis

Contrast venography

Contrast venography is no longer appropriate as the initial diagnostic test in patients exhibiting DVT symptoms, although it remains the "gold standard" for confirmatory diagnosis of **DVT** (Fig. 3). Venography is nearly 100% sensitive

and specific, and provides the ability to investigate the distal and proximal venous system for thrombosis [39]. Venography is still warranted when non-invasive testing is inconclusive or impossible to perform, but its use is no longer widespread due to the need for administration of a contrast medium and the increased availalbility of non-invasive diagnostic strategies. Additional drawbacks of venography include its contraindication in patients with renal insufficiency and its lack of accuracy in recurrent DVT due to the difficulty of visualizing an intralumental defect in veins that have been thrombosed previously.

Ultrasound

Ultrasound is a safe and noninvasive and has a higher specificity than impedance plethysmography for the evaluation of suspected DVT (Fig. 4) [40]. With color flow Doppler and compression ultrasound, a DVT is diagnosed based on the inability to compress the common femoral or popliteal veins. With a first symptomatic DVT, sensitivity is 95% and specificity 96%. The

Table 5
Symptoms in all patients with pulmonary embolism according to age

	≥70 Y N = 53–55 n (%)	<70 Y N = 130–137 n (%)
Dyspnea		
Dyspnea (rest or exertion)	41 (75)	110 (80)
Dyspnea (at rest)[a]	33 (60)	84 (61)
Dyspnea (exertion only)[a]	7 (13)	24 (18)
Orthopnea (≥2-pillow)	17 (31)	52 (39)
Pleuritic pain	18 (33)	71 (52)[b]
Chest pain (not pleuritic)	7 (13)	26 (19)
Cough	24 (44)	58 (43)
Wheezing	13 (25)	45 (33)
Calf or thigh swelling	14 (26)	61 (46)[b]
Calf or thigh pain[b]	15 (28)	62 (46)

[a] Information not available in some.
[b] P < .025 age ≥ 70 years versus < 70 years. All other differences between age groups are not significant.
Data from Stein PD, Beemath A, Matta F, et al. Clinical characteristics of patients with acute pulmonary embolism: data from PIOPED II. Am J Med 2007;120:871–9.

Table 6
Signs in all patients with pulmonary embolism

	≥70 y N = 52–55 n (%)	<70 y N = 130–137 n (%)
General		
Tachypnea (≥20 min)	28 (51)	80 (59)
Tachycardia (>100 min)	11 (21)	38 (28)
Diaphoresis	1 (2)	7 (5)
Cyanosis	0 (0)	1 (1)
Temperature >38.5°C(>101.3°F6)	0 (0)	3 (2)
Cardiac examination (any)	12 (22)	30 (23)
Increased P2[a]	3 (7)	19 (18)
Right ventricular lift[b]	2 (4)	6 (5)
Jugular venous distension	10 (19)	15 (11)
Lung examination (any)	25 (45)	44 (32)
Rales (crackles)	14 (26)	36 (27)
Wheezes	2 (4)	4 (3)
Rhonchi	3 (6)	6 (4)
Decreased breath sounds	16 (29)	24 (18)
Pleural friction rub	1 (2)	1 (1)

All differences between age groups not significant.
[a] Data in 42 patients ≥ 70 years, 103 patients < 70 years.
[b] Data in 45 patients ≥70 years, 110 patients <70 years.
Data from Stein PD, Beemath A, Matta F, et al. Clinical characteristics of patients with acute pulmonary embolism: data from PIOPED II. Am J Med 2007;120:871–9.

diagnosis accuracy of ultrasound in patients with first asymptomatic DVT, recurrent DVT, or isolated calf DVT is less reliable.

The sensitivity of ultrasound improves with serial testing in untreated patients. Repeat testing as 5 to 7 days will identify another 2% of patients with clots not apparent on the first ultrasound [41]. Serial testing can be particularly valuable in ruling out proximal extension of a possible calf DVT. Because the accuracy of ultrasound in diagnosing calf DVT is acknowledged to be lower (81% for DVT below the knee versus 99% for proximal DVT), follow up ultrasounds at 5 to 7 days are reasonable because most calf DVTs that extend proximally will do so within days of the initial presentation [42].

Ultrasound after a non-diagnostic V/Q scan is particularly effective in excluding PE in stable patients. In one study of patients with non-diagnostic V/Q scans, the negative predictive value of serial ultrasound performed at days 3, 7, and 14 was 99.5% [38]. Serial ultrasound after a non-diagnostic V/Q scan can thus reduce the percentage of patients who need angiography from 73% to 29% [43].

Diagnostic testing for pulmonary embolism

Chest xray

Although a chest xray is commonly ordered during the process of evualuating a patient suspected of pulmonary embolism, it is frequently normal (Fig. 5). A normal chest xray in the presence of severe dyspnea or hypoxemia without evidence of bronchospasm or cardiac shunt is strongly suggestive of but not diagnostic of PE [44]. The Hampton hump, which is visible in some xrays, is a classic finding caused by a pleural based abnormality due to pulmonary infarction; its presence, however, is no common and cannot be used to confirm or exclude PE. Chest xray is most useful to rule out other conditions that may mimic PE, such as pneumothorax or pneumonmediastinum [44].

Ventilation-perfusion lung scanning

Ventilation-perfusion (V/Q) lung scanning has long been considered the major test for diagnosing PE (Fig. 6). The Prospective Investigation of Pulmonary Embolism Diagnosis (PIOPED) study evaluated the sensitivity and specificity of V/Q lung scanning in patients with clinically suspected PE (Table 8) [37]. The diagnosis of PE was confirmed by pulmonary angiography or autopsy. The key findings from this study were that PE was present in 96% of patients who had a high pretest PE clinical probability plus a high probability V/Q lung scan, while 40% of patients with a high pretest PE clinical probability and a low probability V/Q lung scan had PE. However, when a high probability V/Q lung scan was associated with a low pretest PE clinical probability, the likelihood of PE was only 56% to 88%. In the group of patients with low clinical suspicion and low probability V/Q scan, only 4% had angiographically confirmed PE. In some clinical scenarios, the ventilation portion of the V/Q lung scan cannot be performed. The value of perfusion scanning alone was also evaluated in the PIOPED study, which revealed that the positive predictive value of a high, intermediate, and low probability perfusion scan did not differ from complete V/Q

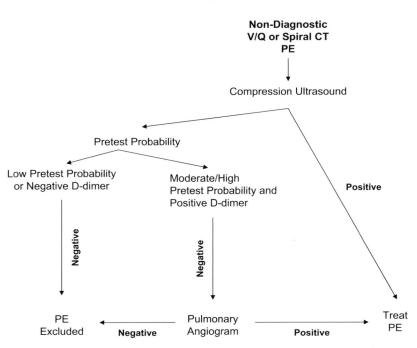

Fig. 2. Algorithm for non-diagnostic V/Q or spiral CT. (*Adapted from* Wells P, Anderson D, Rodger M, et al. Derivation of a simple clinical model to categorize patients with a probability of pulmonary embolism: increasing the models utility with the SimpliRED D-dimer. Thromb Haemost 2000;83:416–20; with permission).

lung scans [37]. The key point when interpreting V/Q scanning is that the combination of clinical suspicion and V/Q results was non-diagnostic in 72% of patients. Therefore additional testing is required to confirm thrombotic events.

Table 7
Pretest probability for pulmonary embolism

Clinical characteristics	Score
1. DVT Symptoms & Signs	3
2. PE as or more likely	3
3. Heart Rate > 100/min	1.5
4. Immobilization/surgery	1.5
5. Previous DVT or PE	1.5
6. Hemoptysis	1.0
7. Malignancy	1.0

Scoring.
>6 points = High Probability.
2–6 points = Moderate Probability.
<2 = Low Probability.
Data from Wells PS, Ginsberg JS, Anderson DR, et al. Use of a clinical model for safe management of patients with suspected pulmonary embolism. Ann Intern Med 1998;129:997–1005.

Single-detector spiral or helical computed tomography angiography (SCTA)

One of the techniques for the diagnosis of PE is contrast-enhanced single detector spiral computed tomography angiography (SCTA) (Fig. 7). SCTA scanning is minimally invasive and widely available, and offers the advantage of imaging any emboli directly within the pulmonary arteries. With regard to sensitivity and specificity, pooled data indicate a sensitivity of about 70% and a specificity of 88% with a positive predictive value of 76% and a negative predictive value of 84% [45]. A recent prospective, multi-center study evaluated helical SCTA as initial testing for PE [46]. In 24% (124/510) PE was diagnosed while 26% (130/510) had an alternative diagnosis such as pneumonia, malignancy, pleural effusion, or heart failure. The remaining 248 patients had negative SCTA scans. These patients had serial lower extremity ultrasounds to ensure lower extremity thrombosis was not missed. SCTA scanning appears to be more accurate in detecting central or lobar PE than segmental PE, and thus a normal SCTA scan cannot be taken to rule out the possibility of subsegmental PE. However, isolated

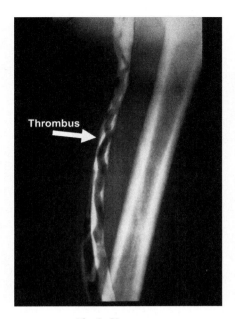

Fig. 3. Venogram.

subsegmental PE is uncommon and this limitation should therefore be kept in perspective. A recent systematic review of the clinical validity of a negative SCTA scan in patient suspected with pulmonary embolism demonatrated that withholding anticoagulation with a negative SCTA was safe and similar to having a negative pulmonary angiogram [47].

Multi-detector spiral computed tomography (MDCT)

Multi-Detector spiral computed tomography (MDCT) technology quickly followed Single Detector Spiral (or Helical) Computed Tomography (SCTA), improving on the same concept (Fig. 8) [48]. With MDCT, multiple detectors are staggered and rotated around the patient as they slide through the CT scanner. Initially, 4 detectors were used for MDCT, but this quickly progressed to 6-, 8-, 10-, 16-, 32-, and 64-detector technology [49]. The use of more detectors shortens the time of the study to <10 seconds and allows for cuts as thin as 0.5 mm to be obtained. This greatly improves the resolution of the study, allowing for imaging out to sixth-order pulmonary arteries [50]. Consequently, MDCT improves the detection of segmental and subsegmental PEs decreasing false-negative results and improving sensitivity [51,52]. The significance of subsegmental PEs, especially those in arteries out to the fifth and sixth generation, is unknown, as is the importance of treating them. Subsegmental PEs may not be acutely dangerous to the patient but may predict the potential for a future, more severe embolism [44,53]. It may also identify patients at risk for the development of pulmonary hypertension [54,55]. Regardless of importance, MDCT does not seem to increase the diagnosis of PE even at the subsegmental level. If the use of MDCT did lead to an increased diagnosis of isolated subsegmental clots, the incidence of PE in MDCT

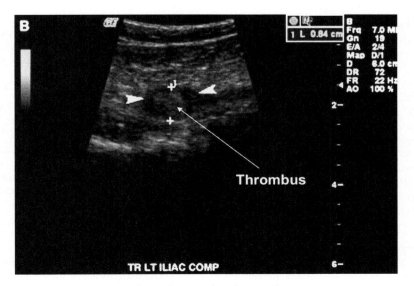

Fig. 4. Compression ultrasound.

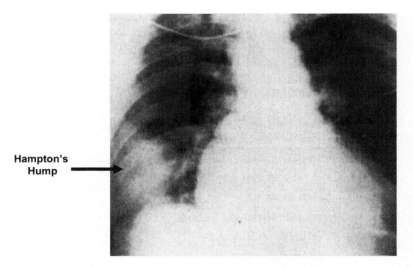

Hampton's Hump →

Fig. 5. Chest Xray.

studies should be higher than those performed with other methods.

As with SCTA, MDCT exposes patients to radiation exposure and the risk of contrast induced nephropathy. It is worth noting that radiation exposure is significantly greater with MDCT. A 4-row MDCT may increase radiation exposure by 30% to 100% when compared with SCTA [50]. In summary, single- or multidetector CT scanning has an excellent specificity for the diagnosis of PE, and patients with a positive study should be treated with confidence.

Magnetic resonance angiography

Recent advances in magnetic resonance imaging (MRI) technology have made imaging of the chest, and particularly the vascular structures, feasible (Fig. 9). Specifically, the development of parallel imaging has greatly decreased the amount of time necessary to complete a study, allowing images to be acquired during a short breath hold of 20 seconds [56]. MRI is attractive since it does not use ionizing radiation and the contrast agent used is less nephrotoxic. The 3 most commonly used MRI techniques are gadolinium-enhanced MRA (Gd-MRA), real-time MRI (RT-MR), and magnetic resonance (MR) perfusion. The accuracy for the evaluation of PE differs with the different techniques.

Gadolinium-enhanced MRA (Gd-MRA)

Gd-MRA is perhaps the most common MRA method currently used to evaluate a patient for PE. In the largest study of Gd-MRA, conducted by Oudkerk and colleagues [57] 118 patients underwent Gd-MRA followed by pulmonary angiography, and 2 independent readers interpreted the Gd-MRAs. Gd-MRA sensitivity was 77% and specificity was 98%. Although Gd-MRA identified all emboli in the central and lobar arteries, its sensitivity was only 40% for isolated subsegmental emboli. Sensitivity improved to 72% when all subsegmental emboli were included. Similar results were reported in smaller studies and in a study that compared Gd-MRA with 16-row MDCT as the reference standard [58–60]. The high specificity of Gd-MRA allows patients with a positive study to be treated for PE with confidence. However, at this time, its sensitivity as a single test is not high enough to reliably exclude PE, particularly in the distal, subsegmental arteries.

Real-time-magnetic resonance imaging (RT-MR)

RT-MR uses technology similar to that used for electrocardiographically gated CT scanners to acquire images of moving organs. When used for the evaluation of PE, RT-MR is timed to take images gated to a patient's respiratory cycle. This modality has 2 advantages. First, it eliminates the need for a breath hold. Second, RT-MR sequences produce T2-weighted images, which allow for imaging of thrombus without the need for contrast [61].

There are few published studies comparing RT-MR with other modalities. In a study by Kluge and colleagues [60] 62 patients with signs

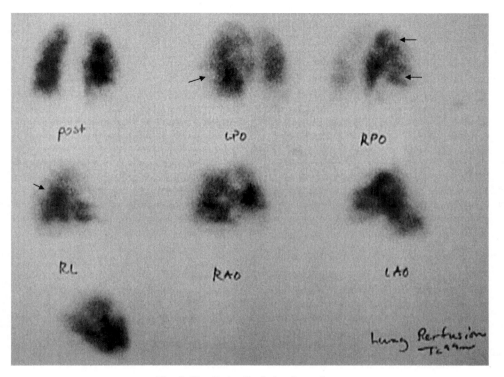

Fig. 6. Ventilation Perfusion Lung Scan.

and symptoms of PE underwent 16-row MDCT (standard), Gd-MRA, RT-MR, and MR perfusion imaging. The incidence of PE was 31% and the sensitivity and specificity of RT-MR were 85% and 98%, respectively. The sensitivity of RT-MR was superior to that of Gd-MRA (77%), and the specificities were essentially the same. Although RT-MR showed continued excellent specificity, its sensitivity was not nearly what might be expected based on the preclinical study and does not appear to be high enough to allow its use as a stand-alone test for the evaluation of PE.

Magnetic resonance perfusion (MR perfusion)

MR perfusion images use contrast agents that cause local disturbances in a magnetic field that can be measured by an MR scanner. Gadolinium is frequently the contrast agent used, and perfusion studies can be performed immediately after Gd-MRA. The patient does need to perform a breath hold for an optimal study. Perfusion images do not directly image vascular structures, but rather generate a signal based on the volume of blood in a region. MR perfusion studies act in

a similar fashion as nuclear medicine perfusion studies, in that areas where blood flow is decreased or absent suggest areas where blood flow is obstructed. This acts as indirect evidence of PE. Although clinical studies of MR perfusion are limited, it is hoped that MR perfusion will perform better with respect to identifying peripheral thrombus in the subsegmental arteries than Gd-MRA and RT-MR. The major concern with MRI for the evaluation of PE is its lack of sensitivity. Although there are few studies of this technique to date, there is already a trend toward a reproducible sensitivity in the range of 75% to 93% [62]. In the future, combining MRI with imaging of the lower extremities may prove to be adequate to rule out PE.

There are contraindications for MRI, the most important of which is the presence of an electronic implanted device. Fatal arrhythmias have been attributed to cardiac pacemaker malfunctions during an MRI, and pacemakers are considered an absolute contraindication. Nerve stimulators, continuous medicine pumps (eg, epoprostanol), cardiac defibrillators, insulin pumps, cochlear implants, and some prosthetic devices should be

Table 8
Clinical assessment and ventilation-perfusion (V/Q) scan probability in the prospective investigation of pulmonary embolism diagnosis (PIOPED) study [adapted from the PIOPED investigators [37]

V/Q lung scan category (probability)	Clinical suspicion of PE		
	High (80%–100%) n/N (%)	Intermediate (20%–79%) n/N (%)	Low (0%–19%) n/N (%)
High	28/29 (96)	70/80 (88)	5/9 (56)
Intermediate	27/41 (66)	66/236 (28)	11/68 (16)
Low	6/15 (40)	30/191 (16)	4/90 (4)
Normal	0/5 (0)	4/62 (6)	1/61 (2)
Total	61/90 (68)	170/569 (30)	21/228 (9)

Abbreviations: n, number of patients with proven PE; N, number of patients with specific V/Q lung scan results; PE, pulmonary embolism.

Data from The PIOPED Investigators. Value of the ventilation/perfusion scan in acute pulmonary embolism: results of the Prospective Investigation of Pulmonary Embolism Diagnosis (PIOPED). JAMA 1990;263(20):2753–59.

considered contraindications as should residual metallic fragments (shrapnel, bullets), which may move during the course of an MRI [63]. Gadolinium-based contrast agents are thought to be less toxic than ionic contrast agents used for fluoroscopy and CT scanning. The incidence of adverse events associated with gadolinium contrast is 1.47% [64]. At least 69% of these reactions are mild in nature. Severe reactions, such as anaphylaxis, occur in 0.0003% of patients. Although gadolinium was thought to be safe for use in patients with renal failure at US Food and Drug Administration (FDA)–approved doses, gadolinium-containing agents recently have been implicated in the development of nephrogenic fibrosing dermopathy (NFD)/nephrogenic systemic fibrosis (NSF). NFD/NSF is a rare condition (only 215 cases have been reported worldwide since 1997) that occurs exclusively in

patients with chronic renal insufficiency, tends to be progressive, and may be fatal [65].

In summary, MRI and MRA of the pulmonary vasculature is a rapidly developing technology for evaluating PE. The accuracy of MR for evaluating PE is dependent on the technique used. When these techniques are used as stand-alone tests, they have a high specificity for diagnosing PE, but sensitivity is not high enough to reliably exclude PE without additional testing. However, when combined to evaluate PE, these techniques have a sensitivity and specificity that rivals 4-row MDCT.

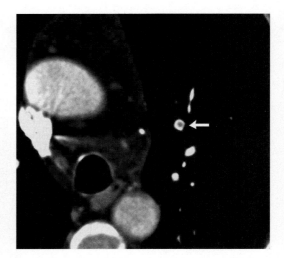

Fig. 8. MDCT through the left upper lobe partial defect in anterior segmental artery. *From* Storto ML, DiCredico A, Guido F, et al. Incidental detection of pulmonary emboli on routine MDCT of the chest. AJR Am J Roentgenol 2005;184:264–7; with permission.

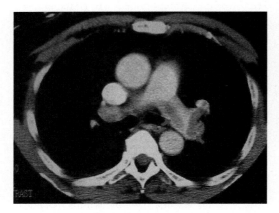

Fig. 7. Helical Computed Tomography.

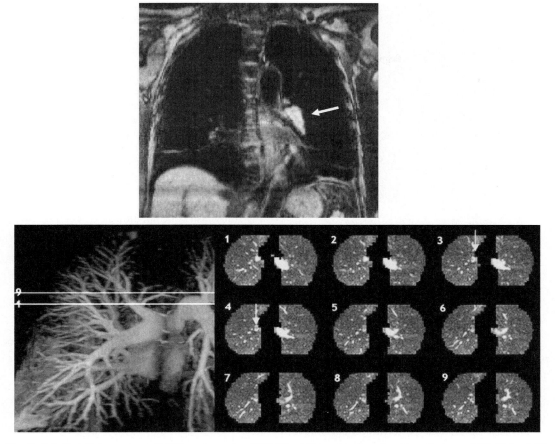

Fig. 9. 3 D Gadolinium enhanced MR angiography. MRI Direct Thrombus Imaging. *From* Pedersen MR, Fisher MT, van Beek EJ. MR imaging of the pulmonary vasculaturedan update. Eur Radiol 2006;16:1374–86; with permission.

Pulmonary angiography

Pulmonary angiography is the gold standard diagnostic test for PE, but it is invasive – a factor responsible for its underuse by clinicians (Fig. 10). The major concern is the estimated 1%–2% risk of major complications that include death, renal failure, cardiac arrhythmias and adverse dye reactions [66]. However, the safety of pulmonary angiography has improved over the last 10 years and the actual risks associated with this test are low compared with cardiac catheterization, which is far more frequently performed, with little hesitation from clinicians. Current recommendations state that pulmonary angiography is the reference standard but should be reserved for patients in whom non-invasive tests have proved inconclusive [67]. A normal angiogram can safely be assumed to rule out suspected PE.

D-dimer

D-dimer is a specific degradation product released into the blood circulation when cross-linked fibrin undergoes endogenous fibrinolysis (Table 9) [68,69]. A number of clinical studies have been performed using either an enzyme-linked immunosorbent assay (ELISA) or a latex agglutination test for D-dimer. A review of the literature comparing D-dimer results and objective diagnostic tests for DVT or PE revealed the following points: (1) results of clinical studies using one manufacturer's D-dimer assay cannot be extrapolated to another; (2) no one D-dimer test has been established as the best; (3) D-dimers have a poor specificity particularly in the settings of hospitalization, pregnancy, cancer, and the postoperative state, and (4) future studies should be more rigorous regarding the definitive presence

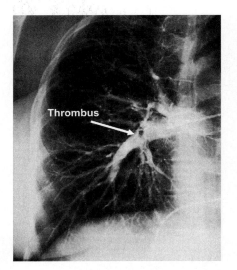

Fig. 10. Pulmonary Angiogram.

had a nondiagnostic lung scan and an intermediate clinical probability of PE, their D-dimer concentration was measured. A normal D-dimer concentration (defined as < 500 μg/L) ruled out PE, while an abnormal concentration (≥ 500 μg/L) was followed by an ultrasound scan. Patients with DVT were classified as having PE. The study revealed that of 147 patients with a nondiagnostic lung scan and an intermediate clinical probability of PE, 53 had PE ruled out as they had normal D-dimer concentrations. No patient with a normal D-dimer concentration experienced a thrombotic event by the 6-month follow-up. The negative predictive value of D-dimer in this this strategy was 99%, while its specificity was 50%. Interestingly, the study also concluded that in a clinical setting without lung scan facilities, normal D-dimer test results could have been used to rule out PE in 32% of patients. These data support the use of D-dimer as part of future algorithms for diagnosis of PE concomitant with objective testing.

D-dimer testing has been the subject of intensive investigation as a candidate for a non-invasive test for DVT and PE. However, the performance of the D-dimer test is highly dependent upon the type of assay used and has some significant limitations, particularly in relation to medical patients. Traditional latex and whole blood agglutination tests, such as the Simplired, have been shown to have a low sensitivity for D-dimer and should not be used to rule out PE [67,73,74]. However, plasma D-dimer, when assayed using a quantitative ELISA or ELISA-based method, is highly sensitive for PE, and a normal D-dimer level (≤ 500 μg/L) safely excludes PE [67,73]. While ELISA-based D-dimer testing has a high negative predictive

or absence of DVT and PE, and should address issues such as the extent of thrombosis, the clinical setting and comorbidity [70,71].

D-dimer testing was examined in a study by Perrier and colleagues [72], which evaluated diagnosis of PE in 308 consecutive patients presenting to the emergency room with suspected PE. All patients had a clinical probability assessment, a V/Q lung scan, and an ELISA plasma D-dimer test. Noninvasive tests were performed sequentially. A normal lung scan was deemed to rule out PE, and a high probability scan established PE. In the case of a nondiagnostic lung scan, the clinical probability was combined with the lung scan results; a low clinical probability ruled out PE and a high probability established PE. If patients

Table 9
Sensitivity and specificity of the D-dimer based on the laboratory technique

	Mean (range)	
	Sensitivity	Specificity
ELISA	95% (85%–100%)	44% (34%–54%)
Rapid quantitative ELISA	95% (83%–100%)	39% (28%–51%)
Rapid semiquantitative ELISA	93% (79%–100%)	36% (23%–50%)
Rapid qualitative ELISA	93% (74%–100%)	68% (50%–87%)
Quantitative latex agglutination	89% (81%–98%)	45% (36%–53%)
Semiquantitative latex agglutination	92% (79%–100%)	45% (31%–59%)
Whole blood agglutination	78% (64%–92%)	74% (60%–88%)

ELISA, enzyme-linked immunosorbent assay.
Data from Stein PD, Hull RD, Patel KC, et al. D-dimer for the exclusion of acute venous thrombosis and pulmonary embolism: a systematic review. Ann Intern Med. 2004;140:589–602.

value, specificity is relatively low because, in addition to VTE, a range of acute illnesses including cancer, inflammation and infection also produce fibrin. The specificity of D-dimer testing is even lower in elderly patients. Overall, D-dimer has proven most useful in the assessment of patients in the emergency care department; D-dimer testing of medical in-patients is still a valid method to rule out PE, but normal levels are seen in less than 10% of patients so the technique must be used in conjunction with other methods such as V/Q lung scanning [67,73].

Summary

This chapter reviews Virchow's Triad to provide clinicians with the pathophysiologic basis for the development of VTE. Armed with this data physicians should be vigilant of the development of VTE when these factors are present. The second clinical point is the appropriate need to evaluate elderly patients for primary or secondary thrombophilia. By using statistical probability and clinical history selected geriatric patients with VTE should be assessed for the etiology of their hypercoagulable state. Finally evaluating symptomatic patients for VTE should be structured to use the appropriate testing to confirm the diagnosis.

References

[1] Anderson FA Jr, Wheeler HB, Goldberg RJ, et al. A population based perspective of the hospital incidence and case fatality rates of deep vein thrombosis and pulmonary embolism. The Worcester DVT Study. Arch Intern Med 1991;151:933–8.

[2] Kim V, Spandorfer J. Epidemiology of venous thromboembolic disease. Emerg Med Clin North Am 2001;19:839–59.

[3] Kahn SR, Ginsberg JS. The post-thrombotic syndrome: current knowledge, controversies, and directions for future research. Blood Rev 2002;16:155–65.

[4] Oger E, Bressollette L, Nonent M, et al. High prevalence of asymptomatic deep vein thrombosis on admission in a medical unit among elderly patients. Thromb Haemost 2002;88:592–7.

[5] Goldhaber SZ, Tapson VF. A prospective registry of 5,451 patients with ultrasound confirmed deep vein thrombosis. Am J Cardiol 2004;93:259–62.

[6] Silverstein MD, Heit JA, Mohr DN, et al. Trends in the incidence of deep vein thrombosis and pulmonary embolism: a 25 year population based study. Arch Intern Med 1998;158:585–9.

[7] Virchow R. Gesammalte abhandlungen zur wissenschaftlichen medtzin. Frankfurt (Germany): Medinger Sohn & Company; 1856.

[8] Ogawa S, Gerlach H, Esposito C, et al. Hypoxia modulates the barrier and coagulant function of cultured bovine endothelium. Increased monolayer permeability and induction of procoagulant properties. J Clin Invest 1990;85:1090–8.

[9] Prins MH, Hirsh J. A critical review of the evidence supporting a relationship between impaired fibrinolytic activity and venous thromboembolism. Arch Intern Med 1991;151:1721–31.

[10] Dittman WA, Majerus PW. Structure and function of thrombomodulin: a natural anticoagulant. Blood 1990;75:329–36.

[11] Esmon CT. The regulation of natural anticoagulant pathways. Science 1987;235:1348–52.

[12] Wiman B, Ljungberg B, Chmielewska J, et al. The role of the fibrinolytic system in deep vein thrombosis. J Lab Clin Med 1985;105:265–70.

[13] Bauer KA, Kass BL, ten Cate H, et al. Factor IX is activated in vivo by the tissue factor mechanism. Blood 1990;76:731–6.

[14] Stewart GJ, Ritchie WG, Lynch PR. Venous endothelial damage produced by massive sticking and emigration of leukocytes. Am J Pathol 1974;74:507–32.

[15] Gordon SG, Franks JJ, Lewis B. Cancer procoagulant A: a factor X activating procoagulant from malignant tissue. Thromb Res 1975;6:127–37.

[16] Bauer KA. The thrombophilias: well defined risk factors with uncertain therapeutic implications. Ann Intern Med 2001;135:367–73.

[17] Perry SL, Ortel TL. Clinical and laboratory evaluation of thrombophilia. Clin Chest Med 2003;24:153–70.

[18] Ridker PM, Miletich JP, Hennekens CH, et al. Ethnic distribution of factor V Leiden in 4047 men and women. Implications for venous thromboembolism screening. JAMA 1997;277:1305–7.

[19] Poort SR, Rosendaal FR, Reitsema PH, et al. A common genetic variation in the 3′ untranslated region of the prothrombin gene associated with elevated plasma prothrombin levels and an increase in venous thrombosis. Blood 1996;88:3698–703.

[20] Arruda VR, Annichiono-Bizzacchi JM, Goncalves MS, et al. Prevalence of the prothrombin gene variant in venous thrombosis and arterial disease. Thromb Haemost 1997;78:1430–3.

[21] Margaglione M, Brancaccio V, Giuliani N, et al. Increased risk for venous thrombosis in carriers of prothrombin gene A20210 gene variant. Ann Intern Med 1998;129:89–93.

[22] Cattaneo M. Hyperhomocyteinemia, atherosclerosis and thrombosis. Thromb Haemost 1999;81:165–76.

[23] Ray JG. Meta-analysis of hyperhomocysteinemia as a risk factor for venous thromboembolic disease. Arch Intern Med 1998;158:2101–6.

[24] van Guldener C, Stehouwer CD. Hyperhomocysteinemia, vascular pathology, and endothelial dysfunction. Semin Thromb Hemost 2000;26:281–9.

[25] Werstuck GH, Lentz SR, Dayal S, et al. Homosysteine-induced endoplasmic reticulum stress

causes dysregulation of the cholesterol and tri-glyceride biosynthetic pathways. J Clin Invest 2001;107:1263–73.

[26] Kluijtmans LA, van den Heuvel LP, Boers GH, et al. Molecular genetic analysis in mild hyperhomocyteinemia: a common mutation in the methylenetetrahydofolate reductase gene is a genetic risk factor for cardiovascular disease. Am J Hum Genet 1996;58: 35–41.

[27] Ma J, Stampfer MJ, Hennekens CH, et al. Methylenetetrahydrofolate reductase polymorphism, plasma folate, homocysteine, and risk of myocardial infarction in US physicians. Circulation 1996;94:2410–6.

[28] O'Donnell T, Abbott W, Athanasoulis C, et al. Diagnosis of deep venous thrombosis in the outpatient by venography. Surg Gynecol Obstet 1980;150: 69–74.

[29] Haeger K. Problems of acute deep venous thrombosis, I. The interpretation of signs and symptoms. Angiology 1969;20:219–23.

[30] Molloy W, English J, O'Dwyer R, et al. Clinical findings in the diagnosis of proximal deep venous thrombosis. Ir Med J 1982;75:119–20.

[31] Wells PS, Hirsh J, Anderson DR, et al. Accuracy of clinical assessment of deep vein thrombosis. Lancet 1995;345:1326–30.

[32] Wells PS, Anderson DR, Bormanis J, et al. Value of assessment of pretest probability of DVT in clinical management. Lancet 1997;300:795–8.

[33] Morpurgo M, Schmid C, Mandelli V. Factors influencing the clinical diagnosis of pulmonary embolism: analysis of 229 postmortem cases. Int J Cardiol 1998;65(Suppl I):S79–82.

[34] Stein PD, Beemath A, Matta F, et al. Clinical characteristics of patients with acute pulmonary embolism: data from PIOPED II. Am J Med 2007;120:871–9.

[35] Wells PS, Ginsberg JS, Anderson DR, et al. Use of a clinical model for safe management of patients with suspected pulmonary embolism. Ann Intern Med 1998;129:997–1005.

[36] Wells P, Anderson D, Rodger M, et al. Derivation of a simple clinical model to categorize patients with a probability of pulmonary embolism: increasing the models utility with the SimpliRED D-dimer. Thromb Haemost 2000;83:416–20.

[37] The PIOPED Investigators. Value of the ventilation/perfusion scan in acute pulmonary embolism: results of the prospective investigation of pulmonary embolism diagnosis (PIOPED). JAMA 1990;263(20): 2753–9.

[38] Chunilal S, Eikelboom J, Attia J, et al. Does this patient have pulmonary embolism? JAMA 2003; 290:2849–58.

[39] Rabinov K, Paulin S. Roentegen diagnosis of venous thrombosis in the leg. Arch Surg 1972;104: 134–44.

[40] Wells PS, Hirsh J, Anderson DR, et al. Comparison of the accuracy of impedance plethysmography and compression ultrasonography in outpatients with clinically suspected deep vein thrombosis. A two center paired design prospective trial. Thromb Haemost 1995;74:1423–7.

[41] Birdwell BG, Raskob GE, Whitsett TL, et al. The clinical validity of normal compression ultrasonography in outpatients suspected of having deep venous thrombosis. Ann Intern Med 1998;128:1–7.

[42] Rose SC, Zwiebel WJ, Nelson BD, et al. Symptomatic lower extremity deep venous thrombosis: accuracy, limitations, and role of color duplex flow imaging in diagnosis. Radiology 1990;175: 639–44.

[43] Stein PD, Hull RD, Pineo G. Strategy that includes serial noninvasive leg tests for diagnosis of thromboembolic disease in patients with suspected acute pulmonary embolism based on data from PIOPED. Prospective investigation of pulmonary embolism diagnosis. Arch Intern Med 1995;155:2101–4.

[44] Morgenthaler TI, Ryu JH. Clinical characteristics of fatal pulmonary embolism in a referral hospital. Mayo Clin Proc 1995;70:417–24.

[45] Stein PD, Hull RD, Pineo GF. The role of newer diagnostic techniques in the diagnosis of pulmonary embolism. Curr Opin Pulm Med 1999;5:212–5.

[46] van Strijen MJ, de Monye W, Schiereck J, et al. Single detector helical computed tomography as the primary diagnostic test in suspected pulmonary embolism: a multicenter clinical management study of 510 patients. Ann Intern Med 2003;138: 307–14.

[47] Quiroz R, Kucher N, Zou KH, et al. Clinical validity of a negative computed tomography scan in patients with suspected pulmonary embolism: a systematic review. JAMA 2005;293:2012–7.

[48] Storto ML, DiCredico A, Guido F, et al. Incidental detection of pulmonary emboli on routine MDCT of the chest. AJR Am J Roentgenol 2005;184:264–7.

[49] Stein PD, Fowler SE, Goodman LR, et al. Multidetector computed tomography for acute pulmonary embolism. N Engl J Med 2006;354:2317–27.

[50] Schoepf UJ. Diagnosing pulmonary embolism: time to rewrite the textbooks. Int J Cardiovasc Imaging 2005;21:155–63.

[51] Schoepf UJ, Holzknecht N, Helmberger TK, et al. Subsegmental pulmonary emboli: improved detection with thin-collimation multi-detector row spiral CT. Radiology 2002;222:483–90.

[52] Brunot S, Corneloup O, Latrabe V, et al. Reproducibility of multi-detector spiral computed tomography in detection of sub-segmental acute pulmonary embolism. Eur Radiol 2005;15:2057–63.

[53] Wood KE. The presence of shock defines the threshold to initiate thrombolytic therapy in patients with pulmonary embolism. Intensive Care Med 2002;28: 1537–46.

[54] Pengo V, Lensing AW, Prins MH, et al. Incidence of chronic thromboembolic pulmonary hypertension

after pulmonary embolism. N Engl J Med 2004;350: 2257–64.

[55] Becattini C, Agnelli G, Pesavento R, et al. Incidence of chronic thromboembolic pulmonary hypertension after a first episode of pulmonary embolism. Chest 2006;130:172–5.

[56] Pedersen MR, Fisher MT, van Beek EJ. MR imaging of the pulmonary vasculature—an update. Eur Radiol 2006;16:1374–86.

[57] Oudkerk M, van Beek EJ, Wielopolski P, et al. Comparison of contrast-enhanced magnetic resonance angiography and conventional pulmonary angiography for the diagnosis of pulmonary embolism: a prospective study. Lancet 2002;359:1643–7.

[58] Meaney JF, Weg JG, Chenevert TL, et al. Diagnosis of pulmonary embolism with magnetic resonance angiography. N Engl J Med 1997;336:1422–7.

[59] Gupta A, Frazer CK, Ferguson JM, et al. Acute pulmonary embolism: diagnosis with MR angiography. Radiology 1999;210:353–9.

[60] Kluge A, Luboldt W, Bachmann G. Acute pulmonary embolism to the subsegmental level: diagnostic accuracy of three MRI techniques compared with 16-MDCT. AJR Am J Roentgenol 2006;187: W7–14.

[61] Kluge A, Muller C, Hansel J, et al. Real-time MR with TrueFISP for the detection of acute pulmonary embolism: initial clinical experience. Eur Radiol 2004;14:709–18.

[62] Clemens S, Leeper KV. Newer modalities for detection of pulmonary emboli. Am J Med 2007;120:S2–12.

[63] Kanal E, Borgstede JP, Barkovich AJ, American College of Radiology, et al. ACR white paper of magnetic resonance (MR) safety: combined papers of 2002 and 2004 [ACR Practice Guidelines and Clinical Standards]. Reston (VA): American College of Radiology; 2004. p. 1005–30.

[64] Niendorf HP, Haustein J, Cornelius I, et al. Safety of gadolinium-DTPA: extended clinical experience. Magn Reson Med 1991;22:222–8.

[65] US Food and Drug Administration, Center for Drug Evaluation and Research. Gadolinium-based contrast agents for magnetic resonance imaging scans [FDA Information for Healthcare Professionals]. Rockville (MD): US Food and Drug Administration; 2006 June; updated December 2006.

[66] Stein PD, Athanasoulis C, Alavi A, et al. Complications and validity of pulmonary angiography in acute pulmonary embolism. Circulation 1992;85(2): 462–8.

[67] The Task Force on Pulmonary Embolism, European Society of Cardiology. Guidelines on the diagnosis and management of acute pulmonary embolism. Eur Heart J 2000;21:1301–36.

[68] Stein PD, Hull RD, Patel KC, et al. D-dimer for the exclusion of acute venous thrombosis and pulmonary embolism: a systematic review. Ann Intern Med 2004;140:589–602.

[69] Bounameaux H, Cirafici P, de Moerloose P, et al. Measurement of D-dimer in plasma as diagnostic aid in suspected pulmonary embolism. Lancet 1991;337:196–200.

[70] Becker DM, Philbrick JT, Bachhuber TL, et al. D-dimer testing and acute venous thromboembolism. A shortcut to accurate diagnosis? Arch Intern Med 1996;156:939–46.

[71] Brotman DJ, Segal JB, Jani JT, et al. Limitations of D-dimer testing in unselected inpatients with suspected venous thromboembolism. Am J Med 2003; 114:276–82.

[72] Perrier A, Bounameaux H, Morabia A, et al. Diagnosis of pulmonary embolism by a decision analysis-based strategy including clinical probability, D-dimer levels, and ultrasonography: a management study. Arch Intern Med 1996;156:531–6.

[73] Tapson VF, Carroll BA, Davidson BL, et al. American Thoracic Society. Clinical practice guideline: the diagnostic approach to acute venous thromboembolism. Am J Respir Crit Care Med 1999;160: 1043–66.

[74] Perrier A, Roy PM, Sanchez O, et al. Multidetector-row computed tomography in suspected pulmonary embolism. N Engl J Med 2005;352: 1760–8.

ELSEVIER
SAUNDERS

Cardiol Clin 26 (2008) 221–234

CARDIOLOGY
CLINICS

Prevention of Venous Thromboembolism in the Geriatric Patient

Daniel J. Brotman, MD[a], Amir K. Jaffer, MD[b],*

[a]Hospitalist Program, The Johns Hopkins Hospital, Park 307, 600 North Wolfe Street, Baltimore, MD 21287, USA
[b]Department of Medicine, Leonard M. Miller School of Medicine, University of Miami, 1120 NW 14th Street, 933 CRB (C216) Miami, FL 33136, USA

Venous thromboembolism (VTE), including deep vein thrombosis (DVT) and pulmonary embolism (PE), is the third leading cause of cardiovascular death after myocardial infarction and stroke in the United States [1]. VTE has an average annual incidence of more than 100 cases per 100,000 person-years [2]. Autopsy studies demonstrate large numbers of silent events [3,4] leading to the widely reported estimates of 2 million DVT cases and up to 200,000 PE deaths annually [5]. Because VTE disproportionately affects the elderly, and in the United States seniors are the fastest growing subset of the population, the number of VTE events and VTE-associated deaths will likely continue to increase [1,6–8].

Epidemiology

The rate ratio for VTE among elderly patients is about 10 to 20 times that of young adults [9], making advanced age an important risk factor for VTE. The mechanisms for the age-dependency of VTE are multiple. With aging, there is an increasing prevalence of chronic conditions that contribute to VTE risk, including malignancy, atherosclerosis, heart failure, and immobility. Compared with younger patients, geriatric patients are more often hospitalized for acute illness and for urgent or elective surgeries. Finally, following acute illness, recovery of mobility may be slower. All of these factors contribute to the high incidence of VTE in the geriatric population. Given these demographic considerations, studies of VTE prevention usually include many elderly patients. Few studies, however, have examined this population specifically. As such, the authors' recommendations pay special attention to VTE prevention in the elderly given their overall increased risk for VTE.

The incidence of VTE is more than 150-fold higher among hospitalized patients compared with community residents [10], and most VTE episodes occur in conjunction with hospitalization or institutionalization [6,11]. Attention to primary VTE prevention should focus on the hospitalized patient. In hospitalized patients, the incidence of venographically detectable DVT is alarmingly high in the absence of thromboprophylaxis, ranging from 10% to 20% in general medical and surgical patients [12,13], to about 60% in those who have undergone joint arthroplasty, and even up to 80% in those with acute spinal cord injury [12,13]. Although many of the venographically apparent VTE found by routine surveillance are distal and small, some are proximal, and sometimes the first presentation of VTE is a fatal PE. Autopsy studies show that VTE remains a leading cause of preventable in-hospital mortality, often undiagnosed before death [14–16]. Thromboprophylactic treatments are effective, but none is foolproof. In general, pharmacologic prophylactic regimens reduce the risk of VTE by about 50% in medical patients [17] and perhaps over 50% in surgical patients [13], but given the high baseline rates of

A version of this article originally appeared in *Clinics in Geriatric Medicine*, volume 22, issue 1.

* Corresponding author.
E-mail address: AJaffer@med.miami.edu (A.K. Jaffer).

thrombosis, breakthrough VTE is still a common problem, even when appropriate antithrombotic regimens are used [12]. All clinicians caring for hospitalized patients should ensure that patients undergo VTE risk factor assessment to help guide appropriate prophylaxis on hospital admission (or following surgery), and an index of suspicion for VTE is maintained, even when a patient is receiving appropriate prophylaxis.

Risk factor assessment and stratification

Three main factors precipitate venous thrombosis: (1) stasis of blood; (2) damage to vascular structures; and (3) disordered hemostasis (transient or chronic hypercoagulability). These factors have been referred to as "Virchow's triad," named for the nineteenth century pathologist, Rudolf Virchow, who showed that pulmonary thrombi generally originated in the deep veins of the systemic circulation and were carried to the pulmonary circulation by venous blood flow (although he was not who originally described the triad that bears his name) [18,19]. Common and important causes of stasis, vascular damage, and altered coagulability in the elderly are shown in Box 1. The more risk factors present, the higher the risk of VTE, and elderly patients are far more likely than younger patients to have multiple risk factors. In general, any immobilized elderly patient admitted to the hospital for a medical condition needs aggressive pharmacologic prophylaxis as outlined in Table 1.

In surgical patients, the overall risk of VTE depends not only on the patient's baseline morbidities and risk factors (obesity, advanced age, prior VTE history, malignancy) but also the nature of the surgery (type of surgery, type and duration of anesthesia) [12,20,21]. Even in the absence of these risk factors, patients over the age of 60 are classified as having a high risk of VTE (rate of proximal DVT up to 8% and clinical PE up to 4% in the absence of prophylaxis) according to a scheme put forth by the American College of Chest Physicians (ACCP) in their most recent evidence-based guidelines published in 2004; (A 2008 update is anticipated). [12]. These numbers are twice as high among patients in the highest risk category, which includes those elderly undergoing cancer surgeries, major joint replacement, or hip fracture repair and those with prior VTE, recent trauma, or spinal cord injury [12]. Virtually all elderly patients are in the high and the highest

---

> **Box 1. Conditions predisposing to VTE in the elderly**
>
> *Stasis of blood*
> Impaired mobility or ambulation
>   (hospitalization or institutionalization)
> Anesthesia
> Valvular incompetence of leg veins
>   (varicose veins)
> Congestive heart failure
>
> *Damage to vessels*
> Surgery
> Falls or fractures
> Vascular catheters
> Prior VTE with or without residual
>   thrombus
> Atherosclerosis
>
> *Altered coagulation*
> Malignancy
> Inflammation (infections, rheumatic
>   disease, tissue trauma)
> Medications (hormone replacement,
>   estrogen receptor modulators,
>   chemotherapy)
> Smoking
> Hereditary or acquired thrombophilia
> Nephrotic syndrome
> Obesity

risk categories and need aggressive pharmacologic prophylaxis as outlined in Table 1.

Prophylaxis in medical patients

The problem of inadequate and omitted prophylaxis for DVT in medical patients has clearly been shown in the DVT Free Registry. This registry was conducted at 183 United States hospitals and included 5451 patients, both inpatients and outpatients, with ultrasound-confirmed DVT. Approximately 2726 (50%) were inpatients (ie, were diagnosed with DVT in the hospital). Of these only 1147 or 42% had received any prophylaxis before diagnosis. The number of medical inpatients overall who received prophylaxis in the 30 days before diagnosis was only 28%; this was lower than the 48% of the surgical patients who received prophylaxis in the 30 days before diagnosis. This suggests that the use of VTE prophylaxis is far from optimal in

Table 1
Recommendations for VTE prophylaxis in the elderly

Condition	Type of prophylaxis	Duration[a]
Medical	UFH 5000 U SC tid or LMWH	Until discharge[b]
General surgery	UFH 5000 U SC tid or LMWH	Until discharge
General surgery for cancer	UFH 5000 U SC tid or LMWH plus IPC or GCS	Up to 28 d
Vascular surgery	UFH 5000 U SC tid or LMWH	Until discharge
Laparoscopic gynecologic surgery >30 min	UFH 5000 U SC tid or LMWH plus IPC or GCS	Until discharge
Major gynecologic surgery	UFH 5000 U SC tid or LMWH plus IPC or GCS	Until discharge
Urologic surgery other than low-risk	UFH 5000 U SC tid or LMWH plus IPC or GCS	Until discharge
Total knee replacement	LMWH or VKA	At least 10 d
Total hip replacement or hip fracture surgery	LMWH or VKA or fondaparinux	28 – 35 d
Neurosurgery		Until discharge
Extracranial	IPC ± GCS ± LMWH or UFH	
Intracranial	IPC ± GCS ± LMWH or UFH	

LMWH dosing: enoxaparin, 40 mg SC daily; dalteparin, 5000 IU SC daily.

Fondaparinux: 2.5 mg SC daily.

Abbreviations: GCS, graded compression stockings; IPC, intermittent pneumatic compression; LMWH, low-molecular-weight heparin; UFH, unfractionated heparin; VKA, vitamin k antagonists (warfarin).

[a] "Until discharge" applies to discharge from the acute care setting. If patients are being discharged to a rehabilitation facility because of functional limitations, then these patients should receive ongoing prophylaxis in the rehabilitation setting.

[b] If patients are >75 years old, have previous history of VTE or active cancer they should receive prophylaxis for 35 days.

hospitalized medical patients at risk for VTE [22]. Despite increasing public awareness of this gap and dissemination of practice guidelines, clinical inertia persists [23].

Mechanical forms of prophylaxis, such as graduated compression stockings, have been evaluated in patients with stroke and myocardial infarction. Intermittent pneumatic compression stockings and venous foot pumps have not been studied in randomized controlled trials in general medical patients. Although there are data supporting the efficacy of these devices in surgical patients (discussed later), the authors discourage their use as solo prophylactic measures in medical patients, except when pharmacologic prophylaxis is contraindicated [12].

The ideal prophylactic agent is one that is cheap, efficacious, has acceptable bleeding risk (and risk of other adverse events), and is well tolerated. Available pharmacologic options for prevention of VTE in medical patients include unfractionated heparin (UFH), low-molecular-weight heparin (LMWH), and the synthetic pentasaccharide fondaparinux. Oral anticoagulants, including vitamin K antagonists (VKAs), have

not been adequately studied in hospitalized medical patients. Because VKAs take a few days to achieve therapeutic anticoagulation, the authors do not recommend using them de novo as VTE prophylaxis. Patients taking oral VKAs in the outpatient setting who have therapeutic international normalized ratios during hospitalization, however, are probably adequately protected from VTE and do not need additional pharmacologic prophylaxis.

Unfractionated heparin

UFH is a heterogenous mixture of repeating polysaccharide chains of varying sizes, averaging about 15 kd. It binds antithrombin III and facilitates antithrombin III–mediated inactivation of factors IIa, Xa, IXa, and XIIa. Of these, IIa and Xa are most responsive to inhibition. Because of its large size, UFH is only partially absorbed from subcutaneous (SC) tissue, and it has a variable anticoagulant response caused by interactions with plasma proteins, macrophages, and endothelial cells [24]. In prophylactic SC doses (5000 units twice or three times daily), monitoring of the activated partial thromboplastin time is not required; in some cases (eg, small frail elderly patients), prophylactic SC doses may prolong the activated partial thromboplastin time slightly. UFH also binds to platelets and platelet factor 4, and may precipitate heparin-induced thrombocytopenia. Three clinical trials [25–27] have compared the efficacy of SC UFH with placebo and found that prophylactic doses of UFH decrease the relative risk of DVT as detected by fibrinogen uptake test by approximately 70% without increasing the risk of bleeding [12]. Additional studies have compared UFH with active treatment (eg, LMWH), as discussed later.

Low-molecular-weight heparins

LMWHs are derived from UFH through a chemical depolymerization or fractionation process. They are about one third the size of UFH, with a molecular weight of approximately 5 kd. These smaller molecules are readily absorbed from the SC tissue, eliciting a more predictable anticoagulant response than UFH. Unlike UFH, LMWHs have only minimal nonspecific binding to plasma proteins, endothelial cells, and monocytes [24], resulting in a predictable dose response, which obviates the need for laboratory monitoring, even when used in full (therapeutic) dosing. The longer plasma half-life of LMWHs compared with UFH allows these drugs to be dosed subcutaneously once or twice daily. LMWHs do not bind platelets as readily as UFH and may carry a lower risk of heparin-induced thrombocytopenia than UFH. Because of their smaller size, LMWHs tend preferentially to inhibit factor Xa, whereas UFH tends to inhibit both factors Xa and IIa equally [24].

LMWHs have also been evaluated in two large placebo-controlled clinical trials for the prevention of VTE in medical patients. In the first trial, called MEDENOX, almost half the patients were older than 75 years (mean age, approximately 73 years). Enoxaparin, 40 mg SC once daily, decreased the rates of VTE by two thirds from 15% to 5% ($P = .0002$) without any increased rate of bleeding or thrombocytopenia compared with placebo [28]. In the second trial (the PREVENT trial), dalteparin, 5000 U, decreased the rate of VTE as detected by compression ultrasound from 5% in the placebo group to 2.8%, a relative risk reduction of 45% ($P = .0015$). Approximately one third of the patients were over the age of 75 (mean age, approximately 68 years). Despite the higher drug-acquisition costs of LMWH,

they may be more cost-effective than UFH for prophylaxis in medical patients because of lower complication rates [29].

Unfractionated heparin versus low-molecular-weight heparin

UFH has been compared with LMWH in six randomized-controlled trials [30–35]. In four out of these six trials the rates of DVT were similar in both groups, but two trials suggested that enoxaparin, 40 mg SC once daily, may be more efficacious than UFH, 5000 U SC every 8 hours [30,33]. Both studies used venography to detect DVT. However, in aggregate, data suggest that LMWH and UFH have similar efficacy in terms of VTE prevention and bleeding complications [36].

New anticoagulants

Fondaparinux is a synthetic analogue of the unique pentasaccharide sequence that mediates the interaction of factor X with antithrombin. It inhibits both free and platelet-bound factor Xa. It binds antithrombin with high affinity, has close to 100% bioavailability, and has a plasma half-life of 17 hours that permits once-daily administration. The drug is excreted unchanged in the urine and is contraindicated in patients with severe renal impairment (ie, creatinine clearance <30 mL/min). It does not bind platelet factor 4 in vitro and should not cause heparin-induced thrombocytopenia. Fondaparinux has been evaluated in medical patients in a randomized-controlled trial called ARTEMIS. In addition, there was a significant reduction in symptomatic VTE with fondaparinux ($P = 0.029$), and there were nonsignificant trends favoring fondaparinux with regard to fatal pulmonary embolism and all-cause mortality [36].

Prophylaxis in surgical patients

In addition to early postoperative ambulation, the authors and others recommend pharmacologic thromboprophylaxis for all but the most minor surgical procedures (eg, cataract surgery, tooth extractions, and other minor outpatient procedures) in the elderly. The choice of prophylaxis, however, remains a subject of continued controversy [37]. Mechanical prophylactic measures include graded compression stockings, intermittent pneumatic compression devices, venous foot pumps, and even inferior vena cava filters. Pharmacologic options include parenteral anticoagulants (heparin products and newer antithrombotic agents, such as fondaparinux), and oral anticoagulants (VKAs, aspirin, and oral direct thrombin inhibitors).

Noninvasive mechanical measures

Mechanical options for VTE prevention (graded compression stockings, intermittent pneumatic compression, and venous foot pumps) are appealing in that they pose no risk of bleeding. This appeal is greatest in surgical patients (as opposed to medical patients), in whom bleeding risk may be substantial. Furthermore, systematic reviews demonstrate that mechanical devices, including intermittent pneumatic compression and graded compression stockings, have efficacy in the prevention of VTE in postoperative patients (general surgery and orthopedic surgery) [37–39], although this finding has not been reproduced in medical patients except with graded compression stockings [40]. Venous foot pumps have been studied to a lesser extent, with mixed findings [41,42]. Finally, dual prophylaxis with pneumatic compression devices plus pharmacologic prophylaxis seems to be better than pharmacologic prophylaxis alone [40,43]. The authors' experience, however, suggests that mechanical devices are often not used optimally: patients and nursing staff may disconnect the devices for comfort, or when the patient goes for diagnostic tests or uses the rest room. The authors question whether mechanical devices in real-world practice have the same efficacy that has been seen in clinical trials. Furthermore, even short periods of limited mobility may lead to delayed recuperation in the elderly, and pneumatic compression devices may discourage ambulation. In contrast, pharmacologic treatments have proven to be highly effective, and compliance with treatment can be readily verified by reviewing medication administration records. Pharmacologic VTE prophylaxis does not limit patient mobility. Given these issues, the authors and others advocate the use of pharmacologic prophylactic measures for most patients, especially the elderly, with or without concurrent use of mechanical devices while the patient is confined to bed [12]. The authors recognize, however, that aggressive mechanical prophylactic measures may be the only suitable option for patients at high risk for bleeding, such as those with recent hemorrhage and those who have undergone surgical procedures associated with an unusually high risk for bleeding complications.

They also recommend ambulation as early as possible after surgery or a medical illness. This is especially important in the elderly, not only to prevent VTE, but also to prevent other complications of immobility, such as decubitus ulcers and loss of functional ability.

Pharmacologic prophylaxis

Aspirin has been evaluated in trials involving various types of surgical patients. In patients with hip fracture, when it was added to routine prophylaxis in the Pulmonary Embolism Prevention Trial it did show a 58% relative risk reduction in PE compared with placebo ($P = .002$) [44]. When used by itself for prophylaxis, however, it has lower efficacy than LMWH [45]. The authors and others do not recommend aspirin for VTE prophylaxis [12]. They do, however, recommend it for prevention of vascular events in the elderly who either have established atherosclerotic disease or are at risk for developing it, provided that there are no contraindications (eg, active peptic ulcer disease).

UFH has been studied extensively in randomized-controlled trials in general surgery patients. Most trials evaluated UFH, 5000 U SC dosed 1 to 2 hours before surgery, and then UFH, 5000 U SC two or three times a day until patients were either ambulating or discharged from the hospital. In a meta-analysis of 46 randomized-controlled trials, UFH decreased the rate of DVT from 22% to 9% (odds ratio, 0.3); symptomatic and fatal PE from 2% to 1.3% and 0.8% to 0.3%, respectively (odds ratio, 0.45); and overall mortality 4.2% to 3.2% (odds ratio, 0.8) [46]. Major bleeding increased a little from 3.8% to 5.9% with UFH (odds ratio, 1.6). The meta-analysis also concluded that UFH three times a day was more efficacious than UFH twice a day without increasing bleeding, but this was based on an indirect comparison [46].

LMWH has also been studied in multiple trials, and has been compared with both placebo and UFH in general surgery patients. Multiple meta-analyses have also been done to evaluate the relative efficacy of UFH versus LMWH, and in general there is little difference in efficacy. One meta-analysis [13] concluded that there was a decreased rate of clinical VTE with LWMH following surgery. This meta-analysis concluded that LMWH dose of <3400 IU daily has comparable efficacy with UFH with less bleeding, whereas doses >3400 IU per day yielded slightly better efficacy but slightly higher bleeding rates [12,13]. In the elderly, given their higher VTE risk, the authors prefer more aggressive prophylaxis and doses equivalent to > 3400 IU/d of LMWH (options in the United States include enoxaparin, 40 mg SC, or dalteparin, 5000 IU SC once daily). The authors also prefer LMWH because of its once-daily dosing and other advantages outlined previously.

In orthopedic patients, LMWH is preferred over UFH mainly because of its improved efficacy and comparable risk of bleeding complications [47–50]. The most commonly prescribed anticoagulant in the United States for prevention of VTE after major joint replacement, however, is the VKA warfarin [51].

VKAs, such as oral warfarin, have been used and studied extensively following orthopedic surgery, but are not generally used following general surgery. Warfarin is a coumarin derivative that exerts its anticoagulant effects by limiting hepatic production of the biologically active vitamin K–dependent clotting factors (factors II, VII, IX, X). Additionally, warfarin interferes with the production of the anticoagulant proteins C and S and can potentially exert a transient pro-coagulant effect following initiation of treatment. In addition, it takes approximately 96 hours to decrease the levels of factor IIa enough to provide a clinical anticoagulant effect, even though depletion of the short-lived factors VII and IX can increase the international normalized ratio in less than 24 hours. The long half-life of warfarin allows surgical hemostasis to develop, and its oral dosing allows it to be continued on discharge. Overall, the VKAs are more effective than placebo or no treatment in reducing DVT in patients with joint replacement (relative risk = 0.56; $P < .01$) [52]. These results were obtained at the cost of a higher rate of wound hematoma (relative risk = 2.9; $P = .03$) [52]. VKAs also seem to be more effective than intermittent pneumatic compression (relative risk = 0.46; $P = .009$) in preventing proximal DVT [52]. In contrast, VKAs were less effective than LMWH in preventing total DVT and proximal DVT (relative risk = 1.51; $P < .001$). There was no significant difference between VKA and LMWH with regards to major hemorrhage [52]. These results suggest that in patients undergoing major orthopedic surgery, VKAs are a little less effective than LMWH, without any significant difference in the bleeding risk except for wound hematomas. Warfarin remains a popular choice among orthopedic surgeons largely based on this reduction in wound hematomas.

It is important to understand the difference in the temporal patterns of clinically symptomatic thromboembolic complications after total hip and total knee arthroplasty, which occur early (median time of diagnosis of VTE is postoperative day 7) after total knee arthroplasty and (median time to diagnosis of VTE is postoperative day 17) after total hip arthroplasty [53]. This suggests that to reduce thromboembolic outcomes further, earlier more intense prophylaxis may be needed for total knee arthroplasty, and more prolonged prophylaxis may be required after total hip arthroplasty. In a case-control study of patients undergoing major joint replacement, warfarin monotherapy initiated postoperatively was strongly associated with early VTE (within the first 5 postoperative days) compared with enoxaparin, 30 mg SC every 12 hours started postoperative day 1 (odds ratio, 11; $P < .0001$) [54]. Even though the ACCP gives warfarin a grade 1A recommendation for prevention of VTE after orthopedic surgery, it is the authors' preference to avoid warfarin monotherapy as VTE prophylaxis after major surgery, especially because the patient is unprotected from thrombosis during the first few days of treatment. In addition, cost-effective analyses [55–57] suggest that enoxaparin is more cost-effective than warfarin for VTE prophylaxis after major joint replacement.

New anticoagulants

Fondaparinux has been studied in four randomized clinical trials involving major knee and hip fracture surgery. A meta-analysis [58] pooled results from these four multicenter, randomized, double-blind trials (N = 7344 and mean age > 65 years) and showed that fondaparinux, SC 2.5 mg once daily starting 6 hours after surgery, was more effective but with more bleeding compared with approved enoxaparin regimens in preventing VTE. The primary efficacy outcome was VTE up to day 11, defined as DVT detected by mandatory bilateral venography or documented symptomatic DVT or PE. The primary safety outcome was major bleeding. Fondaparinux significantly reduced the incidence of VTE by day 11 (182 [6.8%] of 2682 patients) compared with enoxaparin (371 [13.7%] of 2703 patients), with a common odds reduction of 55.2% ($P < .001$); this beneficial effect was consistent across all types of major orthopedic surgery and all subgroups. Although major bleeding occurred more frequently in the fondaparinux-treated group ($P = .008$), the incidence of bleeding resulting in death or re-operation did not differ significantly between groups.

Hip fractures occur predominantly in the elderly and surgery for hip fractures puts patients at high risk for VTE. Of the ACCP recommended agents (fondaparinux, warfarin, LMWH, and low-dose UFH), fondaparinux carries the highest recommendation (1A) and is the only agent that is FDA-approved for VTE prevention after hip fracture surgery. In the PENTHIFRA trial [59] where the mean age of the patients was 77 ± 12, the relative risk reduction compared with enoxaparin, 40 mg SC once daily, was over 50%. The PENTIHIFRA-PLUS trial, which evaluated extended prophylaxis by prolonging prophylaxis for up to 31 days postoperatively, demonstrated a remarkable reduction in VTE relative to nonextended treatment from 35% (77 of 220) to 1.4% (3 of 208), with a relative reduction in risk of 95.9% (95% confidence interval, 87.2%–99.7%; $P < .001$). Similarly, the incidence of symptomatic VTE was significantly lower with fondaparinux (1 of 326; 0.3%) than with placebo (9 of 330; 2.7%). The relative reduction in risk was 88.8% ($P = .02$). There was a trend towards more major bleeding in the fondaparinux group: 2.4% versus 0.6%, $P = 0.06$) [60].

Fondaparinux also has demonstrated efficacy in general surgery patients. The Pentasaccharide in General Surgery Study compared fondaparinux with LMWH in 2927 patients undergoing major abdominal surgery (mean age > 65). The rates of VTE in the fondaparinux and dalteparin groups were 4.6% and 6.1%, respectively ($P = 0.14$). Major bleeding rates were not significantly different at 3.4% and 2.4%, respectively ($P = NS$). For those patients who underwent abdominal cancer surgery (approximately 70% of the overall sample), VTE incidence was significantly lower in fondaparinux recipients compared with dalteparin recipients (4.7% versus 7.7%, $P = .02$).

The clinical studies using fondaparinux demonstrated that selective inhibition of factor Xa is a highly effective approach to the prevention and treatment of venous thromboembolism. This gave further impetus to developing oral direct factor Xa inhibitors for the prevention of VTE. It should, however, be noted that these agents inhibit factor Xa within the assembled prothrombinase complex as well as free factor Xa, while fondaparinux is only able to inhibit the pool of free factor Xa in the blood. The oral direct factor Xa inhibitors that are in clinical development include rivaroxaban (BAY 59-7939), apixaban (BMS), YM150 (Astellas), DU-176b (Daiichi), LY517717 (Lilly), and PRT054021

(Portola). Rivaroxaban (Bay 59-7939) is a nonpeptidic, orally bioavailable, small molecule that directly inhibits factor Xa. It has a rapid onset of action and a half-life of 5–9 hours. Two phase III trials with rivaroxaban have suggested that it may be more effective than enoxaparin in preventing venous thromboembolism (VTE) in patients undergoing major orthopedic surgery. The RECORD-1 and RECORD-2 studies were presented at the American Society of Hematology annual meeting in December, 2007. In both studies, rivaroxaban reduced VTE events to a significantly greater extent than enoxaparin. Bleeding rates were similar between the two drugs. The RECORD-1 and RECORD-2 data complement data from a third study, RECORD-3, which was reported earlier this year and showed similar results. Additionally new oral direct thrombin inhibitors—in the same class as ximelagatran—are in development.

Ximelagatran is an oral direct thrombin inhibitor. It is a prodrug that is rapidly hydrolyzed to melagatran, the active drug that binds thrombin. It is given twice daily in fixed doses. It does not have drug and food interactions like warfarin and is renally cleared. The drug has been shown in phase III trials to be affective for treatment and prevention of a range of venous and arterial thromboembolic disorders [61], and has been shown in orthopedic surgery studies to have comparable safety and efficacy to LMWH when used prophylactically [62–66]. Ximelagatran would have been the first new oral anticoagulant since the introduction of warfarin almost 60 years ago; however, for concerns of hepatotoxicity, the FDA rejected it in 2004. We remain optimistic that new drugs in this class, such as dabigatran become available in the United States, offering fixed-dose oral anticoagulation options for VTE prevention.

Dabigatran etexilate is an oral prodrug that is converted to dabigatran, an oral thrombin inhibitor that has a plasma half-life of 14-17 hours, allowing for once-daily dosing, and is eliminated via the kidneys. The bioavailability of dabigatran etexilate following oral administration is only $\sim$4-5%. The efficacy and safety of dabigatran etexilate has been evaluated in phase II studies in patients undergoing total hip and knee replacement. The RE-MOBILIZE (2600 patients) and RE-MODEL (2000 patients) trials were DVT prophylaxis trials following total knee replacement, while the RE-NOVATE trial (3415 patients) was carried out in patients undergoing total hip replacement. The trials were powered for noninferiority and compared to enoxaparin. The results were recently presented at the International thrombosis and Hemostasis (ISTH) meeting. The RE-NOVATE trial [67] demonstrated that oral dabigatran etexilate once daily, administered for an average of 33 days, was as effective as enoxaparin, also administered for an average of 33 days, in preventing venous thromboembolism (VTE) and all-cause mortality after total hip replacement surgery. For the primary efficacy endpoint of total VTE and death from all-causes, results were similar between all groups, occurring in 8.6%, 6.0%, and 6.7% of patients assigned to 150 mg or 220 mg dabigatran etexilate once daily or 40 mg enoxaparin once daily, respectively. Safety was evaluated for 3463 patients receiving study treatment and no significant difference in major bleeding rates was observed between the groups (1.3%, 2.0%, and 1.6% respectively). The incidence of liver enzyme elevations and acute coronary events during the treatment or during the follow-up period did not differ significantly between the groups. There was a low rate of bleeding associated with dabigatran etexilate with major bleeding rates comparable to enoxaparin. Also presented at ISTH was a pre-specified pooled analysis of major VTE and VTE related death after major orthopaedic surgery across more than 8000 randomized patients that were included in the phase III primary VTE prevention programme (RE-MODELTM, RE-MOBILIZETM and RE-NOVATE studies). The pooled analysis concluded that dabigatran etexilate was efficacious and comparable to enoxaparin in the prevention of major VTE and VTE related mortality after both knee and hip replacement. Major VTE rates for both doses of dabigatran etexilate were similar to enoxaparin – major VTE and VTE related death occurred in 3.8%, of the 150 mg dabigatran etexilate group and 3.0% of the 220 mg dabigatran etexilate group versus 3.3% of the enoxaparin group. Major bleeding events were infrequent, and were similar across all treatment groups (1.1%, 1.4% and 1.4% respectively). As part of the safety analysis, patients were frequently monitored for liver enzyme elevations. Those patients with elevations $> 3 \times$ ULN were infrequent and comparable across all treatment groups. In addition, treatment emergent acute coronary syndromes (ACS) events were infrequent and comparable across treatment groups [68].

Timing of prophylaxis in surgical patients

The optimal timing of pharmacologic prophylaxis remains controversial. In Europe, the practice pattern is to initiate LMWH prophylaxis about 10–12 hours before joint replacement surgery, whereas in the United States the LMWH is usually initiated about 12 to 24 hours after surgery. A systematic review that compared LMWH with VKA observed large risk reduction when the LMWH was dosed at half of the usual dose 2 hours before the procedure or 6 to 8 hours after the surgery. In the studies in which LMWH was started 12 to 24 hours before or after surgery, however, this efficacy advantage was not observed. In addition, starting LMWH close to the time of surgery was also associated with an increased risk of major bleeding [69]. Overall, it seems that early initiation of LMWH prophylaxis may increase efficacy at the expense of bleeding risk.

Special considerations with neuroaxial anesthesia

Neuroaxial anesthesia when used concomitantly with anticoagulation increases the risk of epidural hematomas and subsequent spinal cord injury. Detailed guidelines for the use of anticoagulation in the presence of neuroaxial blockade have been developed by the American Society of Regional Anesthesia and Pain medicine [70]. Specific recommendations include waiting 24 hours after a full dose of LMWH, 12 hours after a prophylactic dose of LMWH, and at least 2 hours after removal of the epidural catheter to dose LMWH.

Special considerations in the elderly

Elderly patients are at higher risk than younger patients for bleeding complications during inpatient and outpatient anticoagulant treatment, and may have concomitant conditions that place them at risk for bleeding complications, such as diabetes, renal impairment, and cardiovascular disease [71–74]. This should in no way preclude the use of aggressive pharmacologic VTE prophylaxis in elderly persons. To the contrary, the authors advocate careful but aggressive pharmacologic VTE prophylaxis in the elderly based on their particularly high risk for VTE.

Special emphasis must be placed on the patient's creatinine clearance and age because both of these affect the drug elimination and pharmacokinetics of anticoagulants, such as fondaparinux and LMWH. This means avoiding fixed-dose fondaparinux in patients with creatinine clearances <30 mL/min, creatinine >2 mg/dL, and in patients weighing less than 50 kg because patients with these characteristics were excluded from the fondaparinux VTE prevention trials. Prophylactic doses of LMWH can be used in patients with creatinine clearances of <30 mL/min but the enoxaparin dose should be reduced to 30 mg SC daily. Dalteparin does not require dose adjustment in patients with renal insufficiency based on current recommendations. Caution is also advised when using fixed-dose LMWH in frail elderly patients weighing less than 45 kg.

Although the elderly have higher bleeding risk when treated with anticoagulants, they also are at much higher risk for VTE. Furthermore, if VTE occurs, the intensity of anticoagulation is much higher than that used for prophylaxis, and the elderly are at particularly high risk for bleeding with full-dose anticoagulants. The authors suggest that pharmacologic VTE prophylaxis be used in all hospitalized elderly patients and that only active bleeding, coagulopathy, or an indwelling epidural catheter should prevent its use, or planned invasive procedure justify its temporary discontinuation.

Inferior vena cava filters

The only purpose of inferior vena cava filters is to prevent thrombi in the leg veins from migrating to the pulmonary circulation. They do not prevent the formation of DVT, and may precipitate lower-extremity thrombosis by impairing venous return from the legs [75]. Furthermore, placement of filters is invasive and requires exposure to intravenous contrast, which may be risky in patients with chronic renal impairment. Finally, there is limited evidence to support the notion that using filters in conjunction with anticoagulation improves clinical outcomes over anticoagulation alone [76], and there may be substantial periprocedural mortality [77]. One population-based study suggested that elderly patients who receive inferior vena cava filters have a particularly high mortality: 16% during hospitalization and 48% at 2 years [78], suggesting that requiring an inferior vena cava filter is a poor prognostic sign in the elderly. Given limited data supporting their use, the authors do not recommend prophylactic

placement of inferior vena cava filters except when full-dose anticoagulation is contraindicated (eg, major hemorrhage, major surgery planned, and recent neurosurgery). If contraindications to anticoagulation are expected to be transient (eg, trauma patients), retrievable filters may be appropriate [79]; however, retrieval of the filter subjects the patient to a second invasive procedure, and the devices themselves are expensive.

Duration of prophylaxis

The risk of VTE does not end when the patient is discharged from the hospital. Patients remain at substantial risk for VTE for a few weeks following discharge, and small thrombi that developed while the patient was hospitalized (but remained subclinical) may propagate if anticoagulation is terminated at the time of hospital discharge. Despite the intuitive appeal of continuing anticoagulation following hospital discharge, this practice is rarely used except during inpatient rehabilitation, and occasionally in the outpatient setting following orthopedic surgery. With few exceptions, there is a lack of demonstrated safety and efficacy of this practice, and there are practical concerns surrounding the implementation of extended VTE prophylaxis following hospital discharge. Specifically, outpatient heparin or LMWH injections may not always be welcomed by patients and caregivers because of out-of-pocket expenses, especially for those without insurance coverage for prescriptions.

Medical patients

The safety and efficacy of postdischarge prophylaxis in medical patients has not yet been defined. To begin to fill this gap, the Extended Clinical Prophylaxis in Acutely Ill Medical Patients (EXCLAIM) trial was conducted to compare extended-duration LMWH prophylaxis with a standard LMWH prophylaxis regimen in acutely ill medical patients using a prospective, multicenter, randomized, double-blind, placebo-controlled design [80]. Patients were eligible for enrollment if they were aged 40 years or older and had recent immobilization (3 days), a predefined acute medical illness, and either level 1 mobility (total bed rest or sedentary state) or level 2 mobility (level 1 with bathroom privileges). The predefined acute medical illnesses consisted of New York Heart Association class III/IV heart failure, acute respiratory insufficiency, or other acute medical conditions, including post-acute ischemic stroke, acute infection without septic shock, and active cancer. All patients received open-label enoxaparin 40 mg subcutaneously once daily for 10 ± 4 days, after which they were randomized to either enoxaparin 40 mg subcutaneously once daily or placebo for an additional 28 ± 4 days.

The primary efficacy end point was the incidence of VTE events, defined as asymptomatic DVT documented by mandatory ultrasonography at the end of the double-blind treatment period (28 ± 4 days) or as symptomatic DVT, symptomatic PE, or fatal PE at any time during the double-blind period. Symptomatic DVT was confirmed by objective tests; PE was confirmed by ventilation-perfusion scan, computed tomography, angiography, or autopsy. Secondary efficacy end points were mortality at the end of the double-blind period, at 3 months, and at 6 months, as well as the incidence of VTE at 3 months. The primary safety outcome measure was the incidence of major hemorrhage during the double-blind period; secondary safety measures were rates of major and minor hemorrhage, minor hemorrhage, HIT, and serious adverse events.

After approximately half of the patients were enrolled, a planned and blinded interim analysis for futility concluded that the study was unlikely to show a statistically significant advantage of enoxaparin over placebo. The trial's steering committee followed the suggestion of its data safety monitoring board to redefine the inclusion criteria to refocus enrollment on patients with a high risk of VTE. A blinded analysis was performed to identify this subgroup. The resulting amended inclusion criteria were the same as above except that level 2 mobility had to be accompanied by at least one of three additional highrisk criteria: (1) age greater than 75 years, (2) history of VTE, or (3) diagnosis of cancer.

The trial's main exclusion criteria were evidence of active bleeding, a contraindication to anticoagulation, receipt of prophylactic LMWH or UFH more than 72 hours prior to enrollment, treatment with an oral anticoagulant within 72 hours of enrollment, major surgery within the prior 3 months, cerebral stroke with bleeding, and persistent renal failure (creatinine clearance < 30 mL/min). The amended study population included 5,105 patients, 5,049 of whom received open-label enoxaparin. Of this group, 2,013 were randomized to active extended prophylaxis with enoxparain and 2,027 to placebo. Baseline characteristics, including level of mobility, were similar between the two groups. VTE events occurred at a statistically significantly higher rate in the placebo arm than in the extended-duration enoxaparin arm, as did asymptomatic proximal DVT and symptomatic VTE. The efficacy of extended prophylaxis with enoxaparin was enduring, as the cumulative incidence of VTE events at day 90 was significantly lower in enoxaparin recipients than in placebo recipients (3.0% vs 5.2%; relative reduction of 42%; $P = .0115$). There was no difference in all-cause mortality at 6 months between the enoxaparin and placebo groups (10.1% vs 8.9%, respectively; $P = .179$). Major hemorrhage was significantly more frequent in the enoxaparin arm, occurring in 0.60% of enoxaparin recipients compared with 0.15% of placebo recipients ($P = .019$). Minor bleeding was also more common with enoxaparin (5.20% vs 3.70%; $P = .024$). Therefore, it is reasonable to consider extended prophylaxis for hospitalized medical patients after identifying these patients' risk factors. In keeping with the trial's amended inclusion criteria, patients older than age 75 and those with cancer or prior VTE should receive special consideration for extended prophylaxis. If a patient is discharged to a rehabilitation facility, the authors recommend continuation of prophylaxis until discharge from this facility. For patients who are discharged to nursing homes (and will remain in a facility indefinitely), it is not recommended to continue VTE prophylaxis beyond the first 2 weeks of institutionalization unless patients meet the criteria outlined above in the Exclaim trial.

Surgical patients

Following hip arthroplasty, extended prophylaxis with oral VKA for 4 weeks following hospital discharge substantially reduces the risk of VTE with low bleeding risk [81]. Evidence also supports extended prophylaxis with LMWH following hip arthroplasty and hip fracture for 4 to 5 weeks [60,82]. There is no proven benefit, however, of extended VTE prophylaxis following knee replacement [82–85]. Postdischarge prophylaxis following other types of surgery has not been well studied except after abdominopelvic cancer surgery. The evidence suggests that patients with cancer undergoing major pelvic or abdominal surgery should receive extended prophylaxis with a LMWH for up to 28 days postoperatively; extended prophylaxis may reduce the risk of postoperative thrombosis by 60% compared with standard prophylaxis that is stopped after 6 to 10 days of treatment, with acceptable bleeding risk [84].

The authors recommend continuation of prophylactic anticoagulants until hospital discharge for surgeries other than hip replacement and abdominopelvic cancer surgery. If individual medical or surgical patients have significant risk factors, such as previous VTE, morbid obesity, cancer, and an acute medical illness, however, and the patient is being discharged to a rehabilitation facility, the authors recommend continuation of VTE prophylaxis throughout the rehabilitation stay.

Summary

Elderly patients who are immobilized because of an acute medical illness or surgery have a very high risk of developing VTE. Aggressive pharmacologic prophylaxis is necessary and should be initiated either at admission for a medical condition or shortly after surgery. Aggressive prophylaxis may result in fewer patients developing VTE in the hospital and ultimately lead to fewer patients requiring full-dose anticoagulation for VTE. Mechanical prophylaxis can be used as an adjunct to an anticoagulant-based regimen but should only be used as primary prophylaxis when there is a contraindication to pharmacologic prophylaxis, such as active bleeding. Recommendations regarding type and duration of prophylaxis for the various conditions are summarized in Table 1. Finally, the authors recommend the clinician carefully evaluate the elderly patient's creatinine clearance and weight before prescribing anticoagulants, particularly when using fixed dosing regimens.

References

[1] National Center for Injury Prevention and ControlInjury Fact Book 2001–2002. Atlanta (GA): Centers for Disease Control and Prevention; 2001.

[2] Silverstein MD, Heit JA, Mohr DN, et al. Trends in the incidence of deep vein thrombosis and pulmonary embolism: a 25-year population-based study. Arch Intern Med 1998;158:585–93.

[3] Havig O. Deep vein thrombosis and pulmonary embolism: an autopsy study with multiple regression analysis of possible risk factors. Acta Chir Scand Suppl 1977;478:1–20.

[4] Lindblad B, Eriksson A, Bergqvist D. Autopsy-verified pulmonary embolism in a surgical department: analysis of the period from 1951 to 1988. Br J Surg 1991;78:849–52.

[5] Hirsh J, Hoak J. Management of deep vein thrombosis and pulmonary embolism: a statement for healthcare professionals. Council on Thrombosis (in consultation with the Council on Cardiovascular Radiology), American Heart Association. Circulation 1996;93:2212–45.

[6] Heit JA, Melton LJ 3rd, Lohse CM, et al. Incidence of venous thromboembolism in hospitalized patients vs community residents. Mayo Clin Proc 2001;76: 1102–10.

[7] Anderson FA Jr, Wheeler HB, Goldberg RJ, et al. A population-based perspective of the hospital incidence and case-fatality rates of deep vein thrombosis and pulmonary embolism. The Worcester DVT Study. Arch Intern Med 1991;151:933–8.

[8] Graves EJ, Owings MF. 1996 summary: national hospital discharge survey. National Center for Health Statistics. Vital Health Stat Series No. 301. 1998.

[9] Stein PD, Hull RD, Kayali F, et al. Venous thromboembolism according to age: the impact of an aging population. Arch Intern Med 2004;164:2260–5.

[10] Kniffin WD Jr, Baron JA, Barret J, et al. The epidemiology of diagnosed pulmonary embolism and deep venous thrombosis in the elderly. Arch Intern Med 1994;154:861–6.

[11] Heit JA, O'Fallon WM, Petterson TM, et al. Relative impact of risk factors for deep vein thrombosis and pulmonary embolism: a population-based study. Arch Intern Med 2002;162:1245–8.

[12] Geerts WH, Pineo GF, Heit JA, et al. Prevention of venous thromboembolism: the Seventh ACCP Conference on Antithrombotic and Thrombolytic Therapy. Chest 2004;126(3 Suppl):338S–400S.

[13] Mismetti P, et al. Meta-analysis of low molecular weight heparin in the prevention of venous thromboembolism in general surgery. Br J Surg 2001;88:913–30.

[14] Morgenthaler TI, Ryu JH. Clinical characteristics of fatal pulmonary embolism in a referral hospital. Mayo Clin Proc 1995;70:417–24.

[15] Attems J, et al. The clinical diagnostic accuracy rate regarding the immediate cause of death in a hospitalized geriatric population; an autopsy study of 1594 patients. Wien Med Wochenschr 2004;154:159–62.

[16] Morpurgo M, Schmid C. The spectrum of pulmonary embolism: clinicopathologic correlations. Chest 1995;107(1 Suppl):18S–20S.

[17] Leizorovicz A, et al. Randomized, placebo-controlled trial of dalteparin for the prevention of venous thromboembolism in acutely ill medical patients. Circulation 2004;110:874–9.

[18] Brotman DJ, et al. Virchow's triad revisited. South Med J 2004;97:213–4.

[19] Virchow RGesammelte abhandlungen zur wissenschaftlichen medicin [Thrombosis and emboli]. Canton (MA): Science History Publications/USA; 1998 [Matzdorff AC, Bell WR, Trans.; original text published 1856.].

[20] Jaffer AK, Barsoum W, Krebs V, et al. Duration of anesthesia and venous thromboembolism following hip and knee arthroplasty. Mayo Clinic Proceedings 2005;80:732–8.

[21] Edmonds MJ, Crichton TJ, Runciman WB, et al. Evidence-based risk factors for postoperative deep vein thrombosis. ANZ J Surg 2004;74:1082–97.

[22] Goldhaber SZ, Tapson VF. A prospective registry of 5,451 patients with ultrasound-confirmed deep vein thrombosis. Am J Cardiol 2004;93:259–62.

[23] Kahn SR, et al. Multicenter evaluation of the use of venous thromboembolism prophylaxis in acutely ill medical patients in Canada. Thromb Res 2007; 119(2):145–55.

[24] Hirsh J, Raschke R. Heparin and low-molecular-weight heparin: the Seventh ACCP Conference on Antithrombotic and Thrombolytic Therapy. Chest 2004;126(3 Suppl):188S–203S.

[25] Cade JF, Andrews JT, Stubbs AE. Comparison of sodium and calcium heparin in prevention of venous thromboembolism. Aust N Z J Med 1982;12:501–4.

[26] Gallus AS, Hirsh J, Tuttle RJ, et al. Small subcutaneous doses of heparin in prevention of venous thrombosis. N Engl J Med 1973;288:545–51.

[27] Belch JJ, Lowe GD, Ward AG, et al. Prevention of deep vein thrombosis in medical patients by low-dose heparin. Scott Med J 1981;26:115–7.

[28] Samama MM, Cohen AT, Darmon JY, et al. A comparison of enoxaparin with placebo for the prevention of venous thromboembolism in acutely ill medical patients. Prophylaxis in Medical Patients with Enoxaparin Study Group. N Engl J Med 1999;341:793–800.

[29] McGarry LJ, Thompson D, Weinstein MC, et al. Cost effectiveness of thromboprophylaxis with a low-molecular-weight heparin versus unfractionated heparin in acutely ill medical inpatients. Am J Manag Care 2004;10:632–42.

[30] Hillbom M, Erila T, Sotaniemi K, et al. Enoxaparin vs heparin for prevention of deep-vein thrombosis in acute ischaemic stroke: a randomized, double-blind study. Acta Neurol Scand 2002;106:84–92.

[31] Kleber FX, Witt C, Vogel G, et al. Randomized comparison of enoxaparin with unfractionated heparin for the prevention of venous thromboembolism in medical patients with heart failure or severe respiratory disease. Am Heart J 2003;145:614–21.

[32] Bergmann JF, Neuhart E. A multicenter randomized double-blind study of enoxaparin compared with unfractionated heparin in the prevention of venous thromboembolic disease in elderly inpatients bedridden for an acute medical illness. The Enoxaparin in Medicine Study Group. Thromb Haemost 1996;76:529–34.

[33] Harenberg J, SU, Flosbach CW, et al. Enoxaparin is superior to unfractionated heparin in the prevention of thromboembolic events in medical inpatients at increased thromboembolic risk. Blood 1999;94:399a.

[34] Lechler E, Schramm W, Flosbach CW. The venous thrombotic risk in non-surgical patients: epidemiological data and efficacy/safety profile of a low-molecular-weight heparin (enoxaparin). The Prime Study Group. Haemostasis 1996;26(Suppl 2):49–56.

[35] Harenberg J, Roebruck P, Heene DL. Subcutaneous low-molecular-weight heparin versus standard heparin and the prevention of thromboembolism in medical inpatients. The Heparin Study in Internal Medicine Group. Haemostasis 1996;26:127–39.

[36] Cohen AT, et al. Efficacy and safety of fondaparinux for the prevention of venous thromboembolism in older acute medical patients: randomised placebo controlled trial. BMJ 2006;332(7537):325–9.

[37] Freedman KB, Brookenthal KR, Fitzgerald RH Jr, et al. A meta-analysis of thromboembolic prophylaxis following elective total hip arthroplasty. J Bone Joint Surg Am 2000;82:929–38.

[38] Amaragiri SV, Lees TA. Elastic compression stockings for prevention of deep vein thrombosis. Cochrane Database Syst Rev 2000;3:CD001484.

[39] Handoll HH, Farrar MJ, McBirnie J, et al. Heparin, low molecular weight heparin and physical methods for preventing deep vein thrombosis and pulmonary embolism following surgery for hip fractures. Cochrane Database Syst Rev 2002;4:CD000305.

[40] Mazzone C, Chiodo GF, Sandercock P, et al. Physical methods for preventing deep vein thrombosis in stroke. Cochrane Database Syst Rev 2004;4: CD001922.

[41] Santori FS, Vitullo A, Stopponi M, et al. Prophylaxis against deep-vein thrombosis in total hip replacement: comparison of heparin and foot impulse pump. J Bone Joint Surg Br 1994;76:579–83.

[42] Norgren L, Toksvig-Larsen S, Magyar G, et al. Prevention of deep vein thrombosis in knee arthroplasty: preliminary results from a randomized controlled study of low molecular weight heparin vs foot pump compression. Int Angiol 1998;17:93–6.

[43] Wille-Jorgensen P, Rasmussen MS, Andersen BR, et al. Heparins and mechanical methods for thromboprophylaxis in colorectal surgery. Cochrane Database Syst Rev 2003;4:CD001217.

[44] Prevention of pulmonary embolism and deep vein thrombosis with low dose aspirin. Pulmonary Embolism Prevention (PEP) trial. Lancet 2000;355: 1295–302.

[45] Gent M, Hirsh J, Ginsberg JS, et al. Low-molecular-weight heparinoid orgaran is more effective than aspirin in the prevention of venous thromboembolism after surgery for hip fracture. Circulation 1996;93: 80–4.

[46] Collins R, Scrimgeour A, Yusuf S, et al. Reduction in fatal pulmonary embolism and venous thrombosis by perioperative administration of subcutaneous heparin: overview of results of randomized trials in general, orthopedic, and urologic surgery. N Engl J Med 1988;318:1162–73.

[47] Colwell CW Jr. Recent advances in the use of low molecular weight heparins as prophylaxis for deep vein thrombosis. Orthopedics 1994;17:5–7.

[48] Colwell CW Jr, Spiro TE, Trowbridge AA, et al. Use of enoxaparin, a low-molecular-weight heparin, and unfractionated heparin for the prevention of deep venous thrombosis after elective hip replacement: a clinical trial comparing efficacy and safety. Enoxaparin Clinical Trial Group. J Bone Joint Surg Am 1994;76:3–14.

[49] Planes A, Vochelle N, Mazas F, et al. Prevention of postoperative venous thrombosis: a randomized trial comparing unfractionated heparin with low molecular weight heparin in patients undergoing total hip replacement. Thromb Haemost 1988;60:407–10.

[50] Prevention of deep vein thrombosis with low molecular-weight heparin in patients undergoing total hip replacement: a randomized trial. The German Hip Arthroplasty Trial (GHAT) Group. Arch Orthop Trauma Surg 1992;111:110–20.

[51] Mesko JW, Brand RA, Iorio R, et al. Venous thromboembolic disease management patterns in total hip arthroplasty and total knee arthroplasty patients: a survey of the AAHKS membership. J Arthroplasty 2001;16:679–88.

[52] Mismetti P, Laporte S, Zufferey P, et al. Prevention of venous thromboembolism in orthopedic surgery with vitamin K antagonists: a meta-analysis. J Thromb Haemost 2004;2:1058–70.

[53] White RH, Romano PS, Zhou H, et al. Incidence and time course of thromboembolic outcomes following total hip or knee arthroplasty. Arch Intern Med 1998;158:1525–31.

[54] Brotman DJ, Jaffer AK, Hurbanek JG, et al. Warfarin prophylaxis and venous thromboembolism in the first 5 days following hip and knee arthroplasty. Thromb Haemost 2004;92:1012–7.

[55] Botteman MF, Caprini J, Stephens JM, et al. Results of an economic model to assess the cost-effectiveness of enoxaparin, a low-molecular-weight heparin, versus warfarin for the prophylaxis of deep vein thrombosis and associated long-term complications in total hip replacement surgery in the United States. Clin Ther 2002;24:1960–86 [discussion; 1938].

[56] Hawkins DW, Langley PC, Krueger KP. A pharmacoeconomic assessment of enoxaparin and warfarin as prophylaxis for deep vein thrombosis in patients undergoing knee replacement surgery. Clin Ther 1998;20:182–95.

[57] Garcia-Zozaya I. Warfarin vs enoxaparin for deep venous thrombosis prophylaxis after total hip and total knee arthroplasty: a cost comparison. J Ky Med Assoc 1998;96:143–8.

[58] Turpie AG, Bauer KA, Eriksson BI, et al. Fondaparinux vs enoxaparin for the prevention of venous thromboembolism in major orthopedic surgery: a meta-analysis of 4 randomized double-blind studies [comment]. Arch Intern Med 2002;162:1833–40.

[59] Eriksson BI, Bauer KA, Lassen MR, et al. Fondaparinux compared with enoxaparin for the prevention of venous thromboembolism after hip-fracture surgery. N Engl J Med 2001;345:1298–304.

[60] Eriksson BI, Lassen MR. Duration of prophylaxis against venous thromboembolism with fondaparinux after hip fracture surgery: a multicenter, randomized, placebo-controlled, double-blind study. Arch Intern Med 2003;163:1337–42.

[61] Weitz JI, Hirsh J, Samama MM. New anticoagulant drugs: the Seventh ACCP Conference on Antithrombotic and Thrombolytic Therapy. Chest 2004; 126(3 Suppl):265S–86S.

[62] Eriksson BI, Bergqvist D, Kalebo P, et al. Ximelagatran and melagatran compared with dalteparin for prevention of venous thromboembolism after total hip or knee replacement: the METHRO II randomised trial. Lancet 2002;360:1441–7.

[63] Eriksson BI, Arfrwidsson AC, Frison L, et al. A dose-ranging study of the oral direct thrombin inhibitor, ximelagatran, and its subcutaneous form, melagatran, compared with dalteparin in the prophylaxis of thromboembolism after hip or knee replacement: METHRO I. MElagatran for THRombin inhibition in Orthopaedic surgery. Thromb Haemost 2002;87:231–7.

[64] Eriksson BI, Agnelli B, Cohen AT, et al. The direct thrombin inhibitor melagatran followed by oral ximelagatran compared with enoxaparin for the prevention of venous thromboembolism after total hip or knee replacement: the EXPRESS study. J Thromb Haemost 2003;1:2490–6.

[65] Eriksson BI, Agnelli B, Cohen AT, et al. Direct thrombin inhibitor melagatran followed by oral ximelagatran in comparison with enoxaparin for prevention of venous thromboembolism after total hip or knee replacement. Thromb Haemost 2003; 89:288–96.

[66] Francis CW, Berkowitz SD, Comp PC, et al. Comparison of ximelagatran with warfarin for the prevention of venous thromboembolism after total knee replacement. N Engl J Med 2003;349:1703–12.

[67] Eriksson BI, Dahl OE, Rosencher N, et al. Dabigatran etexilate is effective and safe for the extended prevention of venous thromboembolism following total hip replacement. Abstract presented at XXIst Congress of the International Society on Thrombosis and Haemostasis in Geneva, Switzerland, July 2007.

[68] Caprini JA, Hwang E, Hantel S, et al. The oral direct thrombin inhibitor dabigatran etexilate is effective and safe for prevention of major venous thromboembolism following orthopaedic surgery. Abstract presented at XXIst Congress of the International Society on Thrombosis and Haemostasis in Geneva, Switzerland, July 2007.

[69] Strebel N, Prins M, Agnelli G, et al. Preoperative or postoperative start of prophylaxis for venous thromboembolism with low-molecular-weight heparin in

elective hip surgery? Arch Intern Med 2002;162: 1451–6.

[70] Horlocker TT, Wedel DJ, Benzon H, et al. Regional anesthesia in the anticoagulated patient: defining the risks (the second ASRA Consensus Conference on Neuraxial Anesthesia and Anticoagulation). Reg Anesth Pain Med 2003;28:172–97.

[71] Beyth RJ, Quinn LM, Landefeld CS. Prospective evaluation of an index for predicting the risk of major bleeding in outpatients treated with warfarin. Am J Med 1998;105:91–9.

[72] Landefeld CS, McGuire E III, Rosenblatt MW. A bleeding risk index for estimating the probability of major bleeding in hospitalized patients starting anticoagulant therapy. Am J Med 1990;89:569–78.

[73] Campbell NR, Hull RD, Brant R, et al. Aging and heparin-related bleeding. Arch Intern Med 1996; 156:857–60.

[74] Wells PS, Forgie MA, Simms M, et al. The outpatient bleeding risk index: validation of a tool for predicting bleeding rates in patients treated for deep venous thrombosis and pulmonary embolism. Arch Intern Med 2003;163:917–20.

[75] Decousus H, Leizorovicz A, Parent F, et al. A clinical trial of vena caval filters in the prevention of pulmonary embolism in patients with proximal deep-vein thrombosis. Prevention du Risque d'Embolie Pulmonaire par Interruption Cave Study Group [see comment]. N Engl J Med 1998;338:409–15.

[76] Streiff MB. Vena caval filters: a review for intensive care specialists. J Intensive Care Med 2003;18:59–79.

[77] Alexander JJ, Yuhas JP, Piotrowski JJ. Is the increasing use of prophylactic percutaneous IVC filters justified? Am J Surg 1994;168:102–6.

[78] Walsh DB, Birkmeyer JD, Barrett JA, et al. Use of inferior vena cava filters in the Medicare population. Ann Vasc Surg 1995;9:483–7.

[79] Offner PJ, Hawkes A, Madayag R, et al. The role of temporary inferior vena cava filters in critically ill surgical patients. Arch Surg 2003;138:591–4 [discussion: 594–5].

[80] Hull RD, Schellong SM, Tapson VF, et al. Extended-duration venous thromboembolism (VTE) prophylaxis in acutely ill medical patients with recent reduced mobility: the EXCLAIM study. Presented at: International Society on Thrombosis and Haemostasis XXIst Congress; July 6–12, 2007; Geneva, Switzerland.

[81] Davidson BL, Berkowitz SD, Lotke PA, et al. Prolonged thromboprophylaxis with oral anticoagulants after total hip arthroplasty: a prospective controlled randomized study. Ann Intern Med 2002;137:648–55.

[82] Eikelboom JW, Quinlan DJ, Douketis JD. Extended-duration prophylaxis against venous thromboembolism after total hip or knee replacement: a meta-analysis of the randomised trials. Lancet 2001;358:9–15.

[83] Kearon C. Duration of therapy for acute venous thromboembolism. Clin Chest Med 2003;24:63–72.

[84] Bergqvist D, Agnelli G, Cohen AT, et al. Duration of prophylaxis against venous thromboembolism with enoxaparin after surgery for cancer. N Engl J Med 2002;346:975–80.

[85] Rasmussen MS. Preventing thromboembolic complications in cancer patients after surgery: a role for prolonged thromboprophylaxis. Cancer Treat Rev 2002;28:141–4.

ELSEVIER
SAUNDERS

Cardiol Clin 26 (2008) 235–250

CARDIOLOGY
CLINICS

Anticoagulant Treatment of Deep Vein Thrombosis and Pulmonary Embolism

Huyen Tran, MBBS, FRACP, FRCPA,
Simon McRae, MB, ChB, FRACP, FRCPA,
Jeffrey Ginsberg, MD, FRCPC*

*Department of Medicine, McMaster University Medical Centre, 1200 Main Street West,
Room 3X28, Hamilton, Ontario L8N 3Z5, Canada*

Venous thromboembolism (VTE), consisting of deep vein thrombosis (DVT) and pulmonary embolism (PE), is a potentially fatal disease with an estimated annual incidence of 0.1% in white populations [1]. The initial aim of treatment of VTE is safely to prevent thrombus extension and new or recurrent PE. Long-term goals are a reduction in the incidence of chronic sequelae including the postthrombotic syndrome, chronic thromboembolic pulmonary hypertension, and recurrent VTE. Anticoagulants have played a central role in therapy for VTE since the seminal trial by Barritt and Jordan [2] in which 35 patients with clinically diagnosed PE were randomized to either intravenous (IV) unfractionated heparin (UFH) therapy or no anticoagulant treatment. Death occurred in 25% of patients who received no treatment with another 25% experiencing nonfatal recurrent PE, whereas no deaths occurred in the patients receiving heparin. Although this study can be criticized because some patients with clinically diagnosed PE probably did not have the disease, it is likely that this would result in an underestimate of the true risk reduction associated with UFH therapy.

VTE is a significant health issue in the elderly because the population incidence increases exponentially with age in both men and women [3–6], from a figure of <5 per 100,000 per year in children <15 years of age to 450 to 600 per 100,000

per year in individuals over the age of 80 [1]. As in younger patients, VTE in elderly patients is often associated with the presence of one or more well-defined risk factors at the time of diagnosis [7,8]. Increased age seems to be a strong predictor of VTE in acutely ill medical patients [9], with one study reporting the prevalence of asymptomatic DVT in medical patients aged >80 years to be 18% at admission compared with 3% in patients aged 55 to 69 years [10].

Treatment of the elderly patient with VTE is complicated by an age-associated increase in the risk of bleeding, the frequent coexistence of other diseases, and the exclusion of older patients from trials examining anticoagulant efficacy and safety. These factors may result in a tendency to treat older patients with inadequate anticoagulant therapy. An increased case-fatality rate of VTE in the elderly emphasizes the need for particularly careful therapy in this subgroup of patients, however, except in the presence of a clear contraindication [3,4]. This article reviews the initial and long-term treatment of VTE, and emphasizes the available data on the efficacy and safety of anticoagulant therapy in the elderly patient. Treatment of uncomplicated PE or DVT is similar, with one condition often silently present when the other clinically manifests [11–14], and the discussion covers the management of either condition except where specified.

Initiation of anticoagulant therapy

Anticoagulant therapy is the standard of care in patients with VTE, and has been shown to

A version of this article originally appeared in *Clinics in Geriatric Medicine*, volume 22, issue 1.

* Corresponding author.

E-mail address: ginsbrgj@mcmaster.ca (J. Ginsberg).

reduce extension and recurrence of symptomatic proximal (involving the popliteal or more proximal veins) and calf DVT [15,16], and reduce mortality in patients with PE [2]. Coumarin derivatives (eg, warfarin) are usually the drugs of choice for long-term anticoagulant therapy, but such drugs have a delayed onset of anticoagulant effect. Initial short-term anticoagulant therapy with alternative drugs is necessary in patients with acute VTE, and failure to do so results in a threefold increase in the rate of recurrent VTE [17]. Initial inpatient treatment with IV UFH is being replaced by outpatient therapy with low-molecular-weight heparin (LMWH) as the most commonly used initial anticoagulant regime. The impact of increased age on dosage, efficacy, and safety of both treatment options is discussed.

Initial treatment with unfractionated heparin

UFH is a sulfated glycosaminoglycan that exerts its anticoagulant effect predominantly by binding to antithrombin, inducing a conformational change that accelerates the rate at which antithrombin inhibits coagulation enzymes [18]. UFH consists of a heterogeneous group of molecules ranging in molecular weight from 3000 to 30,000 d, and only one third of UFH molecules contain the unique pentasaccharide sequence required for binding to antithrombin. This molecular heterogeneity, along with variable charge-related nonspecific binding of UFH to other plasma proteins, such as von Willebrand's factor and platelet factor 4, contributes to the large variability in the anticoagulant response to UFH in individual patients [18].

Route of administration, dosage, and monitoring

UFH is usually administered by continuous IV infusion, a route that has been shown to be effective in reducing thrombus recurrence and extension [15]. Because of reduced bioavailability, larger doses of subcutaneous (SC) UFH are required in comparison with IV UFH for therapeutic anticoagulation to be achieved, and when given in adequate doses, SC UFH is likely to be at least as effective and safe as IV UFH for treatment of acute DVT [19]. Adequate trials to assess the efficacy of SC UFH for treatment of PE have not been performed.

A minimum threshold dose of UFH is probably required for optimal therapeutic efficacy [15].

Individuals vary in anticoagulant response to UFH, and it is standard practice to monitor UFH therapy by measurement of the activated partial thromboplastin time (aPTT). In a study published in 1972, an aPTT result within the therapeutic range of 1.5 to 2.5 times the control value (corresponding at the time to a UFH level of 0.3–0.7 anti–factor Xa IU/mL) was associated with a reduced risk of recurrent VTE [20], and this therapeutic range has been subsequently widely adopted. Over the years, with changes in the reagents and coagulometers used to determine the aPTT, it has become clear that there is wide variation in the relationship between aPTT results and plasma heparin levels among different laboratories [21]. Because plasma heparin levels, rather than aPTT, are the more accurate measures of the biologic effect of UFH therapy [22–24], it is recommended that individual institutions establish their own therapeutic aPTT range that correlates with a therapeutic heparin level of 0.3 to 0.7 IU/mL anti–factor Xa activity [18].

An initial bolus dose of UFH followed by a constant IV infusion is standard practice when treating people for acute VTE. Physician-directed UFH dosing often results in inadequate therapy. In the general adult population, use of a validated nomogram using either fixed initial dosing or dosing according to patient weight (Table 1) is recommended [22,25]. The use of a nomogram results in more rapid achievement of therapeutic aPTT levels and improves outcome, although

Table 1
Weight-based IV unfractionated heparin nomogram

aPTT result[a]	Dose adjustment
Initial dose 80 U/kg bolus, then infusion 18 U/kg/h	
<35 seconds	80 U/kg bolus, then increase infusion by 4 U/kg/h
35–45 seconds	40 U/kg bolus, then increase infusion by 2 U/kg/h
46–70 seconds	No change
71–90 seconds	Decrease infusion rate by 2 U/kg/h
>90 seconds	Hold infusion 1 h, then decrease rate by 3 U/kg/h

aPTT should be checked 6 hours after commencing heparin or a change in infusion rate.
[a] aPTT, activated partial thromboplastin time.
Adapted from Raschke RA, Reilly BM, Guidry JR, et al. The weight-based heparin dosing nomogram compared with a "standard care" nomogram: a randomized controlled trial. Ann Intern Med 1993;119:874–81; with permission.

adjustment according to the sensitivity of local aPTT methods is required [22]. The initial aPTT level should be measured 6 hours after commencing therapy. Up to 25% of patients with acute VTE have heparin resistance, arbitrarily defined as a requirement of > 35,000 U of UFH per day to achieve a therapeutic aPTT [24]. In a randomized trial enrolling 131 patients with heparin resistance, monitoring UFH therapy using anti–factor Xa levels (target range, 0.35–0.67 IU/mL) was as effective and safe as aPTT monitoring and resulted in a lower mean daily dose of UFH [24]. Anti–factor Xa monitoring is recommended in patients with heparin resistance.

Efficacy and safety of unfractionated heparin in the elderly

Overall, approximately 5% of patients with acute VTE treated with IV UFH develop recurrent VTE during the initial period of treatment [18]. Initial treatment with 5 days is as effective as 10 days of IV UFH, both followed by oral anticoagulant therapy, in preventing recurrent VTE [26]. Retrospective subgroup analysis of cohort studies suggested that patients who fail to achieve a therapeutic aPTT in the first 24 hours of treatment have a dramatic increase in the risk of recurrent VTE [27]. Data from two meta-analyses contradicts this finding, however, reporting that there is no relationship between subtherapeutic aPTT results and risk of recurrence in patients treated with a 5000-U bolus followed by a continuous IV infusion of at least 30,000 U per day [28,29].

Although the in-hospital case-fatality rate of VTE is increased in the elderly, it is unclear if this is caused by a higher rate of serious underlying disease, suboptimal treatment caused by a fear of bleeding complications, reduced efficacy of anticoagulant therapy in the aged, or a combination of the three [3]. Subgroup analyses of trials in which patients with VTE were treated with UFH, examining efficacy according to patient age, have not been performed. Advanced age was not an exclusion criterion, however, in trials establishing the efficacy of IV UFH for treatment of VTE [2,15,16].

Bleeding is the most common side effect of anticoagulant therapy. Bleeding episodes are normally defined as major if they are intracranial, and retroperitoneal if they are fatal or lead to hospitalization or transfusion [30]. Major bleeding occurs in approximately 2% of patients treated

with IV UFH for acute VTE [18]. Patient factors, such as recent surgery, trauma, and concurrent aspirin or thrombolytic therapy, have been identified as indicators of increased bleeding risk [30]. Although there is evidence suggesting that supratherapeutic aPTT levels are associated with increased bleeding rates in patients with acute coronary syndromes receiving UFH [31], the evidence is by no means definitive in patients receiving UFH for VTE [30].

Increased age has also been identified as an indicator of increased bleeding risk with anticoagulant therapy. Proposed reasons have included increased drug interactions, increased drug sensitivity, a higher incidence of concurrent disease including renal insufficiency, malnutrition, and increased vascular fragility [32]. In a systematic review, Beyth and Landefeld [32] identified 11 studies that examined age as a risk factor for heparin-related bleeding. Eight of the 11 studies found bleeding to be more frequent in older patients [20,33–39], with on average a threefold increase in risk of bleeding in patients over 60 years of age. It is worth noting that in four of the studies UFH was given by intermittent bolus [33–36], a dose regimen known to be associated with an increased risk of bleeding in comparison with continuous IV infusion. Four studies included patients with indications other than VTE [33–35,37], in one study age only increased bleeding risk in postsurgical patients [20], and no study used weight-adjusted dosing of UFH. In a subsequent study, patients with VTE received either 30,000 or 40,000 U of UFH per day by continuous infusion. Increased age was found to be a risk factor for bleeding, independent of gender, weight, and perceived baseline bleeding risk; major bleeding occurred in 3.1% of patients younger than 72 years, and 11.1% aged 72 years or older [40]. In the same trial, the elderly required lower doses of UFH to achieve therapeutic aPTT levels. It was postulated that alterations in the level of heparin-binding proteins with age and reduced renal clearance of UFH, which is only important at high heparin levels [18], contributed to the observed difference in aPTT response.

There is evidence that elderly patients have a moderately increased risk of bleeding with UFH therapy, although this has not been demonstrated when weight-based dosing regimes are used. Age by itself should not be a contraindication to IV UFH, although careful consideration of other bleeding risk factors and monitoring of therapy is required in this population.

Initial treatment with low-molecular-weight heparin

LMWH preparations are produced by either enzymatic or chemical depolymerization of UFH (Table 2) [18,41]. They have a mean molecular weight of approximately 5000 d. Because heparin must bind both antithrombin and thrombin simultaneously to catalyze thrombin inhibition, a process that requires a chain length of 18 saccharides, the reduced molecular size results in a reduced capability of LMWH to inhibit thrombin in comparison with UFH [18]. Factor Xa inhibition only requires binding of the pentasaccharide moiety to antithrombin and not a minimum chain length. LMWH has an increased ratio of Xa to IIa (thrombin) inhibitory activity [41]. Compared with UFH, the reduced size of LMWH also produces decreased charge-related nonspecific protein binding, resulting in improved subcutaneous bioavailability, a more predictable anticoagulant response, and predominantly dose-independent renal clearance [41]. These qualities have made outpatient management of DVT using unmonitored, weight-based SC LMWH feasible.

Dosage and monitoring

LMWH products differ in their method of production, molecular weight, and anticoagulant effect (see Table 2) [41]. Few trials have directly compared different LMWH preparations for treatment of acute VTE, and definitive conclusions with regard to comparative efficacy and safety cannot be made [42–44]. Dosage regimens differ for the various LMWH formulations; those used for treatment of VTE are shown in Table 2. A meta-analysis comparing once-daily with twice-daily SC LMWH for treatment of symptomatic DVT found efficacy and safety to be equivalent, although the statistical confidence was limited by sample size [45].

Because the antithrombotic response to weight-based dosing of LMWH is predictable, laboratory monitoring during treatment is usually unnecessary in patients with VTE [18]. When laboratory monitoring is performed, the anti–factor Xa assay is most commonly used for monitoring LMWH therapy, despite concerns with regards to the clinical relevance of results [46]. Levels are usually performed on blood samples drawn 4 hours after SC injection and therapeutic ranges of 0.6 to 1 U/mL for twice-daily administration and 1 to 2 U/mL for once-daily treatment have been proposed [18].

Because clearance of LMWH is primarily renal it is expected that patients with renal impairment have an increased risk of accumulation of drug (and anti–factor Xa levels). Most pharmacokinetic studies of LMWH in patients with renal failure have found this to be true with some variation among LMWH products seen [47,48]. Current guidelines have recommended that IV UFH be used for initial anticoagulant therapy in patients with a creatinine clearance of <30 mL/min, or if LMWH is used, that anti–factor Xa levels be closely monitored [18]. The authors of a recent review concluded that a clear threshold of creatinine clearance at which patients showed an increased risk of accumulation could not be identified, and the role of laboratory monitoring in patients with renal impairment is unclear [47]. Although individual LMWH products have shown predictable dose responses in obese patients, measuring anti–factor Xa levels on at least one occasion in this patient group seems to be prudent [18].

Table 2
Characteristics of selected low-molecular-weight heparins

Drug name	Mean molecular weight	Anti-Xa:anti-IIa ratio	Therapeutic dose[a]
Enoxaparin	4200	3.8	100 IU/kg twice daily[b] or 150 IU/kg once daily[c]
Dalteparin	5800	2.8	100 IU/kg twice daily[d] or 200 IU/kg once daily[d]
Tinzaparin	5800	1.5–2	175 IU/kg once daily[b]

[a] Doses are in anti-FXa international units.
[b] Current approved FDA dose for treatment of acute VTE.
[c] FDA approved for inpatient treatment.
[d] Regimen used in other countries, but not FDA approved.

Efficacy and safety of low-molecular-weight heparin in the elderly

Two separate meta-analyses reported unmonitored, fixed-dose SC LMWH to be as effective and safe as adjusted-dose IV UFH for the treatment of acute VTE, with both analyses finding a significant difference in mortality favoring LMWH, likely caused by improved survival in patients with malignancy [42,49]. Patients with acute VTE treated as outpatients with LMWH seem to do as well as those receiving inpatient treatments [42]. The suitability of administering outpatient therapy makes LMWH more cost-effective than IV UFH in most health care settings. Patients with extensive iliofemoral DVT have often been excluded from LMWH trials, and extended-duration (ie, >5 days) IV UFH therapy is often administered to such patients.

Concern is often expressed with regards to use of LMWH in the elderly because of the fall in glomerular filtration rate with age, resulting in the perceived risk of accumulation of anticoagulant activity and resulting hemorrhage. Unfortunately, the trial data with regards to bleeding risk in elderly patients with VTE treated with LMWH are limited because advanced age was often used as an exclusion criterion. Pharmacokinetic data for elderly patients given LMWH is available for nadroparin, enoxaparin, and tinzaparin. In a study of nadroparin given at a dose of 180 anti–factor Xa U/kg for 6 to 10 days, evidence of accumulation of anti–factor Xa activity was seen in both healthy elderly volunteers and elderly patients with VTE (mean age in both groups, 65) [50]. Significant correlation was seen between creatinine and drug clearances. Similar evidence of accumulation and impact of renal function was seen in a small study of 18 patients with renal impairment (mean age, 75 years) administered enoxaparin, 1 mg/kg every 12 hours [51]. In contrast, tinzaparin, 175 IU/kg for 10 days, showed no evidence of accumulation of anti–factor Xa or IIa activity in 30 inpatients with VTE, a median age of 87 years, and a creatinine clearance range of 20 to 72 mL/min [52]. It has been suggested that the larger mean molecular weight of tinzaparin results in a lower contribution of the kidneys to clearance of this compound.

Two prospective trials have examined the safety of LMWH in the geriatric population [53,54]. In a study of 200 inpatients with VTE (mean age, 85.2 years), the rate of major bleeding was comparable with that in all adult patients at 1.5%. All patients had a creatinine clearance of >20 mL/min, and received a fixed dose of tinzaparin, 175 IU/kg once daily [53]. In a second prospective registry of 334 patients receiving enoxaparin or tinzaparin for a number of indications (mean age, 85 years) the major bleeding rate was 7%, although overdosage contributed to some bleeding episodes [54].

On the basis of these data, it seems reasonable to use full-dose LMWH (particularly tinzaparin) in elderly patients with VTE and a creatinine clearance of >30 mL/min. Monitoring of anti–factor Xa levels should be considered in patients with impaired renal function [55]. In patients with severe (creatinine clearance <30 mL/min) renal impairment, IV UFH is preferred. Dose reduction of LMWH in the elderly has not been examined in trials, and there is a concern that this may reduce treatment efficacy. Further randomized trials evaluating LMWH in the elderly are needed.

Initial treatment with fondaparinux

Fondaparinux is a synthetic analogue of the critical pentasaccharide sequence required for binding of heparin molecules to antithrombin [56,57]. Chemically engineered, it has minor modifications from the natural pentasaccharide moiety, improving stability and resulting in enhanced binding to antithrombin [56]. Given SC, fondaparinux demonstrates 100% bioavailability with peak plasma concentrations occurring 1.7 hours after dosing [58]. Clearance is predominantly renal, with approximately 70% of the initial dose recovered in the urine in an unchanged form [58]. Patients with reduced creatinine clearance, such as the elderly, show higher peak drug levels and longer drug half-life and may require dose adjustment [58,59].

Two trials have evaluated fondaparinux for initial treatment of VTE [60,61]. In the Matisse-DVT trial, once-daily SC fondaparinux (5 mg daily if weight <50 kg, 7.5 mg daily if weight 50–100 kg, 10 mg daily if weight >100 kg) was compared with enoxaparin, 1 mg/kg twice daily, for the initial treatment of symptomatic proximal DVT. After 3 months, symptomatic recurrence occurred in 3.9% and 4.1% in the fondaparinux and enoxaparin groups, respectively, with low and similar rates of major bleeding in both groups. Fondaparinux was judged to be noninferior to enoxaparin with regards to both efficacy and safety. In the Matisse-PE trial [61], patients with symptomatic PE were randomized to initial treatment with either fondaparinux (5, 7.5, or 10 mg according to weight) SC daily or continuous IV UFH. Recurrent VTE developed in 3.8% and 5% of patients receiving fondaparinux and UFH, respectively. The rates of major bleeding were low and not significantly different between treatment arms. The investigators concluded that fondaparinux seems to be as effective and safe as UFH for treatment of PE. The mean age of patients in both trials was >60 years. Patients with renal impairment (serum creatinine >2 mg/dL) were excluded from both trials, however, meaning care should be taken in extrapolating these results to those elderly patients who are likely to have renal impairment.

Heparin-induced thrombocytopenia

Heparin-induced thrombocytopenia is a non-hemorrhagic complication of UFH and LMWH therapy, manifesting typically with thrombocytopenia and, in many, with new thrombosis [62]. For early detection of heparin-induced thrombocytopenia, platelet count monitoring is recommended every other day until Day 14 in patients receiving therapeutic UFH, but is not routinely recommended in patients with acute VTE treated with LMWH because of an extremely low incidence of heparin-induced thrombocytopenia in such patients [63]. Readers are referred to the recent American College of Chest Physicians guidelines for further information on the manifestations and management of heparin-induced thrombocytopenia [63].

Thrombolytic therapy for venous thromboembolism in the elderly

The role of thrombolytic therapy in patients with VTE remains controversial. Although thrombolytic therapy results in increased rates of early leg vein patency after DVT, it has not been conclusively shown to decrease the subsequent rate of postthrombotic syndrome, and outside of life-threatening limb ischemia caused by massive thrombosis, thrombolysis is not recommended in patients with DVT [64].

Patients with massive PE presenting with circulatory collapse have a mortality rate as high as 30%, and the potential benefits of thrombolysis in this patient subgroup normally outweigh the 2% to 3% risk of intracranial hemorrhage [65,66].

In two case series of patients with massive PE, outcome and bleeding rates were similar in elderly and nonelderly patients [67,68], although another study found increasing age to be a major risk factor for hemorrhage after thrombolysis [69]. Careful consideration on a case-by-case basis of the risks and benefits of thrombolysis is required.

Long-term treatment of venous thrombosis

After the initial period of treatment with heparin (UFH or LMWH), the preferred long-term treatment of VTE for most patients is warfarin or another coumarin derivative (eg, acenocoumarol). Warfarin is usually continued until the benefits of treatment no longer outweigh its risks. In essence, this is a balance between the risk of recurrent VTE if anticoagulation is stopped and the risk of major bleeding if treatment is continued. Because there are many factors involved, the decision to prolong or stop anticoagulation needs to be individualized. Patient preference should be taken into consideration if it is concluded that the benefit of continuing anticoagulation is minimal or unclear.

In this section, issues related to long-term warfarin therapy, including the optimal duration, intensity of treatment, and risks of major hemorrhage, and alternatives to warfarin for the treatment of VTE, such as LMWH, are discussed. The impact of increased age on dosage, efficacy, and safety of treatment options is emphasized.

Coumarin derivatives (warfarin)

For an in-depth review on the pharmacology of coumarin derivatives, readers are referred to the recent American College of Chest Physicians guidelines [70].

Warfarin started within 24 to 48 hours of initiating heparin with a goal of achieving international normalized ratio (INR) results between 2 and 3 as secondary thromboprophylaxis for 3 months reduces the risk of recurrent VTE by 90% as compared with placebo [71]. A higher target INR of 3 to 4 is associated with more bleeding but no better efficacy [72]. Although this latter range was previously thought to be necessary in patients with antiphospholipid antibody syndrome who developed thrombosis [73,74], two recent randomized studies reported that conventional-intensity warfarin therapy (INR, 2–3) was as effective as high-intensity (INR, 3.1–4) in preventing recurrent VTE

[75,76]. Another recent randomized trial comparing low-intensity warfarin therapy (target INR, 1.5–1.9) with conventional-intensity warfarin therapy (target INR, 2–3) for the long-term treatment of unprovoked VTE demonstrated that low-intensity warfarin therapy was less effective at preventing recurrent VTE (1.9% versus 0.7% per patient-year; odds ratio, 2.8; 95% confidence interval, 1.1–7) and was associated with the similar rates of major bleeding as conventional-intensity therapy (INR 2–3) [77]. In all of these studies, the average age of patients involved was less than 65 years. Based on these results, warfarin adjusted to a target INR of 2 to 3 seems optimal for the treatment of VTE.

Warfarin doses are adjusted according to the prothrombin time, expressed as the INR. In two separate randomized trials, Harrison and co-workers [78] and Crowther and coworkers [79] showed that the practice of initiating warfarin starting with an average maintenance dose of 5 mg warfarin and adjusting the dose according to the INR usually results in a value of at least 2 in 4 to 5 days. A 5-mg starting dose of warfarin (rather than 10 mg) reduced the likelihood of early excessive anticoagulation, ameliorated a precipitous decline in protein C, and did not delay achievement of a therapeutic INR. Kovacs and colleagues [80] demonstrated that 10 mg of warfarin in the first 2 days of therapy for outpatients with acute VTE allows more rapid achievement of a therapeutic INR than does a 5-mg dosage, producing effective anticoagulation without an increase in supratherapeutic INR results (greater than 5). Although a 5-mg warfarin starting dose is appropriate for most patients [81], it is reasonable to use 10 mg in select outpatients. Starting doses of 5 mg or less might be appropriate in the elderly [82,83]; patients with liver disease, nutritional deficiency, at high risk of bleeding [84,85]; or patients who are more sensitive to warfarin [86]. In the elderly, the dose of warfarin needed to maintain the patient in the target INR range is decreased, possibly reflecting a reduction in the clearance of the drug with age [87]. Several other factors may influence the response to anticoagulation in the elderly, including an increased likelihood of other medical illnesses, concurrent drug use, and decreased compliance in taking or monitoring of warfarin therapy.

INR monitoring can be performed daily or every other day until the results are in the therapeutic range for at least 24 hours. With the advent of routine outpatient treatment of VTE with LMWHs, which do not require monitoring of their anticoagulant effect, there has been a push to develop warfarin-dosing regimens that reduce the need for initial INR monitoring. Smaller doses of warfarin reduce the need for more frequent INR monitoring because fewer patients develop INR values greater than 3 in the early days of warfarin therapy. Kovacs and colleagues [80,81] demonstrated that algorithm-guided warfarin initiation in outpatients that requires INR measurements only on Days 3 and 5 is safe.

After initial dosing, warfarin can be monitored two or three times per week for 1 to 2 weeks, and then less frequently, depending on the stability of INR results, up to intervals as long as 4 to 6 weeks. If dose adjustment is needed, such as when medications that can interact with warfarin are introduced, the cycle of more frequent monitoring is repeated until a stable dose response is again achieved. Because of the factors that can alter the response to warfarin in the elderly (discussed previously), more frequent monitoring of the INR is advisable in older patients to optimize INR control, thereby minimizing the risk of bleeding.

Risk of bleeding during warfarin therapy

The risk of major bleeding when the INR is adjusted to achieve a target range of 2 to 3 in patients receiving long-term warfarin ranges from 1% to 3% per year [77,88,89]. The risk of bleeding seems to be highest soon after starting treatment, or if anticoagulation is difficult to control [90–92]. Landefeld and Goldman [84] reported that the rate of major bleeding decreased from 3% per month during the first month of warfarin therapy, to 0.8% per month for the rest of the first year and 0.3% per month thereafter. A recent randomized study by Kearon and colleagues [77] reported that the annual risk of major bleeding beyond the first 6 months of anticoagulation (INR, 2–3) was approximately 1% per year. In a meta-analysis of 33 prospective studies to determine how often major episodes of bleeding during warfarin therapy in patients with VTE (INR, 2–3) were fatal, the overall case-fatality rate was 13% [93]. Although the risk of major bleeding seems higher during the early course of anticoagulant therapy, similar case-fatality rates were observed during the acute and long-term phases of treatment.

The risk of major bleeding among patients varies depending on such individual characteristics as age; comorbidities (eg, diabetes, hypertension, renal insufficiency, previous gastrointestinal bleeding, or the presence of cancer); and the use of concomitant drugs, in particular antiplatelet therapy [30]. The association between increasing age and anticoagulant-related bleeding is controversial. Pengo and colleagues [94] reported that major bleeding occurred more frequently in patients older than 75 years than younger patients (5.1% per year versus 1% per year). Multivariate analysis in this study identified age > 75 as the only independent variable related to primary bleeding. Although results of early studies have suggested that older age is not associated with an increased risk of major bleeding [95–97], more recent studies support the association reported by Pengo and coworkers [83,90,98,99]. Older patients whose anticoagulation is carefully managed (eg, anticoagulant clinics) probably have a similar risk of bleeding as younger patients [100]. Although it is not known how aging might increase the risk of anticoagulant-related bleeding, this issue is important as the world population ages and older patients are more likely to have medical illnesses that warrant anticoagulation. An increased case-fatality rate of VTE in the elderly means that optimal therapy in this subgroup of patients is important unless a clear contraindication is present [3,4]. Warfarin should not be withheld because of age; instead, smaller starting dosages should be used, and INR carefully monitored to maximize the time in the therapeutic range.

A variety of programs has been developed aimed at increasing the time in the therapeutic range. These programs include anticoagulant monitoring clinics with dedicated personnel, the use of point-of-care monitors that allow patients to self-test and self-manage dose adjustments, and use of computerized programs to assist in dose adjustments [101–107]. Home monitoring of warfarin therapy is accurate, feasible, and associated with a greater time in the therapeutic range and improved quality of life for the patient, but it requires special patient education and training to implement and should be overseen by a knowledgeable provider. In elderly patients, such intense patient involvement may not be practical.

Two prediction rules to assess outpatients receiving warfarin at increased risk of major bleeding have been prospectively validated. Beyth and colleagues [85] identified age > 65 years, history of gastrointestinal tract bleeding, history of stroke, and one or more of four specific comorbid conditions (recent myocardial infarction, renal impairment, anemia, and diabetes) as independent risk factors for bleeding, and reported that the cumulative rate of bleeding at 2 years of follow-up was 3% in the low-risk group (no risk factors); 12% in the moderate-risk group (one or two risk factors); and 53% in the high-risk group (three or four risk factors). Kuijer and coworkers [108] used age, sex, and the presence of malignancy in their prediction model, and reported that the rates of major bleeding after 3 months of therapy in the low-, middle-, and high-risk groups were 1%, 4%, and 7%, respectively. Although it seems reasonable to use these models to weigh the risk and benefits of warfarin therapy to modify the duration of therapy and adjust the intensity or frequency of monitoring, they should not be used to decide whether or not to initiate anticoagulation.

Alternatives to coumarin derivatives

Low-molecular-weight heparin

Therapeutic doses of LMWH are indicated in patients with VTE and cancer [109], for patients in whom warfarin is impractical or contraindicated, and those who develop recurrent VTE while being treated with appropriate doses of oral anticoagulants. In a randomized trial involving patients with cancer-related VTE (DVT, PE, or both), the dose of LMWH was safely reduced to 75% of the initial, weight-based dose after 1 month of treatment without an increased risk of recurrent VTE [109]. Patients who were receiving LMWH had one half the rate of recurrent VTE as those who were taking warfarin during 6 months of treatment (9% versus 17%). The bleeding rates associated with both medications were similar (6% versus 4%), and patients found the daily injections of LMWH acceptable.

For patients with acute VTE and in whom warfarin is impractical or contraindicated, long-term (3–6 months) LMWH seems to be as effective as warfarin in the prevention of recurrent VTE. In a randomized controlled trial comparing tinzaparin, 175 IU/kg SC daily, with IV UFH followed by warfarin for 3 months in patients with DVT, LMWH was as effective as warfarin for long-term treatment in preventing recurrent VTE, and LMWH was associated with a lower rate of bleeding, in particular minor bleeding [110]. A meta-analysis of randomized controlled trials that compared LMWH with warfarin as secondary thromboprophylaxis in patients with acute DVT reported that the rates of recurrent VTE and major bleeding were similar with the two regimens [111].

The long-term use of LMWH (≥3 months) in elderly patients with VTE seems to be effective and safe. In a randomized trial involving 100 patients aged >75 years with DVT, patients receiving fixed-dose enoxaparin (4000 anti–factor Xa units once daily) for 3 months had similar rates of recurrent VTE and major bleeding to those who were treated with warfarin (INR, 2–3) [112]. The authors are not aware of any randomized study assessing the long-term use of LMWH in patients with PE alone. Because PE and DVT are manifestations of the same disease, however, it seems reasonable to extrapolate the results from studies involving patients with DVT to those with PE, with or without concurrent DVT. Although LMWH is a safe alternative for some patients, such as those who live in geographically inaccessible places or who are reluctant to visit thrombosis services regularly, its cost, the inconvenience of daily injection, and the risk of osteoporosis associated with long-term treatment limits its routine use as secondary prophylaxis.

Therapeutic strategies used to manage patients who develop symptomatic recurrent VTE while receiving conventional-intensity warfarin include UFH; LMWH; higher- intensity warfarin (eg, INR range, 3–4); or insertion of a vena caval filter. In a recent case-series consisting of 887 patients with acute VTE, 3 of 32 patients who developed recurrent VTE while receiving warfarin developed further recurrent events when treated with dalteparin, 200 IU/kg SC daily (9%; 95% confidence interval, 2%–25%) [113]. The optimal management of such patients is unknown, because no randomized studies have been performed.

Vena caval filters

Inferior vena caval filters can be considered in patients who have contraindications to, or develop major bleeding while receiving, anticoagulant therapy, or those who develop recurrent VTE while receiving adequate treatment. In a randomized trial comparing anticoagulant therapy either alone or with a filter among 400 patients with acute DVT, the incidence of PE at Day 12 was lower in patients with a filter compared with those without. This benefit did not persist at 2 years, however, and was offset by an almost doubling in the risk of recurrent DVT. Further, filters did not reduce early or late survival [114]. This suggests that anticoagulant therapy should be used concurrently if safe to do so to prevent recurrent DVT.

Oral direct thrombin inhibitors

Coumarin derivatives, such as warfarin, have long been the only available oral anticoagulant for patients who need long-term anticoagulation. Their drawbacks, however, include a narrow therapeutic index, need for careful routine monitoring, and consequent dose adjustments to avoid overdosing and underdosing, with associated risks of hemorrhage and thrombosis, respectively. Ximelagatran is an oral direct thrombin inhibitor that does not require monitoring for the anticoagulant effect. When used as long-term treatment (≥6 months) in patients with VTE, ximelagatran has been demonstrated in randomized trials to be as effective as warfarin in preventing recurrent VTE [115,116]. Elevation in liver enzymes (especially alanine aminotransferases) has been reported in 5% to 10% of patients with long-term use, however, the clinical implications of which are unclear because levels may decrease to normal with continued treatment. Ximelagatran has not been approved by the Food and Drug Administration for clinical use.

Indirect factor Xa inhibitors

Idraparinux is a novel synthetic pentasaccharide with a substantially long half-life that inhibits activated factor X. Two randomized clinical trials comparing the efficacy and safety of idraparinux versus standard therapy involving patients with DVT and PE have been performed [117]. Once-weekly subcutaneous idraparinux for 3 or 6 months demonstrated similar efficacy compared with heparin followed with coumarin derivatives among patients with DVT. However, among patients with pulmonary embolism, idraparinux was less efficacious than standard therapy. Possible reasons for differences between results of DVT and PE trials include:

- Chance (LMWH performed much better than historical controls).
- DVT and PE are different diseases.
- LMWH/coumarin derivatives group in PE study performed exceptionally well compared with the DVT trial and historical LMWH/coumarin derivatives controls.
- The idraparinux group in the PE trial is less efficacious and needs change in early anticoagulation.

There were no differences in the rates of major or clinically relevant bleeding in both the DVT and PE studies.

Compression stockings

The use of below-knee graduated compression stockings for 2 years following acute DVT have been reported to halve the rate of postthrombotic syndrome, but does not reduce the risk of recurrent VTE [118–120].

Duration of anticoagulant therapy

Patients with symptomatic proximal DVT or PE should be treated for at least 3 months. Kearon and coworkers [121] compared 1 month with 3 months of warfarin therapy (target INR, 2–3) in patients whose VTE was associated with a transient risk factor. The rate of recurrent VTE after stopping treatment was 3.2% per patient-year in patients who received 3 months compared with 6.8% per patient-year in patients who received 1 month of treatment. This result is consistent with previous randomized trials in which patients with VTE who were treated for 4 to 6 weeks had a doubling in the risk of recurrence compared with those who were treated for 3 months [122,123].

The optimal duration of treatment for patients whose VTE was unprovoked is controversial. Such patients who are treated with warfarin for 3 months have a 10% to 27% risk of developing recurrence during the 12 months after anticoagulant therapy is stopped [88,89,124]. With 6 months of anticoagulant therapy, the risk of recurrence in the first year after stopping is approximately 10% [124,125]. Although extending treatment beyond 6 months reduces the risk of recurrent VTE, the benefit is lost after warfarin is discontinued [89,126]. In patients whose VTE developed in association with minor risk factors (eg, air travel, pregnancy, within 6 weeks of estrogen therapy, less serious leg injury, or immobilization) the risk of recurrence is probably lower than 10% [125].

Thrombophilia has been reported to be associated with an increased risk of recurrent VTE. The most convincing association is the presence of an antiphospholipid antibody (lupus anticoagulant or anticardiolipin antibody), which is associated with a twofold increase in the risk of recurrence [127–129]. Deficiencies of antithrombin, protein C and protein S [130,131], and homozygous factor V Leiden [132], and elevated levels of homocysteine [133], have also been reported to be associated with an increased risk of recurrence. Opposing this view, Baglin and colleagues [125] reported that testing for heritable thrombophilia does not allow prediction of recurrent VTE in the first 2 years after anticoagulant therapy is stopped; instead, assessment of clinical risk factors associated with the first episode of VTE predicted risk of recurrence. Further, there

are no randomized trials assessing different duration of anticoagulation in patients with VTE and thrombophilia to determine the risk of recurrence. The assumption that anticoagulation should be prolonged in such patients to reduce recurrent VTE has not been proved and thrombophilia testing need not be routinely performed, especially among older patients.

Evidence regarding the effect of age on recurrence is conflicting: some studies have reported a lower relative risk of recurrence with age [88,134], whereas others have reported a higher relative risk of recurrence [135]. Currently, most experts do not consider age to be a risk factor for recurrent VTE [136].

The decision to extend anticoagulant therapy beyond 3 months should be determined to balance the risk of recurrent VTE with the risk of bleeding. The annual risk of major bleeding when warfarin is adjusted to achieve a target INR of 2 to 3 is 1% to 3% [77,88,89,137]. Case-fatality rates of 10% for major bleeding in patients who

Table 3
Recommended duration of anticoagulation for patients with symptomatic DVT or PE

VTE scenario	Duration of treatment
Major transient risk factor[a]	3 mo
Associated with minor risk factors, no high-risk thrombophilia[b]	6 mo
Unprovoked, with or without low-risk thrombophilia[c]	≥ 6 mo[e]
Unprovoked with high-risk thrombophilia[d]	Indefinite
Cancer or persistent risk factor	Indefinite

Abbreviations: DVT, deep vein thrombosis; PE, pulmonary embolism.

[a] Major transient risk factors include major surgery (requiring anesthesia for >30 minutes); major trauma (eg, lower limb fracture requiring casting); major medical illness.

[b] Examples of minor risk factors include nonspecific transient illnesses, a history of air travel, estrogen-containing oral contraception, or hormone-replacement therapy [124].

[c] Examples of low-risk thrombophilia include heterozygosity for factor V Leiden and prothrombin gene mutations, hyperhomocysteinemia.

[d] Examples of high-risk thrombophilia include the presence of antiphospholipid antibodies; homozygosity for factor V Leiden or prothrombin gene mutation or combined heterozygosity for both; and deficiencies of antithrombin, protein C, or protein S.

[e] Consider prolonging therapy if risk of major bleeding is low or preferred by patient.

received treatment for more than 3 months [93] and 5% for recurrences have been reported [138]. In patients whose VTE was associated with a transient risk factor, treatment for 3 months is generally adequate because the risk of fatal recurrent VTE is lower than the risk of fatal bleeding if warfarin is prolonged. Among patients with unprovoked VTE, prolonged warfarin therapy greater than 6 months can be considered because the risk of fatal hemorrhage is counterbalanced by the risk of fatal recurrence. The argument to prolong therapy in these patients is stronger in the case of a high-risk thrombophilia, such as antiphospholipid antibody; homozygous factor V Leiden; deficiency of antithrombin, protein C, or protein S; or combined heterozygous state for factor V Leiden and the prothrombin gene mutation [139]. In patients whose VTE developed in the setting of minor risk factors or who are at high risk of bleeding, therapy for 6 months or less seems appropriate [136]. Indefinite therapy (preferably with LMWH) should be considered in patients with cancer-related VTE if the risk of bleeding is not high because the risk of recurrent VTE is >10% in the first year after stopping anticoagulation (Table 3).

Summary

Venous thrombosis is a common disease. As the mean age of the population increases, so does the incidence of VTE. Anticoagulant therapy is equally effective in young and older patients, and can substantially reduce the associated morbidity and mortality. When considering long-term oral anticoagulant therapy in older patients, however, careful ongoing evaluation is imperative to ensure that the risk of bleeding does not outweigh the antithrombotic benefits.

References

[1] White RH. The epidemiology of venous thromboembolism. Circulation 2003;107(Suppl 1):I4–8.

[2] Barritt DW, Jordan SC. Anticoagulant drugs in the treatment of pulmonary embolism: a controlled trial. Lancet 1960;1:1309–12.

[3] Anderson FA Jr, Wheeler HB, Goldberg RJ, et al. A population-based perspective of the hospital incidence and case-fatality rates of deep vein thrombosis and pulmonary embolism. The Worcester DVT Study. Arch Intern Med 1991;151:933–8.

[4] Heit JA, Silverstein MD, Mohr DN, et al. The epidemiology of venous thromboembolism in the community. Thromb Haemost 2001;86:452–63.

[5] Kierkegaard A. Incidence of acute deep vein thrombosis in two districts: a phlebographic study. Acta Chir Scand 1980;146:267–9.

[6] Oger E. Incidence of venous thromboembolism: a community-based study in Western France. EPI-GETBP Study Group. Groupe d'Etude de la Thrombose de Bretagne Occidentale. Thromb Haemost 2000;83:657–60.

[7] Anderson FA Jr, Spencer FA. Risk factors for venous thromboembolism. Circulation 2003; 107(Suppl 1):9–16.

[8] Kniffin WD Jr, Baron JA, Barrett J, et al. The epidemiology of diagnosed pulmonary embolism and deep venous thrombosis in the elderly. Arch Intern Med 1994;154:861–6.

[9] Alikhan R, Cohen AT, Combe S, et al. Risk factors for venous thromboembolism in hospitalized patients with acute medical illness: analysis of the MEDENOX Study. Arch Intern Med 2004; 164(9):963–8.

[10] Oger E, Bressollette L, Nonent M, et al. High prevalence of asymptomatic deep vein thrombosis on admission in a medical unit among elderly patients. Thromb Haemost 2002;88:592–7.

[11] Huisman MV, Buller HR, ten Cate JW, et al. Unexpected high prevalence of silent pulmonary embolism in patients with deep venous thrombosis. Chest 1989;95:498–502.

[12] Doyle DJ, Turpie AG, Hirsh J, et al. Adjusted subcutaneous heparin or continuous intravenous heparin in patients with acute deep vein thrombosis: a randomized trial. Ann Intern Med 1987;107: 441–5.

[13] Girard P, Musset D, Parent F, et al. High prevalence of detectable deep venous thrombosis in patients with acute pulmonary embolism. Chest 1999;116:903–8.

[14] Hull RD, Hirsh J, Carter CJ, et al. Pulmonary angiography, ventilation lung scanning, and venography for clinically suspected pulmonary embolism with abnormal perfusion lung scan. Ann Intern Med 1983;98:891–9.

[15] Hull RD, Raskob GE, Hirsh J, et al. Continuous intravenous heparin compared with intermittent subcutaneous heparin in the initial treatment of proximal-vein thrombosis. N Engl J Med 1986; 315:1109–14.

[16] Lagerstedt CI, Olsson CG, Fagher BO, et al. Need for long-term anticoagulant treatment in symptomatic calf-vein thrombosis. Lancet 1985;2: 515–8.

[17] Brandjes DP, Heijboer H, Buller HR, et al. Acenocoumarol and heparin compared with acenocoumarol alone in the initial treatment of proximal-vein thrombosis. N Engl J Med 1992;327:1485–9.

[18] Hirsh J, Raschke R. Heparin and low-molecular-weight heparin: the Seventh ACCP Conference on Antithrombotic and Thrombolytic Therapy. Chest 2004;126(3 Suppl):188S–203S.

[19] Hommes DW, Bura A, Mazzolai L, et al. Subcutaneous heparin compared with continuous intravenous heparin administration in the initial treatment of deep vein thrombosis: a meta-analysis. Ann Intern Med 1992;116:279–84.

[20] Basu D, Gallus A, Hirsh J, et al. A prospective study of the value of monitoring heparin treatment with the activated partial thromboplastin time. N Engl J Med 1972;287:324–7.

[21] Brill-Edwards P, Ginsberg JS, Johnston M, et al. Establishing a therapeutic range for heparin therapy. Ann Intern Med 1993;119:104–9.

[22] Raschke RA, Reilly BM, Guidry JR, et al. The weight-based heparin dosing nomogram compared with a "standard care" nomogram: a randomized controlled trial. Ann Intern Med 1993;119:874–81.

[23] Chiu HM, Hirsh J, Yung WL, et al. Relationship between the anticoagulant and antithrombotic effects of heparin in experimental venous thrombosis. Blood 1977;49:171–84.

[24] Levine MN, Hirsh J, Gent M, et al. A randomized trial comparing activated thromboplastin time with heparin assay in patients with acute venous thromboembolism requiring large daily doses of heparin. Arch Intern Med 1994;154:49–56.

[25] Cruickshank MK, Levine MN, Hirsh J, et al. A standard heparin nomogram for the management of heparin therapy. Arch Intern Med 1991;151:333–7.

[26] Hull RD, Raskob GE, Rosenbloom D, et al. Heparin for 5 days as compared with 10 days in the initial treatment of proximal venous thrombosis. N Engl J Med 1990;322:1260–4.

[27] Hull RD, Raskob GE, Brant RF, et al. Relation between the time to achieve the lower limit of the APTT therapeutic range and recurrent venous thromboembolism during heparin treatment for deep vein thrombosis. Arch Intern Med 1997;157:2562–8.

[28] Anand SS, Bates S, Ginsberg JS, et al. Recurrent venous thrombosis and heparin therapy: an evaluation of the importance of early activated partial thromboplastin times. Arch Intern Med 1999;159:2029–32.

[29] Anand S, Ginsberg JS, Kearon C, et al. The relation between the activated partial thromboplastin time response and recurrence in patients with venous thrombosis treated with continuous intravenous heparin. Arch Intern Med 1996;156:1677–81.

[30] Levine MN, Raskob G, Beyth RJ, et al. Hemorrhagic complications of anticoagulant treatment: the Seventh ACCP Conference on Antithrombotic and Thrombolytic Therapy. Chest 2004;126 (3 Suppl):287S–310S.

[31] Anand SS, Yusuf S, Pogue J, et al. Relationship of activated partial thromboplastin time to coronary events and bleeding in patients with acute coronary syndromes who receive heparin. Circulation 2003; 107:2884–8.

[32] Beyth RJ, Landefeld CS. Anticoagulants in older patients: a safety perspective. Drugs Aging 1995; 6:45–54.

[33] Jick H, Slone D, Borda IT, et al. Efficacy and toxicity of heparin in relation to age and sex. N Engl J Med 1968;279:284–6.

[34] Walker AM, Jick H. Predictors of bleeding during heparin therapy. JAMA 1980;244:1209–12.

[35] Vieweg WV, Piscatelli RL, Houser JJ, et al. Complications of intravenous administration of heparin in elderly women. JAMA 1970;213:1303–6.

[36] Glazier RL, Crowell EB. Randomized prospective trial of continuous vs intermittent heparin therapy. JAMA 1976;236:1365–7.

[37] Nelson PH, Moser KM, Stoner C, et al. Risk of complications during intravenous heparin therapy. West J Med 1982;136:189–97.

[38] Holm HA, Abildgaard U, Kalvenes S. Heparin assays and bleeding complications in treatment of deep venous thrombosis with particular reference to retroperitoneal bleeding. Thromb Haemost 1985;53:278–81.

[39] Mant MJ, O'Brien BD, Thong KL, et al. Haemorrhagic complications of heparin therapy. Lancet 1977;1:1133–5.

[40] Campbell NR, Hull RD, Brant R, et al. Aging and heparin-related bleeding. Arch Intern Med 1996; 156:857–60.

[41] Weitz JI. Low-molecular-weight heparins. N Engl J Med 1997;337:688–98.

[42] Dolovich LR, Ginsberg JS, Douketis JD, et al. A meta-analysis comparing low-molecular-weight heparins with unfractionated heparin in the treatment of venous thromboembolism: examining some unanswered questions regarding location of treatment, product type, and dosing frequency. Arch Intern Med 2000;160:181–8.

[43] White RH, Ginsberg JS. Low-molecular-weight heparins: are they all the same? Br J Haematol 2003;121:12–20.

[44] van der Heijden JF, Prins MH, Buller HR. For the initial treatment of venous thromboembolism: are all low-molecular-weight heparin compounds the same? Thromb Res 2000;100:V121–30.

[45] Couturaud F, Julian JA, Kearon C. Low molecular weight heparin administered once versus twice daily in patients with venous thromboembolism: a meta-analysis. Thromb Haemost 2001;86:980–4.

[46] Greaves M. Limitations of the laboratory monitoring of heparin therapy. Scientific and Standardization Committee Communications: on behalf of the Control of Anticoagulation Subcommittee of the Scientific and Standardization Committee of the International Society of Thrombosis and Haemostasis. Thromb Haemost 2002;87:163–4.

[47] Nagge J, Crowther M, Hirsh J. Is impaired renal function a contraindication to the use of low-molecular-weight heparin? Arch Intern Med 2002; 162:2605–9.

[48] Gouin-Thibault I, Pautas E, Siguret V. Safety profile of different low-molecular weight heparins used at therapeutic dose. Drug Saf 2005;28:333–49.

[49] Gould MK, Dembitzer AD, Doyle RL, et al. Low-molecular-weight heparins compared with unfractionated heparin for treatment of acute deep venous thrombosis: a meta-analysis of randomized, controlled trials. Ann Intern Med 1999;130:800–9.

[50] Mismetti P, Laporte-Simitsidis S, Navarro C, et al. Aging and venous thromboembolism influence the pharmacodynamics of the anti-factor Xa and anti-thrombin activities of a low molecular weight heparin (nadroparin). Thromb Haemost 1998;79:1162–5.

[51] Chow SL, Zammit K, West K, et al. Correlation of antifactor Xa concentrations with renal function in patients on enoxaparin. J Clin Pharmacol 2003;43:586–90.

[52] Siguret V, Pautas E, Fevrier M, et al. Elderly patients treated with tinzaparin (Innohep) administered once daily (175 anti-Xa IU/kg): anti-Xa and anti-IIa activities over 10 days. Thromb Haemost 2000;84:800–4.

[53] Pautas E, Gouin I, Bellot O, et al. Safety profile of tinzaparin administered once daily at a standard curative dose in two hundred very elderly patients. Drug Saf 2002;25:725–33.

[54] Cestac P, Bagheri H, Lapeyre-Mestre M, et al. Utilisation and safety of low molecular weight heparins: prospective observational study in medical inpatients. Drug Saf 2003;26:197–207.

[55] Siguret V, Pautas E, Gouin I. Low molecular weight heparin treatment in elderly subjects with or without renal insufficiency: new insights between June 2002 and March 2004. Curr Opin Pulm Med 2004;10:366–70.

[56] Walenga JM, Jeske WP, Bara L, et al. Biochemical and pharmacologic rationale for the development of a synthetic heparin pentasaccharide. Thromb Res 1997;86:1–36.

[57] Choay J, Lormeau JC, Petitou M, et al. Structural studies on a biologically active hexasaccharide obtained from heparin. Ann N Y Acad Sci 1981;370:644–9.

[58] Donat F, Duret JP, Santoni A, et al. The pharmacokinetics of fondaparinux sodium in healthy volunteers. Clin Pharmacokinet 2002;41(Suppl 2):1–9.

[59] Boneu B, Necciari J, Cariou R, et al. Pharmacokinetics and tolerance of the natural pentasaccharide (SR90107/Org31540) with high affinity to antithrombin III in man. Thromb Haemost 1995;74:1468–73.

[60] Buller HR, Davidson BL, Decousus H, et al. Fondaparinux or enoxaparin for the initial treatment of symptomatic deep venous thrombosis: a randomized trial. Ann Intern Med 2004;140:867–73.

[61] Buller HR, Davidson BL, Decousus H, et al. Subcutaneous fondaparinux versus intravenous unfractionated heparin in the initial treatment of pulmonary embolism. N Engl J Med 2003;349:1695–702.

[62] Warkentin TE. Heparin-induced thrombocytopenia: pathogenesis and management. Br J Haematol 2003;121:535–55.

[63] Warkentin TE, Greinacher A. Heparin-induced thrombocytopenia: recognition, treatment, and prevention: the Seventh ACCP Conference on Antithrombotic and Thrombolytic Therapy. Chest 2004;126(3 Suppl):311S–37S.

[64] Forster AJ, Wells PS. The rationale and evidence for the treatment of lower-extremity deep venous thrombosis with thrombolytic agents. Curr Opin Hematol 2002;9:437–42.

[65] Dalen JE, Alpert JS, Hirsh J. Thrombolytic therapy for pulmonary embolism: is it effective? Is it safe? When is it indicated? Arch Intern Med 1997;157:2550–6.

[66] Jerjes-Sanchez C, Ramirez-Rivera A, de Lourdes Garcia M, et al. Streptokinase and heparin versus heparin alone in massive pulmonary embolism: a randomized controlled trial. J Thromb Thrombolysis 1995;2:227–9.

[67] Meneveau N, Bassand JP, Schiele F, et al. Safety of thrombolytic therapy in elderly patients with massive pulmonary embolism: a comparison with non-elderly patients. J Am Coll Cardiol 1993;22:1075–9.

[68] Gisselbrecht M, Diehl JL, Meyer G, et al. Clinical presentation and results of thrombolytic therapy in older patients with massive pulmonary embolism: a comparison with non-elderly patients. J Am Geriatr Soc 1996;44:189–93.

[69] Mikkola KM, Patel SR, Parker JA, et al. Increasing age is a major risk factor for hemorrhagic complications after pulmonary embolism thrombolysis. Am Heart J 1997;134:69–72.

[70] Ansell J, Hirsh J, Poller L, et al. The pharmacology and management of the vitamin K antagonists: the Seventh ACCP Conference on Antithrombotic and Thrombolytic Therapy. Chest 2004;126(3 Suppl):204S–33S.

[71] Prins MH, Hutten BA, Koopman MM, et al. Long-term treatment of venous thromboembolic disease. Thromb Haemost 1999;82:892–8.

[72] Hull R, Hirsh J, Jay R, et al. Different intensities of oral anticoagulant therapy in the treatment of proximal-vein thrombosis. N Engl J Med 1982;307:1676–81.

[73] Khamashta MA, Cuadrado MJ, Mujic F, et al. The management of thrombosis in the antiphospholipid-antibody syndrome. N Engl J Med 1995;332:993–7.

[74] Rosove MH, Brewer PM. Antiphospholipid thrombosis: clinical course after the first thrombotic event in 70 patients. Ann Intern Med 1992;117:303–8.

[75] Crowther MA, Ginsberg JS, Julian J, et al. A comparison of two intensities of warfarin for the prevention of recurrent thrombosis in patients with the antiphospholipid antibody syndrome. N Engl J Med 2003;349:1133–8.

[76] Finazzi G, Marchioli R, Brancaccio V, et al. A randomized clinical trial of high-intensity warfarin vs. conventional antithrombotic therapy for the prevention of recurrent thrombosis in patients with the antiphospholipid syndrome (WAPS). J Thromb Haemost 2005;3:848–53.

[77] Kearon C, Ginsberg JS, Kovacs MJ, et al. Comparison of low-intensity warfarin therapy with conventional-intensity warfarin therapy for long-term prevention of recurrent venous thromboembolism. N Engl J Med 2003;349:631–9.

[78] Harrison L, Johnston M, Massicotte MP, et al. Comparison of 5-mg and 10-mg loading doses in initiation of warfarin therapy. Ann Intern Med 1997;126:133–6.

[79] Crowther MA, Ginsberg JB, Kearon C, et al. A randomized trial comparing 5-mg and 10-mg warfarin loading doses. Arch Intern Med 1999; 159:46–8.

[80] Kovacs MJ, Rodger M, Anderson DR, et al. Comparison of 10-mg and 5-mg warfarin initiation nomograms together with low-molecular-weight heparin for outpatient treatment of acute venous thromboembolism: a randomized, double-blind, controlled trial. Ann Intern Med 2003; 138:714–9.

[81] Kovacs MJ, Cruickshank M, Wells PS, et al. Randomized assessment of a warfarin nomogram for initial oral anticoagulation after venous thromboembolic disease. Haemostasis 1998;28:62–9.

[82] O'Connell MB, Kowal PR, Allivato CJ, et al. Evaluation of warfarin initiation regimens in elderly inpatients. Pharmacotherapy 2000;20:923–30.

[83] Gage BF, Fihn SD, White RH. Management and dosing of warfarin therapy. Am J Med 2000;109: 481–8.

[84] Landefeld CS, Goldman L. Major bleeding in outpatients treated with warfarin: incidence and prediction by factors known at the start of outpatient therapy. Am J Med 1989;87:144–52.

[85] Beyth RJ, Quinn LM, Landefeld CS. Prospective evaluation of an index for predicting the risk of major bleeding in outpatients treated with warfarin. Am J Med 1998;105:91–9.

[86] Ageno W, Turpie AG. Exaggerated initial response to warfarin following heart valve replacement. Am J Cardiol 1999;84:905–8.

[87] Mungall D, White R. Aging and warfarin therapy. Ann Intern Med 1992;117:878–9.

[88] Kearon C, Gent M, Hirsh J, et al. A comparison of three months of anticoagulation with extended anticoagulation for a first episode of idiopathic venous thromboembolism. N Engl J Med 1999;340: 901–7.

[89] Agnelli G, Prandoni P, Santamaria MG, et al. Three months versus one year of oral anticoagulant therapy for idiopathic deep venous thrombosis. Warfarin Optimal Duration Italian Trial Investigators. N Engl J Med 2001;345:165–9.

[90] Palareti G, Leali N, Coccheri S, et al. Bleeding complications of oral anticoagulant treatment: an inception-cohort, prospective collaborative study (ISCOAT). Italian Study on Complications of Oral Anticoagulant Therapy. Lancet 1996;348: 423–8.

[91] Landefeld CS, Beyth RJ. Anticoagulant-related bleeding: clinical epidemiology, prediction, and prevention. Am J Med 1993;95:315–28.

[92] White RH, Beyth RJ, Zhou H, et al. Major bleeding after hospitalization for deep-venous thrombosis. Am J Med 1999;107:414–24.

[93] Linkins LA, Choi PT, Douketis JD. Clinical impact of bleeding in patients taking oral anticoagulant therapy for venous thromboembolism: a meta-analysis. Ann Intern Med 2003;139:893–900.

[94] Pengo V, Legnani C, Noventa F, et al. Oral anticoagulant therapy in patients with nonrheumatic atrial fibrillation and risk of bleeding. A Multicenter Inception Cohort Study. Thromb Haemost 2001;85:418–22.

[95] Gurwitz JH, Goldberg RJ, Holden A, et al. Age-related risks of long-term oral anticoagulant therapy. Arch Intern Med 1988;148:1733–6.

[96] Wickramasinghe LS, Basu SK, Bansal SK. Long-term oral anticoagulant therapy in elderly patients. Age Ageing 1988;17:388–96.

[97] Forfar JC. Prediction of hemorrhage by during long-term oral coumarin anticoagulation by excessive prothrombin ratio. Am Heart J 1982;103: 445–6.

[98] Launbjerg J, Egeblad H, Heaf J, et al. Bleeding complications to oral anticoagulant therapy: multivariate analysis of 1010 treatment years in 551 outpatients. J Intern Med 1991;229:351–5.

[99] Wittkowsky AK, Whitely KS, Devine EB, et al. Effect of age on international normalized ratio at the time of major bleeding in patients treated with warfarin. Pharmacotherapy 2004;24:600–5.

[100] McCormick D, Gurwitz JH, Goldberg RJ, et al. Long-term anticoagulation therapy for atrial fibrillation in elderly patients: efficacy, risk, and current patterns of use. J Thromb Thrombolysis 1999;7: 157–63.

[101] Ryan PJ, Gilbert M, Rose PE. Computer control of anticoagulant dose for therapeutic management. BMJ 1989;299:1207–9.

[102] Wyld PJ, West D, Wilson TH. Computer dosing in anticoagulant clinics: the way forward? Clin Lab Haematol 1988;10:235–6.

[103] Ryan PJ, Gilbert M, Rose PE. Computer control of anticoagulant dose for therapeutic management. BMJ 1989;299:1207–9.

[104] Poller L, Wright D, Rowlands M. Prospective comparative study of computer programs used for management of warfarin. J Clin Pathol 1993;46: 299–303.

[105] Poller L, Shiach CR, MacCallum PK, et al. Multicentre randomised study of computerised

anticoagulant dosage. European Concerted Action on Anticoagulation. Lancet 1998;352:1505–9.

[106] Cromheecke ME, Levi M, Colly LP, et al. Oral anticoagulation self-management and management by a specialist anticoagulation clinic: a randomised cross-over comparison. Lancet 2000;356:97–102.

[107] Ansell J, Hirsh J, Dalen J, et al. Managing oral anticoagulant therapy. Chest 2001;119(1 Suppl): 22S–38S.

[108] Kuijer PM, Hutten BA, Prins MH, et al. Prediction of the risk of bleeding during anticoagulant treatment for venous thromboembolism. Arch Intern Med 1999;159:457–60.

[109] Lee AY, Levine MN, Baker RI, et al. Low-molecular-weight heparin versus a coumarin for the prevention of recurrent venous thromboembolism in patients with cancer. N Engl J Med 2003;349:146–53.

[110] Hull R, Pineo GF, Mah A. A randomized trial evaluating long-term low-molecular-weight heparin therapy for three months versus intravenous heparin followed by warfarin sodium [abstract]. Blood 2002;100:148a.

[111] van der Heijden MH, Hutten BA, Buller H, et al. Vitamin K antagonists or low-molecular-weight heparin for the long term treatment of systematic venous thromboembolism. Cochrane Database Syst Rev 2001;3:CD002001.

[112] Veiga F, Escriba A, Maluenda MP, et al. Low molecular weight heparin (enoxaparin) versus oral anticoagulant therapy (acenocoumarol) in the long-term treatment of deep venous thrombosis in the elderly: a randomized trial. Thromb Haemost 2000;84:559–64.

[113] Luk C, Wells PS, Anderson D, et al. Extended outpatient therapy with low molecular weight heparin for the treatment of recurrent venous thromboembolism despite warfarin therapy. Am J Med 2001;111:270–3.

[114] Decousus H, Leizorovicz A, Parent F, et al. A clinical trial of vena caval filters in the prevention of pulmonary embolism in patients with proximal deep-vein thrombosis. Prevention du Risque d'Embolie Pulmonaire par Interruption Cave Study Group. N Engl J Med 1998;338:409–15.

[115] Schulman S, Wahlander K, Lundstrom T, et al. Secondary prevention of venous thromboembolism with the oral direct thrombin inhibitor ximelagatran. N Engl J Med 2003;349:1713–21.

[116] Fiessinger JN, Huisman MV, Davidson BL, et al. Ximelagatran vs low-molecular-weight heparin and warfarin for the treatment of deep vein thrombosis: a randomized trial. JAMA 2005;293:681–9.

[117] Buller HR, Cohen AT, Davidson B, et al. Idraparinux versus standard therapy for venous thromboembolic disease. N Engl J Med 2007;357(11):1094–104.

[118] Brandjes DP, Buller HR, Heijboer H, et al. Randomised trial of effect of compression stockings in patients with symptomatic proximal-vein thrombosis. Lancet 1997;349:759–62.

[119] Prandoni P. Below-knee compression stockings for prevention of the post-thrombotic syndrome: a randomized study [abstract]. Pathophysiol Haemost Thromb 2002;32(Suppl 2):72.

[120] Prandoni P, Lensing AW, Prins MH, et al. Below-knee elastic compression stockings to prevent the post-thrombotic syndrome: a randomized, controlled trial. Ann Intern Med 2004;141:249–56.

[121] Kearon C, Ginsberg JS, Anderson DR, et al. Comparison of 1 month with 3 months of anticoagulation for a first episode of venous thromboembolism associated with a transient risk factor. J Thromb Haemost 2004;2:743–9.

[122] Sudlow MF, Campbell IA, Angel JH, et al. Optimum duration of anticoagulation for deep-vein thrombosis and pulmonary embolism. Research Committee of the British Thoracic Society. Lancet 1992;340:873–6.

[123] Levine MN, Hirsh J, Gent M, et al. Optimal duration of oral anticoagulant therapy: a randomized trial comparing four weeks with three months of warfarin in patients with proximal deep vein thrombosis. Thromb Haemost 1995;74:606–11.

[124] Pinede L, Ninet J, Duhaut P, et al. Comparison of 3 and 6 months of oral anticoagulant therapy after a first episode of proximal deep vein thrombosis or pulmonary embolism and comparison of 6 and 12 weeks of therapy after isolated calf deep vein thrombosis. Circulation 2001;103:2453–60.

[125] Baglin T, Luddington R, Brown K, et al. Incidence of recurrent venous thromboembolism in relation to clinical and thrombophilic risk factors: prospective cohort study. Lancet 2003;362:523–6.

[126] Agnelli G, Prandoni P, Becattini C. Extended oral anticoagulant therapy after a first episode of pulmonary embolism. Ann Intern Med 2003;139:19–25.

[127] Schulman S, Svenungsson E, Granqvist S. Anticardiolipin antibodies predict early recurrence of thromboembolism and death among patients with venous thromboembolism following anticoagulant therapy. Duration of Anticoagulation Study Group. Am J Med 1998;104:332–8.

[128] Schulman S, Granqvist S, Holmstrom M, et al. The duration of oral anticoagulant therapy after a second episode of venous thromboembolism. The Duration of Anticoagulation Trial Study Group. N Engl J Med 1997;336:393–8.

[129] Levine JS, Branch DW, Rauch J. The antiphospholipid syndrome. N Engl J Med 2002;346:752–63.

[130] Prandoni P, Lensing AW, Cogo A, et al. The long-term clinical course of acute deep venous thrombosis. Ann Intern Med 1996;125:1–7.

[131] Kearon C, Crowther M, Hirsh J. Management of patients with hereditary hypercoagulable disorders. Annu Rev Med 2000;51:169–85.

[132] Lindmarker P, Schulman S, Sten-Linder M, et al. The risk of recurrent venous thromboembolism in carriers and non-carriers of the G1691A allele in the coagulation factor V gene and the G20210A

allele in the prothrombin gene. DURAC Trial Study Group. Duration of Anticoagulation. Thromb Haemost 1999;81:684–9.

[133] Eichinger S, Stumpflen A, Hirschl M, et al. Hyperhomocysteinemia is a risk factor of recurrent venous thromboembolism. Thromb Haemost 1998;80:566–9.

[134] White RH, Zhou H, Romano PS. Length of hospital stay for treatment of deep venous thrombosis and the incidence of recurrent thromboembolism. Arch Intern Med 1998;158:1005–10.

[135] Heit JA, Mohr DN, Silverstein MD, et al. Predictors of recurrence after deep vein thrombosis and pulmonary embolism: a population-based cohort study. Arch Intern Med 2000;160:761–8.

[136] Kearon C. Long-term management of patients after venous thromboembolism. Circulation 2004; 110(Suppl 1):I10–8.

[137] Ridker PM, Goldhaber SZ, Danielson E, et al. Long-term, low-intensity warfarin therapy for the prevention of recurrent venous thromboembolism. N Engl J Med 2003;348:1425–34.

[138] Douketis JD, Kearon C, Bates S, et al. Risk of fatal pulmonary embolism in patients with treated venous thromboembolism. JAMA 1998;279:458–62.

[139] Simioni P, Prandoni P, Lensing AW, et al. Risk for subsequent venous thromboembolic complications in carriers of the prothrombin or the factor V gene mutation with a first episode of deep-vein thrombosis. Blood 2000;96:3329–33.

CARDIOLOGY
CLINICS

Cardiol Clin 26 (2008) 251–265

Antithrombotic and Thrombolytic Therapy for Ischemic Stroke

Oriana Cornett, MD[a], Lenore C. Ocava, MD[b,c], Manjeet Singh, MD[b],
Samit Malhotra, MD[a], Daniel M. Rosenbaum, MD[a,*]

[a]Department of Neurology, SUNY Downstate, 450 Clarkson Avenue, Brooklyn, NY 11203, USA
[b]Department of Neurology, Kennedy Center, Room 303, Albert Einstein College of Medicine,
1410 Pelham Parkway South, Bronx, NY 10461, USA
[c]Stroke Center, Jacobi Medical Center, Room 2 East 8, 1410 Pelham Parkway South, Bronx, NY 10461, USA

Stroke is the leading cause of severe disability in the adult population. More than 700,000 Americans have a stroke each year, of which approximately 200,000 are recurrent events. The risk for stroke increases exponentially with age. Approximately 29% of people aged 65 years or older die within 1 year, making stroke the third leading cause of death [1,2]. At any one time, 4.7 million people in the United States have had strokes, which results in stroke-related health care costs in excess of $18 billion per year, in addition to the cost of lost wages. Because the number of individuals aged older than 65 years is rapidly growing, there is an overwhelming need to develop therapies aimed at the prevention and treatment of this disease. The number of individuals aged older than 65 years is projected to increase from 39 million in 1995 to 69 million, or 20% of the total population, in 2030 [3].

Primary prevention of stroke

Preventing the elderly from having their first stroke requires a comprehensive multidisciplinary approach. The first objective is to identify and modify stroke risk factors, including

hypertension, diabetes mellitus, myocardial infarction, atrial fibrillation, hyperlipidemia, and asymptomatic carotid stenosis, and lifestyle factors, including smoking, alcohol use, and sedentary lifestyle. The guidelines for risk reduction have recently been reviewed [4].

In addition to lifestyle modification, recent attention has focused on the role of aspirin in reducing the risk for stroke, given its well-established efficacy in the prevention of myocardial infarction [5]. Aspirin reduces stroke by approximately 25% in patients who have clinically manifest atherosclerosis [6]. For people without clinically known vascular disease, the data are scant regarding aspirin's protective effects. A meta-analysis of five randomized trials, totaling more than 50,000 patients, found no difference in the incidence of stroke between low-risk patients randomized to receive aspirin or placebo during an average follow-up of 4.6 years. Regular use of aspirin did significantly increase the rate of intracranial hemorrhage by a relative risk factor of 1.35 [7]. The mean age of the patients in these trials, however, was 57 years. The long-term effects of aspirin for primary prevention of vascular events in the elderly remain unknown. No randomized trials have specifically investigated this question in the geriatric population. At the present time, no evidence exists to recommend aspirin for the prevention of stroke in a low-risk asymptomatic elderly population. Other studies, however, have found that aspirin may be beneficial in middle-aged women with specific stroke subtypes. A prospective observational study found

A version of this article originally appeared in *Clinics in Geriatric Medicine*, volume 22, issue 1.

* Corresponding author.
E-mail address: daniel.rosenbaum@downstate.edu (D.M. Rosenbaum).

that women aged 34 to 59 years taking one to six aspirins per week (325 mg) followed over 14 years had a lower risk for large-artery occlusive infarction compared with women who reported no aspirin use [8]. Women who took higher doses (more than 15 tablets per week), however, were approximately twice as likely to have subarachnoid hemorrhage. Current understanding of the pathophysiology of stroke is consistent with these results. Large-artery occlusive stroke is caused by in situ thrombosis, with a risk factor profile similar to coronary artery disease, for which aspirin has been shown to be protective. The authors of the study noted, however, that approximately 80% of the respondents took aspirin for headache or musculoskeletal pain, which may be irrelevant to stroke risk reduction. Whether the results of this trial apply to men and the elderly awaits further study. Randomized trials are currently underway to address more adequately the effects of aspirin on the primary prevention of stroke.

The use of warfarin in primary prevention of thromboembolic events is discussed elsewhere in this issue.

Secondary prevention of stroke

Stroke prevention after cardioembolic stroke or transient ischemic attack

Individuals at high risk for recurrent cardioembolic stroke are managed with anticoagulants. Patients who have atrial fibrillation, the most common cause of cardioembolic stroke, should receive oral anticoagulation in the form of warfarin to reach an international normalized ratio (INR) range of 2 to 3, unless there are contraindications to warfarin. Warfarin inhibits the synthesis of vitamin K–dependent factors (VII, IX, X, and II) that are fundamental components of the "intrinsic pathway" of clotting. A recent meta-analysis found warfarin superior to aspirin for stroke prevention in patients who had atrial fibrillation and a recent transient ischemic attack (TIA) or minor stroke [9]. For patients with contraindications to warfarin, aspirin is an alternative therapy.

Warfarin is also appropriate for patients with several other high-risk sources of cardiogenic emboli who have had a previous TIA or stroke; however, randomized trials have not been conducted for every specific etiology. High-risk sources include mechanical prosthetic heart valves, recent myocardial infarction, left ventricular thrombus, and dilated cardiomyopathies [10]. Anticoagulation is contraindicated, however, in patients who have infective endocarditis. Further studies are necessary to evaluate the efficacy of anticoagulation for those patients not at high risk for recurrent stroke.

The Patent Foramen Ovale (PFO) in Cryptogenic Stroke Study was a multicenter study that evaluated transesophageal echocardiographic findings in patients randomly assigned to warfarin or aspirin in the Warfarin Aspirin Recurrent Stroke Study (WARSS). The PFO in Cryptogenic Stroke Study evaluated the results of the transesophageal echocardiographic findings of the 2206 (28%) patients in the WARSS who were randomly assigned to take warfarin (mean INR = 2.02) or aspirin. A total of 34% of the patients were found to have a PFO (36% large and 64% small). After 2 years of follow-up, there was no significant difference among those with no PFO, a small PFO, or a large PFO, with event rates of 15.4%, 18.5%, and 9.5%, respectively. In the presence of an associated atrial septal aneurysm, the 2-year events rates were not significantly different from those with a PFO alone (15.9% versus 14.5%) [11].

Of note, the correlation between a PFO and cryptogenic stroke is only in patients younger than 55 years of age [12] and is not valid in older age groups, which may have many additional risk factors and potential causes that could lead to a stroke. The risk for major bleeding during warfarin therapy was reported to be higher in older patients, especially those older than 75 years of age, when the INR is greater than therapeutic levels [13,14].

Although it was previously suggested that a lower intensity of anticoagulation decreases the risk for warfarin-related bleeding in elderly patients who have atrial fibrillation [15], a recent retrospective study showed that INRs less than 2 were not associated with lower risk for intracranial hemorrhage compared with INRs between 2 and 3 [16].

Stroke prevention after atherothrombotic stroke or transient ischemic attack

Recurrent ischemic events in patients who have had a stroke or TIA need to be prevented. According to longitudinal studies of patients who have had an ischemic stroke, 1-year mortality rates range from 15% to 25% and 5-year mortality rates range from 40% to 60%. The rate of stroke recurrence ranges from 5% to 14% in the first year and from 25% to 40% within 5 years [17]. The medical management of patients who have had a prior stroke or TIA but are not candidates for surgical intervention is discussed next.

Stroke in patients with cardiomyopathy and reduced ejection fraction

Patients who have heart failure are a well-established cohort at risk for ischemic stroke. Second to atrial fibrillation, cardiomyopathy and a low ejection fraction (EF) is the leading cause of cardiogenic ischemic stroke with a proposed mechanism of cardioembolism [18]. Analogous to clot formation in a dilated fibrillating atria, it is proposed that mural thrombus may form in a dilated ventricle, especially one with focal wall motion abnormality after myocardial ischemia. The association of a low EF with ischemic stroke led to several studies whose goal was to determine the best drug for secondary stroke prevention in these patients.

The Warfarin and Antiplatelet Therapy in Chronic Heart Failure (WATCH) trial was designed to investigate the efficacy of warfarin (goal INR: 2.5–3.0) versus aspirin at a dosage of 162 mg/d or clopidogrel at a dosage of 75 mg/d in preventing ischemic stroke and all-cause mortality in patients who have heart failure and an EF of 35% or less. This study was ended 18 months prematurely because of poor enrollment, which resulted in a lack of power to demonstrate the study objectives [19]. This left the question of appropriate antithrombotic medications with a low EF open for further study.

The National Institutes of Health funded a randomized double-blind clinical trial that hopes to determine the appropriate antithrombotic therapy in patients with a reduced cardiac EF. The Warfarin Versus Aspirin in Patients with Reduced Cardiac Ejection Fraction [WARCEF] trial enrolled 2860 patients from 70 North American and 70 European sites [18]. In the warfarin-treated patients, the target INR was 2.5 to 3.0, and the aspirin-treated patients received aspirin at a dosage of 325 mg/d. The primary objective was to determine the superiority of aspirin or warfarin in preventing all-cause mortality and all strokes, with ischemic and hemorrhagic strokes being considered in patients with a left ventricular EF of 30% or less. The trial is ongoing, but preliminary data suggest that warfarin is superior to aspirin in preventing ischemic stroke in the study population.

Antiplatelet agents

Studies have supported the efficacy and safety of antiplatelet therapy in reducing atherothrombotic stroke recurrence. Large randomized trials have shown the benefit of four different agents: (1) aspirin, (2) ticlopidine, (3) clopidogrel, and (4) dipyridamole (Fig. 1). Recent trials have also looked into the benefits of combination antiplatelet agents. Selecting the optimal antiplatelet therapy to prevent stroke recurrence, however, remains the subject of debate and controversy. In clinical practice, physicians select individual agents based on relative efficacy, availability, cost, and adverse side effects (Table 1).

Aspirin. Aspirin is the most widely used and studied antiplatelet agent. It inhibits platelet aggregation by irreversibly blocking cyclooxygenase, which is essential for the synthesis of thromboxane A2, which promotes platelet activation and vasoconstriction.

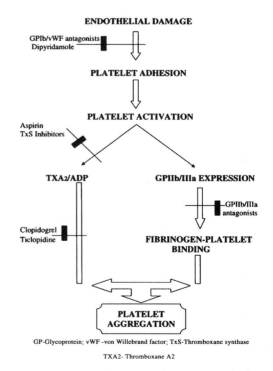

GP-Glycoprotein; vWF -von Willebrand factor; TxS-Thromboxane synthase

TXA2- Thromboxane A2

Fig. 1. Target sites of antiplatelet therapy. ADP, adenosine diphosphate; GP, glycoprotein; TxA2, thromboxane A2; TxS, thromboxane synthase; vWF, von Willebrand's factor.

Table 1
Antithrombotic agents in cerebral ischemia

Atherothrombotic stroke	Aspirin, 50–1300 mg/d	Aspirin, 25 mg + ER dipyridamole, 200 mg bid
		Clopidogrel, 75 mg/d
		Ticlopidine, 250 mg bid
Atherothrombotic stroke and aspirin-intolerant or recurrent stroke during aspirin therapy	Aspirin, 25 mg, + ER dipyridamole, 200 mg bid	Ticlopidine, 250 mg bid
		Clopidogrel, 75 mg/d
		Warfarin (INR: 2–3)
		Aspirin, 50–1300 mg/d
Cardioembolic stroke	Warfarin (INR: 2–3)	If warfarin is contraindicated, then aspirin, 325 mg/d

Abbreviations: bid, twice daily; ER, extended release.

Several trials support the benefits of aspirin in patients who are at risk for stroke. The Swedish Aspirin Low Dose Trial randomized 1360 patients who had a minor stroke or TIA to aspirin at a dosage of 75 mg/d or placebo [20]. Patients in the aspirin group were found to have an 18% relative reduction in stroke plus all death. A meta-analysis of 10 trials comparing aspirin with placebo for the prevention of vascular events in patients who have cerebrovascular disease found an overall statistically significant relative risk reduction of 13% [21], which equates to 36 patients who must be treated for 2 years to avoid one vascular event.

The optimal dose of aspirin for stroke prevention has been the subject of extensive debate [22]. No clear evidence favors one dose over another. Two studies have directly compared aspirin doses. The United Kingdom Transient Ischemic Attack study, which compared aspirin at a dosage of 300 mg/d versus a dosage of 1200 mg/d versus placebo, found no differences in vascular events between the two doses [23]. The Dutch Transient Ischemic Attack Trial of 3131 patients who had a minor stroke similarly corroborated the lack of differences in vascular events between groups receiving 30 mg/d and 283 mg/d [24]. A meta-analysis by the Antiplatelet Trialists showed equivalent efficacy of high-dose (500–1500 mg/d) and medium-dose (75–325 mg/d) aspirin in preventing the composite end point of nonfatal myocardial infarction, nonfatal stroke, or vascular death [6]. A more recent meta-analysis also could find no dose-dependent relation for the efficacy of aspirin in patients who had a prior stroke or TIA [21]. These studies, and others, suggest no important differences in doses between 30 and 1200 mg for stroke prevention and a modest dose-related incidence of adverse events. Based on the results of these studies, the American College of Chest Physicians recommends the use of aspirin at a dosage of 50 to 325 mg/d [25]. There is no evidence to suggest that increasing the dose provides additional benefits to patients who have an ischemic event while taking aspirin, an occurrence commonly referred to as "aspirin failure." The typical practice is to place these patients on another antiplatelet agent or warfarin, although there are no studies directly supporting this decision.

Ticlopidine. Ticlopidine hydrochloride inhibits ADP, which participates in platelet aggregation and fibrinogen binding to the glycoprotein IIb-IIIa receptor [26]. In the Canadian American Stroke Study, ticlopidine was shown to be 30.2% more effective than placebo in preventing recurrent vascular events (including stroke) in patients who experienced a recent thromboembolic stroke [27]. The Ticlopidine Aspirin Stroke Study showed that ticlopidine at 250 mg administered twice daily is more effective than aspirin at 650 mg administered twice daily in preventing a second thromboembolic event, following patients who experienced a TIA [28]. The ticlopidine group had a 21% greater relative risk reduction for fatal and nonfatal stroke compared with the aspirin group, which translates into a number-needed-to-treat of 34 patients. Clinically relevant adverse effects noted in these trials were neutropenia, thrombocytopenia, diarrhea, and rash. Ticlopidine is also associated with thrombotic thrombocytopenic purpura [29]. It has been recommended that complete blood cell counts with differentials be monitored every 2 weeks for the first 3 months of therapy to detect blood dyscrasias. In a post hoc analysis of the Ticlopidine Aspirin Stroke Study, certain subgroups of patients were particularly benefited by the use of ticlopidine [30]. The risk-benefit profile was shown to be more favorable for nonwhites, women, and patients who have intracranial disease, in terms of a better relative risk reduction for stroke and death and fewer adverse outcomes.

The African American Antiplatelet Stroke Prevention Study (AAASPS) was specifically designed to target a population that is particularly burdened by stroke. It compared the efficacy of aspirin at 325 mg administered twice daily with ticlopidine at 250 mg administered twice daily in preventing a composite end point of stroke, myocardial infarction, and vascular death among African-American patients who have had a recent noncardioembolic ischemic stroke. The study was terminated prematurely after analysis concluded that there was a less than 1% probability that ticlopidine would be superior to aspirin in the prevention of the primary end point [31]. The AAASPS demonstrated that the number of subjects who reached the primary outcome end point did not differ between the groups assigned to ticlopidine and aspirin. There was also a nonsignificant trend for reduction of fatal and nonfatal strokes in patients treated with aspirin.

Clopidogrel. Clopidogrel is an ADP inhibitor belonging to the same chemical family as ticlopidine. The Clopidogrel versus Aspirin in Patients at Risk of Ischemic Events (CAPRIE) study evaluated its antithrombotic effects. Unlike earlier antiplatelet trials that solely involved patients who had a stroke and TIA, however, the CAPRIE study evaluated 19,185 patients who had a previous ischemic stroke, myocardial infarction, or atherosclerotic peripheral arterial disease, comparing clopidogrel at a dosage of 75 mg/d with aspirin at a dosage of 325 mg/d [32]. Efficacy was determined by the subsequent occurrence of ischemic stroke, myocardial infarction, or vascular death. The incidence of any one of these outcomes was 5.32% per year in the clopidogrel group compared with 5.83% per year in the aspirin group, a small but statistically significant difference. A total of 200 more patients need to be treated with clopidogrel to prevent one more vascular event. For the stroke group of 6431 patients, no statistically significant benefit was found for clopidogrel over aspirin for the defined end point or for recurrent stroke alone. These results suggest that clopidogrel is at least as effective as aspirin in the prevention of secondary thromboembolic events. The CAPRIE trial showed a better side effect profile for clopidogrel. The clopidogrel-treated group had a 0.1% incidence of neutropenia and a 0.26% incidence of thrombocytopenia. No major differences in gastrointestinal symptoms were found between clopidogrel and aspirin, but clopidogrel did cause rash and diarrhea more

frequently than aspirin. More recently, however, thrombotic thrombocytopenic purpura has been shown to occur after the initiation of clopidogrel therapy [33]. Based on existing data, it is the authors' opinion that there is no clear indication to prescribe clopidogrel over aspirin for the prevention of recurrent atherothrombotic stroke unless the patient is aspirin-intolerant.

Combination of antiplatelet agents

Individual antiplatelet agents with different mechanisms of action have been proved safe and effective in preventing recurrent ischemic events, albeit with modest benefits. Despite a lack of scientific evidence, many physicians use combinations of these agents, assuming greater benefit from the combination than when using each agent alone. The clinical studies that address this practice are discussed next.

Aspirin and dipyridamole. The fixed-dose combination of aspirin (25 mg) and extended-release dipyridamole (200 mg) combines two antiplatelet agents with different mechanisms of action. Dipyridamole inhibits platelet aggregation by inhibiting the uptake of adenosine and phosphodiesterase. Although previous studies found no benefit of adding dipyridamole (immediate-release) to aspirin, a fourth study did find benefit. In the European Stroke Prevention Study-2 of 6602 patients who had a prior ischemic stroke or TIA, aspirin and extended-release dipyridamole were found to be twice as effective as either agent alone in the prevention of a second stroke after 2 years [34]. Extended-release dipyridamole (200 mg administered twice daily) and aspirin (25 mg administered twice daily) were both found to afford significant reductions in stroke recurrence (16% and 18%, respectively) compared with placebo, whereas the combination of aspirin and extended-release dipyridamole resulted in a 37% risk reduction. When combined with the previous trials of dipyridamole and aspirin, the combination reduces the risk for stroke by 23% compared with aspirin alone [35]. The absolute risk reduction of the combination in the European Stroke Prevention Study-2 was 3% at the end of 2 years. The most common adverse event with aspirin and extended-release dipyridamole was headache (39.2%), which was more frequent at the onset of therapy, with a tendency to diminish over days as tolerance to dipyridamole develops. The incidence of dyspepsia with aspirin and extended-release dipyridamole was similar to that with aspirin alone (18.4% versus 18.1%), whereas the incidence of gastrointestinal bleeding was comparable to that with aspirin (4.1% versus 3.2%). Post hoc analysis of the European Stroke Prevention Study-2 data reports no increased risk for angina pectoris or myocardial infarction in those patients who had ischemic heart disease at baseline [36].

Aspirin and clopidogrel. The efficacy of the combination of aspirin and clopidogrel was first described in the Clopidogrel in Unstable Angina to Prevent Recurrent Events trial. This trial enrolled 12,562 patients who had unstable angina or suspected myocardial infarction, who were randomized to clopidogrel at a dosage of 75 mg/d or placebo for a duration of 3 to 12 months. All the patients received aspirin at a dosage of 75 mg/d to 325 mg/d [37]. The primary outcome measure consisted of cardiovascular death, nonfatal myocardial infarction, and stroke. The primary outcome event occurred in 9.3% of patients in the clopidogrel-aspirin group and in 11.4% of patients taking aspirin alone, yielding a relative risk reduction of 20%. This equates to 48 patients who must be treated to avoid one primary outcome event. There was a higher rate of major bleeding in the clopidogrel-aspirin group (3.7% versus 2.7%), which equates to a 1% absolute excess of major bleeding complications. Minor bleeding complications were also twice as common in the clopidogrel-aspirin group (5.1% versus 2.4%). Although the Clopidogrel in Unstable Angina to Prevent Recurrent Events trial demonstrated increased efficacy of the combination of clopidogrel and aspirin against vascular events, some of its benefits are counteracted by the associated increased bleeding risk. It is also notable that the rate of stroke as the outcome event is rather low for both groups (1.2% with clopidogrel-aspirin versus 1.4% with aspirin alone).

The superiority of the combination of clopidogrel and aspirin in stroke prevention was evaluated in the Management of Atherothrombosis with Clopidogrel in High-Risk Patients with Recent TIA or Ischemic Stroke trial. This trial enrolled 7599 high-risk patients within 90 days of having had a TIA or ischemic stroke and at least one additional vascular risk factor. Patients were randomized to clopidogrel alone at a dosage of 75 mg/d or to a combination of clopidogrel and aspirin at a dosage of 75 mg/d [38]. The study did not show any significant benefit of taking the combination over clopidogrel alone. A total of

15.7% of patients taking clopidogrel and aspirin reached the primary outcome event of cardiovascular death, nonfatal myocardial infarction, stroke, or rehospitalization for an acute ischemic event, whereas 16.7% of those taking clopidogrel alone experienced an outcome event. More concerning is a statistically significant excess of life-threatening hemorrhage, up to a 1.3% absolute risk increase, in patients taking the clopidogrel-aspirin combination (2.6% versus 1.3% in the clopidogrel-alone group).

The Prevention Regimen for Effectively Avoiding Second Strokes [PRoFESS] trial is designed to evaluate whether aspirin plus extended-release dipyridamole is superior to clopidogrel in preventing stroke in patients who have had an ischemic stroke or TIA [39]. The trial is also designed to compare telmisartan, an angiotensin receptor inhibitor, with placebo to assess whether its addition further reduces stroke risk. The primary outcome is time to repeated event. The study is taking place in 35 countries and 720 centers, with enrollment of more than 20,000 patients. This makes it the largest secondary stroke prevention trial ever undertaken. It is expected to conclude in 2008.

The European/Australian Stroke Prevention in Reversible Ischemia Trial is an ongoing international, multicenter, randomized, nonblind, controlled trial to compare the safety and prophylactic efficacies of mild anticoagulants—aspirin in conjunction with dipyridamole and aspirin alone—against future vascular events in patients who have atherosclerotic cerebral ischemia. This trial is to be divided into three subprotocols: (1) scheme A is going to compare anticoagulants, aspirin combined with dipyridamole, and aspirin alone; (2) scheme B is going to compare aspirin in conjunction with dipyridamole with aspirin alone; and (3) scheme C is going to compare aspirin with anticoagulants. This study is going to include patients who present within 6 months of an atherosclerotic TIA or nondisabling stroke (Rankin Scale score ≤3) and is to be randomized into one of the three schemes. The mean follow-up is planned to be 3 years. The primary outcome is the composite of vascular death, stroke, myocardial infarction, or major bleeding. Outcome assessment is blinded [40].

Any of the antiplatelet agents are acceptable as first-line therapy. When deciding which agent to choose, many experts have made indirect comparisons, keeping in mind that each study had a different study design, patient population, analytic method, and inclusion-exclusion criteria [41,42]. For the prevention of stroke, myocardial infarction, or vascular death during 2 years of therapy, 10 events would be avoided with clopidogrel, an estimated 25 with ticlopidine, and approximately 35 with the aspirin and extended-release dipyridamole combination. In light of the new data from the AAASPS and the Management of Atherothrombosis with Clopidogrel in High-Risk Patients with Recent TIA or Ischemic Stroke trial, however, the only treatment that has been demonstrated to be more effective than aspirin in the prevention of recurrent stroke is the combination of aspirin at 50 mg/d and extended-release dipyridamole at 400 mg/d. The authors recommend that the aspirin-dipyridamole combination be considered when the primary treatment goal is prevention of recurrent stroke rather than myocardial infarction; however, its higher cost might prohibit its use as initial therapy.

Oral anticoagulation

Anticoagulation has been available clinically since 1937 [43], but the indications for its use and its efficacy in treating ischemic stroke remain controversial despite numerous clinical trials. Most of the studies were performed in the 1960s, before CT became available, and were not conducted in a randomized double-blind fashion [44]. Their results and interpretation may have been subjected to criticism. Current clinical trials aimed to address this same issue have failed to show the benefit of using warfarin over aspirin in preventing recurrent ischemic stroke.

The Stroke Prevention in Reversible Ischemia Trial, which compared high-intensity oral anticoagulation (INR: 3–4.5) with aspirin at a dosage of 30 mg/d in patients who had a recent TIA or minor stroke, was terminated prematurely because of a high rate of major hemorrhage in the warfarin group [45]. More recent trials have compared lower intensity anticoagulation with aspirin.

The WARSS was a multicenter, double-blind, randomized trial that enrolled a total of 2206 patients between the ages of 30 and 85 years who had an ischemic stroke in the past 30 days with a Glasgow Coma Scale score of 3 or more, and randomized these patients to take warfarin to an INR of 1.8 to 2.4 or aspirin at a dosage of 325 mg/d [46]. These patients had to be acceptable candidates for warfarin therapy and did not have a high-risk cardioembolic source or an indication for endarterectomy. The primary end points in this study were death or a recurrent ischemic event. The study demonstrated that warfarin is not superior to aspirin, with the end point events occurring in 17.8% of patients treated with warfarin and in 16% of patients treated with aspirin. The incidence of major hemorrhage was found to be low, with a rate of 2.22 per 100 patient-years in the patients treated with warfarin and 1.49 per 100 patient-years in the patients treated with aspirin.

The antiphospholipid antibodies and subsequent thrombo-occlusive events in patients with ischemic stroke study is a prospective cohort within the WARSS that included 1770 (80%) of 2206 WARSS patients tested for antiphospholipid within 90 days of their event and before randomization [47]. A total of 41% of these patients were classified as antiphospholipid-positive. The trial did not show an increased risk for death or subsequent vascular occlusive events over 2 years in antiphospholipid-positive patients (24.2% in antiphospholipid-positive patients and 24% in antiphospholipid-negative patients) or any difference in the response to treatment with warfarin or aspirin in antiphospholipid-positive patients (26.2% in the warfarin group versus 22.2% in the aspirin group). The authors of the report advised that the results of the study cannot definitively state that no such relation exists for younger patients who have a stroke, who may have other features of the antiphospholipid syndrome, or with multiple cerebrovascular events. The result of this trial has been criticized because of the use of low-intensity INR. A double-blind randomized trial, however, did not demonstrate lower event rates, with INRs of 3 to 4 compared with INRs of 2 to 3 [48].

Another clinical trial comparing the efficacy of warfarin with aspirin was the Warfarin Aspirin in Symptomatic Intracranial Disease trial, a prospective, double-blind, multicenter trial that specifically studied a population with angiographically proved symptomatic intracranial stenosis. Patients were treated with warfarin at a dose adjusted to maintain an INR between 2 and 3 or with aspirin at a daily dose of 1300 mg. The primary end point was ischemic stroke, brain hemorrhage, or death from vascular causes other than stroke. The study was prematurely stopped in July 2003, however, when 569 patients had been randomized, and the average length of follow-up was 1.8 years on the recommendation of the external Performance and Safety Monitoring Committee [49]. The study found that the adverse events (eg, death, major hemorrhage, myocardial infarction), or sudden death, were significantly higher in patients treated with warfarin (9.7%, 8.3%, and 7.3%, respectively) when compared with the aspirin-treated group, in which adverse events were comparatively lower (4.3%, 3.2%, and 2.9%, respectively). The rates of death occurring from vascular causes and death occurring from nonvascular causes were 5.9% and 3.8%, respectively, in the warfarin-treated group as compared with the aspirin-treated group, which showed rates of 3.2% and 1.1%, respectively. Finally, the primary end points, such as ischemic stroke, brain hemorrhage, or death from vascular causes other than stroke, occurred in 22.1% of patients on aspirin and in 21.8% of those treated with warfarin. The data strongly suggested an adverse outcome in patients treated with warfarin when compared with aspirin, and this was the reason for the early termination of this study.

Warfarin should not be routinely prescribed as a first-line agent in patients who have ischemic stroke without a definite cardioembolic source of emboli. For patients who have prothrombotic disorders, oral anticoagulation with warfarin may be superior to antiplatelet agents to prevent recurrent ischemic events [50].

Acute stroke treatment with thrombolytics, anticoagulants, antiplatelet agents, neuroprotection, and mechanical devices

Acute stroke therapy is targeted at restoring perfusion to ischemic tissue by thrombolysis of an obstructing clot or limiting the ischemic cascade of biochemical events by means of neuroprotective agents. The former has demonstrated relative success; the latter has yet to achieve clinical efficacy in human patients.

Thrombolytic agents

The approval of the use of intravenous recombinant tissue plasminogen activator (rt-PA) by the United States Food and Drug Administration (FDA) for thrombolysis in patients within the first 3 hours of acute ischemic stroke came as a result of large multicenter, randomized, double-blind, placebo-controlled trials, which investigated its efficacy.

In 1995, the National Institute of Neurological Disorders and Stroke (NINDS) published the result of a clinical trial that used rt-PA to treat ischemic stroke within 3 hours from the onset of symptoms [51]. This study consisted of 625 patients assigned randomly to placebo or intravenous rt-PA at dose of 0.9 mg/kg (maximum dose of 90 mg). Although no significant early benefit was noticed within the first 24 hours of treatment, there was an 11% absolute increase in the number of patients with little or no deficits among those receiving rt-PA compared with those receiving placebo at 3 months. Furthermore, during 12 months of follow-up, the patients who received rt-PA were more likely to have minimal or no disability than the patients given placebo [52].

Although the treatment window is 3 hours long, treatment should be initiated as early as possible for optimal results. Patients treated within 90 minutes from the onset of symptoms have better outcomes than those treated within 90 to 180 minutes from the onset of symptoms. The benefit of rt-PA persisted despite the greater rate of symptomatic intracerebral hemorrhage in the first 36 hours among rt-PA recipients (6.4% versus 0.6%). Despite the increased risk for hemorrhage, there was no statistically significant difference in mortality at 3 months between the two groups.

The European Cooperative Acute Stroke Study (ECASS) randomized 620 patients who had an ischemic stroke to receive a higher dose of intravenous rt-PA (1.1 mg/kg) or placebo within 6 hours of stroke onset [53]. There was no significant benefit of rt-PA over placebo with regard to neurologic outcome, and rt-PA recipients had a significantly higher incidence of parenchymal hemorrhage (19.8% versus 6.5%), although there was no statistical difference in mortality at 30 days. The ECASS II randomized 800 patients who had an ischemic stroke to receive intravenous rt-PA at a dose of 0.9 mg/kg or placebo within 6 hours of symptom onset. The results showed no significant benefit for patients treated with rt-PA at the end of 90 days. Subsequent post hoc analysis, however, suggested benefit in patients treated within 3 hours of stroke onset. The incidence of rt-PA–related parenchymal hemorrhage was similar to that found in the earlier NINDS trial [54].

The Alteplase ThromboLysis for Acute Noninterventional Therapy in Ischemic Stroke study randomized 547 patients to treatment with intravenous rt-PA at a dose of 0.9 mg/kg or placebo within 3 to 5 hours after symptom onset [55]. There was no significant benefit of rt-PA treatment versus placebo with regard to excellent neurologic recovery, but there was a significantly increased risk for symptomatic intracerebral hemorrhage (7% versus 1.1%).

The Standard Treatment with Alteplase to Reverse Stroke trial subsequently confirmed the clinical benefit of rt-PA shown in the NINDS trial and the ability of community physicians to administer rt-PA to patients who have an acute stroke safely [56]. Strict adherence to the guidelines of the NINDS protocol is essential for safe rt-PA administration. Unfortunately, only a small fraction of patients who have an acute ischemic stroke currently meet the NINDS criteria for thrombolysis. Efforts have been directed toward public and professional education and establishing systems of organized evaluation and treatment of patients who have an acute stroke.

Conditions like migraine and seizure, which may mimic stroke, and occlusive small artery disease, large-artery atherosclerosis without thrombosis, and arterial dissections do not benefit from rt-PA but, instead, unnecessarily increase the risk for intracerebral hemorrhage. Such a risk has prompted many physicians first to document occlusive lesions with vascular imaging (MRI or magnetic resonance angiography) in addition to brain imaging before administering rt-PA [57].

Another concern that may have an impact on the safety and effectiveness of rt-PA is age. In the NINDS trial, increasing age was not an independent predictor of intracerebral hemorrhage. Age, however, did emerge as a predictor of parenchymal bleeding in post hoc analysis in the ECASS trial [58]. A retrospective study of 189 patients older than the age of 80 years examined whether rt-PA poses an increased risk to the elderly and found no differences in the incidence of bleeding or functional outcome in such patients compared with their counterparts younger than 80 years of age. The study was limited by the low sample number, the absence of long-term follow-up, and a selective patient population primarily managed by stroke specialists, however [59]. Larger prospective studies are needed to verify these findings. Although rt-PA may pose no additional risks to the elderly for the treatment of stroke, increasing evidence suggests that it does increase the rate of intracerebral hemorrhage for the treatment of myocardial infarction in this patient group.

The Desmoteplase in Acute Ischemic Stroke trial is a promising therapeutic option that may allow a longer treatment window and, possibly, fewer hemorrhagic side effects because of the highly fibrin-specific nature of desmoteplase. This trial was a placebo-controlled, double-blind, randomized, dose-finding phase II trial that included 104 patients within 3 to 9 hours of their ischemic stroke, with National Institutes of Health Stroke Scale (NIHSS) scores of 4 to 20 and MRI evidence of perfusion-diffusion mismatch [60]. In part 1 of the trial, 47 patients were randomized to fixed doses of desmoteplase (25, 37.5, or 50 mg) or placebo; this phase was terminated because of high rates of symptomatic intracranial hemorrhage with desmoteplase (26.7%). Lower weight-adjusted doses escalating through 62.5, 90, and 125 µg/kg were then subsequently investigated in 57 patients (referred to as part 2). The safety end point was the rate of symptomatic intracranial hemorrhage, whereas the efficacy end points were the rate of reperfusion on MRI after 4 to 8 hours and clinical outcome as assessed by the NIHSS, modified Rankin Scale, and Barthel Index at 90 days. Part 2 demonstrated a symptomatic intracranial hemorrhage rate of only 2.2%, whereas the reperfusion rate was up to 71.4% with the 125-µg/kg dose in patients treated with desmoteplase as compared with only 19.2% in patients treated with placebo. In a dose-response manner, a higher favorable 90-day clinical outcome was observed in patients treated with desmoteplase at 125 µg/kg (60%) versus 62.5 µg/kg (13.3%) compared with 22.2% of patients treated with placebo. Early reperfusion correlated favorably with clinical outcome. A favorable outcome occurred in 52.5% of patients experiencing reperfusion versus 24.6% of patients without reperfusion.

Intra-arterial thrombolytic therapy

There are no drugs currently approved by the FDA for intra-arterial treatment of acute ischemic stroke, and such therapy is not standard. At present, this technique is used most commonly for patients who have an occlusive disease of a major anterior (internal carotid or middle cerebral) artery or the basilar artery. Trials have been performed to evaluate the efficacy of the urokinase precursor prourokinase. The Prolyse in Acute Cerebral Thromboembolism I trial was a phase 2 prospective, randomized, double-blind, placebo-controlled study to evaluate intra-arterial administration of recombinant prourokinase for treatment of acute ischemic stroke caused by middle cerebral artery occlusion [61]. Significant recanalization was achieved with prourokinase treatment, although 15% of the treated patients experienced intracerebral hemorrhage compared with 7% of control patients, which was not significant. The Prolyse in Acute Cerebral

Thromboembolism II trial, a phase 3 trial, also showed significant improvement in outcome with prourokinase treatment [61]. Because of nonavailability of urokinase and prourokinase in the US market, however, most medical centers have been using rt-PA for intra-arterial stroke therapy. This use is primarily based on its easy availability and its acceptance as an intravenous therapy for acute stroke.

Recently, the efficacy and safety of a combined intravenous and intra-arterial treatment approach in patients who have an acute ischemic stroke were demonstrated in the Interventional Management of Stroke Study. This study was a multicenter, open-label, single-arm pilot study that treated 80 patients with a median baseline NIHSS score of 18 with intravenous rt-PA within the first 3 hours of symptom onset and with an additional intra-arterial dose of rt-PA delivered at the site of angiographically proved thrombus [62]. The intravenous–intra-arterial approach was found to be equally safe and effective as the intravenous approach. Patients in the Interventional Management of Stroke Study had a better 90-day outcome compared with the patients in the placebo arm of the NINDS trial. A randomized trial of combined intravenous–intra-arterial recanalization compared with standard intravenous rt-PA is planned.

Anticoagulants

Many patients who miss the therapeutic window period of 3 hours or do not meet the criteria for thrombolytic therapy are sometimes treated with intravenous heparin to prevent stroke progression or recurrence. Recent trials have evaluated the efficacy and risks related to treatment with heparin, heparinoids, and low-molecular-weight heparin in these patients who have an acute ischemic stroke.

The International Stroke Trial was a large, multicenter, randomized, open trial of 19,435 patients treated within 48 hours of the onset of ischemic stroke. Patients were randomized to receive one of the four treatment regimens: (1) aspirin alone at a dose of 300 mg, (2) subcutaneous heparin at two doses (5000 U or 12,500 U) twice a day, (3) aspirin plus heparin, or (4) no aspirin and no heparin. Treatment was continued during their hospitalization, up to 14 days [63]. Outcome was determined by telephone interview at 6 months. None of the treatments offered significant benefit in the two primary outcomes:

death from any cause during the treatment period or death or dependency at 6 months. The International Stroke Trial came under a lot of criticism because of flaws in the study design that may have created a bias against heparin, including possible inclusion of patients who have a hemorrhagic stroke, because a CT scan was not an entry requirement (only 67% of patients obtained a CT scan), increased attention to possible bleeding in patients receiving heparin because treatment allocation was open, and the lack of monitoring of coagulation parameters in patients receiving heparin [64].

The Trial of ORG 10,172 in Acute Stroke Treatment was a prospective, multicenter, double-blind, placebo-controlled study of 1280 patients who had an ischemic stroke comparing the efficacy of the low-molecular heparinoid danaparoid with placebo [65]. Patients were randomized within 24 hours of symptom onset to receive intravenous danaparoid or placebo for 7 days. Daily dose adjustments were made based on factor Xa measurements. The primary outcome was based on the assessment of the modified Barthel Index and the Glasgow Outcome Scale at 3 months. Results showed no clear benefit of danaparoid therapy over placebo. Danaparoid therapy did not reduce the risk for stroke progression, which was seen in 10% of patients treated with danaparoid versus 9.9% of patients treated with placebo. Danaparoid treatment also conferred an increased risk for extracranial bleeding. Subgroup analysis of individual stroke subtypes showed a statistically significant benefit of danaparoid treatment in patients who had large-artery atherosclerosis. Favorable outcomes at 7 days were also statistically more likely in patients with a cardioembolic stroke subtype, but this did not maintain statistical significance at 3 months [66].

The initial Hong Kong trial of the low-molecular-weight heparin fraxiparine showed no significant benefit at 3 months compared with placebo, but a favorable outcome was realized at 6 months [67]. To clarify this, the Fraxiparine in Ischemic Stroke Study, a larger multicenter trial using a similar study design, was conducted. The results showed no benefit in the treatment group, with an associated higher rate of intracerebral hemorrhage [68].

At present, the benefit of anticoagulation in acute stroke therapy remains uncertain, as depicted by the numerous previously mentioned trials and because of the potential complications of hemorrhagic transformation of infarction, intracranial and extracranial bleeding, and thrombocytopenia. Specifically, older patients have been found to have a higher risk for heparin-related bleeding complications [69]. The current use of heparin in practice is based on the clinical judgment of the treating physician, after weighing the potential decrease in thromboembolism against the potential increase in bleeding risk.

Antiplatelet therapy

Although the effectiveness of heparin therapy has not been demonstrated by clinical studies, other trials support the efficacy of aspirin in acute stroke. Results from two major studies, the International Stroke Trial [63] and the Chinese Acute Stroke Trial [70], suggest that aspirin started within 48 hours of stroke onset reduces the risk for stroke recurrence and mortality. The randomized International Stroke Trial of 19,435 patients, who received aspirin or placebo for 2 weeks after acute stroke, found mortality rates of 9% and 9.4% and recurrent stroke rates of 2.8% and 3.9% in the aspirin and placebo groups, respectively. The incidence of hemorrhagic strokes did not differ between the two groups. The Chinese Acute Stroke Trial, in which 21,106 patients were randomized to receive aspirin at a dosage of 160 mg/d or placebo for up to 4 weeks, found mortality rates of 3.3% and 3.9% and recurrent stroke rates of 1.6% and 2.1% in the aspirin and placebo groups, respectively. Both trials demonstrated a small net benefit without any increased risk for intracerebral hemorrhage if aspirin is started promptly after the onset of suspected ischemic stroke. If the patient receives rt-PA, however, aspirin should be delayed for at least 24 hours. Meta-analysis of these megatrials further showed aspirin's beneficial effect in a wide range of patients. No differences in stroke reduction were found with respect to age, gender, blood pressure, stroke subtype, or the presence of atrial fibrillation. The absolute benefits of aspirin were the same for the elderly compared with a younger population [71]. Many diverse mechanisms could explain aspirin's apparent beneficial effects on the ischemic brain. Aspirin not only exerts antithrombotic effects, but its antipyretic action may protect neurons subjected to ischemic injury [72]. It remains unknown whether other antiplatelet agents with their own unique mechanisms of action reduce stroke recurrence in the acute setting.

Glycoprotein IIb-IIIa is the most important platelet membrane receptor that mediates the process of platelet aggregation and thrombus formation. Newer drugs that block this receptor play an important role in the treatment of acute coronary syndromes, whereas previous trials in patients who have had a stroke have been disappointing. An ongoing clinical trial, the Abciximab in Emergent Stroke Treatment Trial-II, is evaluating the efficacy and safety of abciximab, a monoclonal antibody against the platelet glycoprotein IIb-IIIa receptor, in the treatment of acute ischemic stroke. Some of the advantages of this trial over previous studies are the longer duration of therapeutic intervention (6 hours from the onset of symptoms) and inclusion of patients who wake from sleep with stroke symptoms in whom the planned treatment initiation is within 3 hours of awakening. Patients are randomized to receive abciximab or placebo given as a bolus (0.25 mg/kg), followed by a 12-hour infusion (0.125 µg/kg/min [10-µg/min maximum]).

Neuroprotection

Intravenous tissue plasminogen activator (t-PA) is the only treatment approved by the FDA for acute ischemic stroke. Unfortunately, it is well accepted that only a few patients are able to receive this treatment because of delays in presentation. As a result, trials have been undertaken whose goal is to lengthen the "therapeutic window" safely and provide neuroprotection in patients who have an acute ischemic stroke.

One such trial sought to reproduce the promise of the free-radical trapping agent NXY-059 as a neuroprotective agent when used in combination with intravenous t-PA in the first 6 hours after ischemic stroke. This study was conceived as a result of the Stroke-Acute Ischemic NXY Treatment I (SAINT I) trial, which demonstrated a positive trend toward reducing disability in patients who has an acute ischemic stroke who received NXY-059 within the first 6 hours after symptom onset [73]. The larger NXY-059 for the Treatment of Acute Ischemic Stroke trial, the report of which was published August 2007 in the *New England Journal of Medicine*, is a placebo-controlled trial that enrolled 3306 patients with acute ischemic stroke. It was designed to demonstrate that coadministration of intravenous t-PA and NXY-059 within 6 hours of ischemic stroke reduced the frequency of symptomatic and asymptomatic intracerebral hemorrhage. The

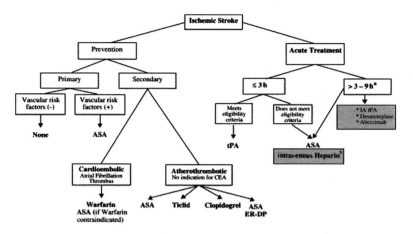

Fig. 2. Prevention and treatment of ischemic stroke. [a]Experimental or ongoing trials. [b]Used in clinical practice for specific stroke syndromes. ASA, aspirin; ER-DP, extended-release dipyridamole; IA tPA, intra-arterial tissue plasminogen activator; Ticlid, ticlopidine.

trial, however, did not validate the efficacy of NXY-059 for this purpose, because there was no statistically significant difference between this agent and placebo [73].

Mechanical embolectomy

Although intravenous t-PA is the only FDA-approved medicine for acute ischemic stroke in patients who present within 3 hours of onset, the fact remains that many stroke patients are not candidates for t-PA because of delayed presentation. The thrust in treatment of acute stroke is to provide recanalization of occluded vessels, especially in patients with large-vessel occlusion, who are not candidates for intravenous t-PA. To fill this void and treat a greater number of patients who have acute stroke, the Mechanical Embolus Removal trial in Cerebral Ischemia (MERCI) was conceived [74]. The trial attempted recanalization in patients up to 8 hours after symptom onset using the MERCI device. The trial was a single-armed prospective study that enrolled a total of 151 patients with an aim to demonstrate that the rate of recanalization in the MERCI exceeded that of spontaneous recanalization. Patients who were candidates for intravenous t-PA were excluded from this trial. Outcome and mortality were measured in this study, with good outcome corresponding to a modified Rankin Scale score of 2 and all-cause mortality. The study demonstrated that overall mortality was 44%, which is believed to be partially attributable to the fact that patients with a higher average National Institutes of Health Stroke Score (NIHSS) than in

other acute stroke trials were included. It also revealed a greater recanalization rate of 48% in patients in whom the device was used.

The Multi MERCI trial followed the MERCI trial with a newer generation device that demonstrated higher recanalization rates compared with the initial device and lower mortality and is currently extending acute stroke treatment up to 8 hours [75].

Summary

Thrombolytic and antithrombotic agents form the cornerstone of stroke treatment and prevention (Fig. 2). rt-PA, the only FDA-approved thrombolytic agent for ischemic stroke to date, improves the outcome in patients treated within 3 hours of stroke onset. The risk-benefit ratio is narrow because of an increased risk for bleeding, but studies do not support a higher risk in the geriatric population. Emerging trials are directed to extend the therapeutic window and identify agents that could provide better safety profiles. Large randomized trials have also highlighted the effectiveness and safety of early and continuous antiplatelet therapy in reducing atherothrombotic stroke recurrence. Aspirin has become the antiplatelet treatment standard against which several other antiplatelet agents (ticlopidine, clopidogrel, and aspirin-dipyridamole) have been shown to be more effective. The prevention of cardioembolic stroke is best accomplished with oral anticoagulation, barring any contraindications.

References

[1] Broderick J, Brott T, Kothari R, et al. The Greater Cincinnati/Northern Kentucky Stroke Study: preliminary first-ever and total incidence rates of stroke among blacks. Stroke 1998;29:415–21.

[2] National Stroke Association. Stroke/brain attack briefing. Englewood (CO): Post-Graduate Institute for Medicine; 1996.

[3] Day JC. Population projections of the US by age, sex, race, and Hispanic origin 1945 to 2050. Washington, DC: US Bureau of the Census, US Government Printing Office; 1996.

[4] Gorelick PB, Sacco RL, Smith DB, et al. Prevention of a first stroke: a review of guidelines and a multidisciplinary consensus statement from the National Stroke Association. JAMA 1999;281:1112–20.

[5] Bronner LL, Kanter DS, Manson JE. Primary prevention of stroke. N Engl J Med 1995;333:1392–400.

[6] Antiplatelet Trialists' Collaboration Collaborative overview of randomized trials of antiplatelet therapy—I: prevention of death, myocardial infarction, and stroke by prolonged antiplatelet therapy in various categories of patients. BMJ 1994;308: 81–106.

[7] Hart RG, Halperin JL, McBride R, et al. Aspirin for the primary prevention of stroke and other major vascular events: meta-analysis and hypotheses. Arch Neurol 2000;57:326–32.

[8] Iso H, Hennekens CH, Stampfer MJ, et al. Prospective study of aspirin use and risk of stroke in women. Stroke 1999;30:1764–71.

[9] Hart RG, Benavente O, McBride R, et al. Antithrombotic therapy to prevent stroke in patients with atrial fibrillation: a meta-analysis. Ann Intern Med 1999;131:492–501.

[10] Cerebral Embolism Task Force. Cardiogenic brain embolism. Arch Neurol 1986;43:71–84.

[11] Homma S, Sacco RL, Di Tullio MR, et al, for the PFO in Cryptogenic Stroke Study (PICSS) Investigators. Effect of medical treatment in stroke patients with patent foramen ovale. Patent Foramen Ovale in Stroke Study. Circulation 2002;105:2625–31.

[12] Cabanes L, Mas J-L, Cohen A, et al. Atrial septal aneurysm and patent foramen ovale as risk factors for cryptogenic stroke in patients less than 55 years of age: a study using transesophageal echocardiography. Stroke 1993;24:1865–73.

[13] Hylek E, Singer DE. Risk factors for intracranial haemorrhage in outpatients taking warfarin. Ann Intern Med 1994;120:897–902.

[14] Stroke Prevention in Atrial Fibrillation Investigators. Bleeding during antithrombotic therapy in patients with atrial fibrillation. Arch Intern Med 1996; 156:409–16.

[15] Yamaguchi T. Optimal intensity of warfarin therapy for secondary prevention of stroke in patients with nonvalvular atrial fibrillation: a multicenter, prospective, randomized trial. Japanese Nonvalvular Atrial Fibrillation-Embolism Secondary Prevention Cooperative Study Group. Stroke 2000;31:817–21.

[16] Fang MC, Chang Y, Hylek EM, et al. Advanced age, anticoagulation intensity, and risk for intracranial hemorrhage among patients taking warfarin for atrial fibrillation. Ann Intern Med 2004;141: 745–52.

[17] Sacco RL. Risk factors, outcomes, and stroke subtypes for ischemic stroke. Neurology 1997;49 (Suppl 4):S39–44.

[18] Pullicino P, Thompson J, Barton B, et al. Warfarin Versus Aspirin in Patients with Reduced Cardiac Ejection Fraction (WARCEF): rationale, objectives, and design. J Card Fail 2006;1(1):39–46.

[19] Massie BM, Kroll WF, Ammon SE, et al. The Warfarin and Antiplatelet Therapy in Heart Failure trial (WATCH): rationale, design, and baseline patient characteristics. J Card Fail 2004;10(2):101–12.

[20] The Swedish Aspirin Low-Dose Trial (SALT) of 75 mg aspirin as secondary prophylaxis after cerebrovascular ischemic events. The SALT Collaborative Group. Lancet 1991;338:1345–9.

[21] Albers GW, Tijssen JG. Antiplatelet therapy: new foundations for optimal treatment decisions. Neurology 1999;53(Suppl 4):S25–31.

[22] Hart RG, Harrison MJ. Aspirin wars: the optimal dose of aspirin prevent stroke. Stroke 1996;27: 585–7.

[23] The UK-TIA Study Group. United Kingdom Transient Ischemic Attack (UK-TIA) Aspirin trial final results. J Neurol Neurosurg Psychiatr 1991;54: 1044–54.

[24] The Dutch TIA Trial Study Group. A comparison of two doses of aspirin (30 mg vs. 283 mg a day) in patients after a transient ischemic attack on minor ischemic stroke. N Engl J Med 1991;325:1261–6.

[25] Sachdev GP, Ohlrogge KD, Johnson CL. Review of the Fifth American College of Chest Physicians Consensus Conference on Antithrombotic Therapy: outpatient management for adults. Am J Health Syst Pharm 1999;56:1505–14.

[26] Harker LA, Bruno JJ. Ticlopidine's mechanism of action on platelets. In: Hass WK, Easton JD, editors. Ticlopidine, platelets and vascular diseases. New York: Springer-Verlag; 1993. p. 41–59.

[27] Gent M, Blakely JA, Easton JD, et al. The Canadian American Ticlopidine Study (CATS) in thromboembolic stroke. Lancet 1989;1:1215–20.

[28] Hass WK, Easton JD, Adams HP, et al. A randomized trial comparing ticlopidine hydrochloride with aspirin for the prevention of stroke in high-risk patients. Ticlopidine Aspirin Stroke Study Group. N Engl J Med 1989;321:501–7.

[29] Steinhubl SR, Tan WA, Foody JM, et al. Incidence and clinical course of thrombotic thrombocytopenic purpura due to ticlopidine following coronary stenting. EPISTENT Investigators. Evaluation of platelet IIb/IIIa inhibitor for stenting. JAMA 1999;281: 806–10.

[30] Grotta JC, Norris JW, Kamm B. Prevention of stroke with ticlopidine: who benefits most? TASS Baseline and Angiographic Data Subgroup. Neurology 1992;42:111–5.

[31] Gorelick PB, Richardson De J, Kelly M, et al, for the African American Antiplatelet Stroke Prevention Study (AAASPS) Investigators. Aspirin and ticlopidine for prevention of recurrent stroke in black patients: a randomized trial. JAMA 2003; 289:2947–57.

[32] CAPRIE Steering Committee. A randomised, blinded trial of clopidogrel versus aspirin in patients at risk of ischaemic events (CAPRIE). Lancet 1996; 348:1329–39.

[33] Bennett CL, Connors JM, Carwile JM, et al. Thrombotic thrombocytopenic purpura associated with clopidogrel. N Engl J Med 2000;342:1773–7.

[34] Diener HC, Cunha L, Forbes C, et al. European Stroke Prevention Study. 2. Dipyridamole and acetylsalicylic acid in the secondary prevention of stroke. J Neurol Sci 1996;143(1–2):1–13.

[35] Wilterdink JL, Easton D. Dipyridamole plus aspirin in cerebrovascular disease. Arch Neurol 1999;56: 1087–92.

[36] Diener HC, Darius H, Bertrand-Hardy JM, et al. Cardiac safety in the European Stroke Prevention Study 2 (ESPS2). Int J Clin Pract 2001;55:162–3.

[37] Yusuf S, Zhao F, Mehta SR, et al. Effects of clopidogrel in addition to aspirin in patients with acute coronary syndromes without ST-segment elevation. N Engl J Med 2001;345:494–502.

[38] Diener HC, Bogousslavsky J, Brass LM, et al. Aspirin and clopidogrel compared with clopidogrel alone after recent ischaemic stroke or transient ischaemic attack in high-risk patients (MATCH): randomized, double-blind, placebo-controlled trial. Lancet 2004; 364:331–7.

[39] ESPIRIT Group. Major ongoing stroke trials. Stroke 2004;35:e359–68.

[40] Gorelick PB, Born GV, D'Agostino RB, et al. Therapeutic benefit: aspirin revisited in light of the introduction of clopidogrel. Stroke 1999;30:1716–21.

[41] Diener SC, Sacco R, Yusuf S. Rationale, design and baseline data of a randomized, double-blind, controlled trial comparing two antithrombotic regimens (a fixed-dose combination of extended-release dipyridamole plus ASA with clopidogrel) and telmisartan versus placebo in patients with strokes: the Prevention Regimen for Effectively Avoiding Second Strokes Trial (PRoFESS). Cerebrovasc Dis 2007; 23(5–6):368–80.

[42] Harbison JW. Clinical considerations in selecting antiplatelet therapy in cerebrovascular disease. Am J Health Syst Pharm 1998;55(Suppl 1):S17–20.

[43] Levine W. Anticoagulant, antithrombotic and thrombolytic drugs. In: Goodman LS, Gilman A, Kodle GB, editors. The pharmacological basis of therapeutics. New York: MacMillan; 1975. p. 1350–68.

[44] Dyken ML. Controversies in stroke: past and present. The Willis Lecture. Stroke 1993;24:1251–8.

[45] The Stroke Prevention in Reversible Ischemia Trial (SPIRIT) Study Group. A randomized trial of anticoagulants versus aspirin after cerebral ischemia of presumed arterial origin. Ann Neurol 1997;42: 857–65.

[46] Mohr JP, Thompson JLP, Lazar RM, et al. A comparison of warfarin and aspirin for the prevention of recurrent ischemic stroke. N Engl J Med 2001;345: 1444–51.

[47] Investigators APASS. Antiphospholipid antibodies and subsequent thrombo-occlusive events in patients with ischemic stroke. JAMA 2004;291:576–84.

[48] Crowther MA, Ginsberg JS, Julian J, et al. A comparison of two intensities of warfarin for the prevention of recurrent thrombosis in patients with the antiphospholipid antibody syndrome. N Engl J Med 2003;349:1133–8.

[49] Chimowitz M, Lynn M, Howlett-Smith H, et al. Comparison of warfarin and aspirin for symptomatic intracranial arterial stenosis. N Engl J Med 2005;352:1305–16.

[50] Albers GW, Amarenco P, Easton JD, et al. Antithrombotic and thrombolytic therapy for ischemic stroke: the Seventh ACCP Conference on Antithrombotic and Thrombolytic Therapy. Chest 2004; 126(3 Suppl):483S–512S.

[51] The National Institute of Neurological Disorders and Stroke rt-PA Stroke Study Group. Tissue plasminogen activator for acute ischemic stroke. N Engl J Med 1995;333:1581–7.

[52] Kwiatkowski TG, Libman RB, Frankel M, et al. Effects of tissue plasminogen activator for acute ischemic stroke at one year. National Institute of Neurological Disorders and Stroke Recombinant Tissue Plasminogen Activator Stroke Study Group. N Engl J Med 1999;340:1781–7.

[53] Hacke W, Kaste M, Fieschi C, et al. Intravenous thrombolysis with recombinant tissue plasminogen activator for acute hemispheric stroke. The European Cooperative Acute Stroke Study (ECASS). JAMA 1995;274:1017–25.

[54] Hacke W, Kaste M, Fieschi C, et al. Randomised double-blind placebo-controlled trial of thrombolytic therapy with intravenous alteplase in acute ischaemic stroke (ECASS II). Second European-Australasian Acute Stroke Study Investigators. Lancet 1998;352:1245–51.

[55] Clark WM, Wissman S, Albers GW, et al. Recombinant tissue-type plasminogen activator (Alteplase) for ischemic stroke 3 to 5 hours after symptom onset. The ATLANTIS study: a randomized controlled trial. JAMA 1999;282:2019–26.

[56] Albers GW, Bates VE, Clark WM, et al. Prospective, monitored, multicenter, post-approval experience with intravenous t-PA for treatment of acute stroke: the Standard Treatment with Alteplase to Reverse Stroke (STARS) study. JAMA 2000;283:1145–50.

[57] Caplan LR, Mohr JP, Kistler JP, et al. Should thrombolytic therapy be the first-line treatment for acute ischemic stroke? Thrombolysis: not a panacea for ischemic stroke. N Engl J Med 1997;337:1309–10 [discussion: 1313].

[58] Larrue V, von Kummer R, del Zoppo G, et al. Hemorrhagic transformation in acute ischemic stroke: potential contributing factors in the European Cooperative Acute Stroke Study. Stroke 1997;28: 957–60.

[59] Tanne D, Gorman MJ, Bates VE, et al. Intravenous tissue plasminogen activator for acute ischemic stroke in patients aged 80 years and older: the tPA stroke survey experience. Stroke 2000;31:370–5.

[60] Hacke W, Albers G, Al-Rawi Y, et al. The Desmoteplase in Acute Ischemic Stroke Trial (DIAS): a phase II MRI-based 9-hour window acute stroke thrombolysis trial with intravenous desmoteplase. Stroke 2005;36:66–73.

[61] Furlan A, Higashida R, Wechsler L, et al. Intraarterial prourokinase for acute ischemic stroke. The PROACT II study: a randomized controlled trial. JAMA 1999;282:2003–11.

[62] IMS-Study Investigators. Combined intravenous and intra-arterial recanalization for acute ischemic stroke: the Interventional Management of Stroke Study. Stroke 2004;35:904–11.

[63] The International Stroke Trial (IST). A randomized trial of aspirin, subcutaneous heparin, both, or neither among 19435 patients with acute ischaemic stroke. International Stroke Trial Collaborative Group. Lancet 1997;349:1569–81.

[64] Bousser MG. Aspirin or heparin immediately after a stroke? Lancet 1997;349:1564–5.

[65] The Publications Committee for the Trial of ORG 10172 in Acute Stroke Treatment (TOAST) Investigators. Low molecular weight heparinoid, ORG 10172 (danaparoid), and outcome after acute ischemic stroke: a randomized controlled trial. The Publications Committee for the Trial of ORG 10172 in

Acute Stroke Treatment (TOAST) Investigators. JAMA 1998;279:1265–72.

[66] Chamorro A, Vila N, Ascaso C, et al. Heparin in acute stroke with atrial fibrillation: clinical relevance of very early treatment. Arch Neurol 1999;56: 1098–102.

[67] Kay R, Wong KS, Yu YL, et al. Low-molecular-weight heparin for the treatment of acute ischemic stroke. N Engl J Med 1995;333:1588–93.

[68] Hommel M, for the FISS bis Investigators Group. Fraxiparine in Ischemic Stroke Study (FISS bis). Presented at the 7th European Stroke Conference 1998. Edinburgh, UK. Cerebrovasc Dis (Suppl 4):19.

[69] Campbell NR, Hull RD, Brant R, et al. Aging and heparin-related bleeding. Arch Intern Med 1996; 156:857–60.

[70] CAST. Randomised placebo-controlled trial of early aspirin use in 20,000 patients with acute ischaemic stroke. CAST (Chinese Acute Stroke Trial) Collaborative Group. Lancet 1997;349:1641–9.

[71] Chen ZM, Sandercock P, Pan HC, et al. Indications for early aspirin use in acute ischemic stroke: a combined analysis of 40 000 randomized patients from the Chinese Acute Stroke Trial and the International Stroke Trial. On behalf of the CAST and IST collaborative groups. Stroke 2000;31:1240–9.

[72] Correia M, Silva M, Veloso M. Cooling therapy for acute stroke. Cochrane Database Syst Rev 2000;2: CD001247.

[73] Lees KR, Zivin JA, Ashwood T, et al. NXY-057 for acute ischemic stroke. N Engl J Med 2006;354:588–600.

[74] Smith WS, Sung G, Starkman S, et al. Safety and efficacy of mechanical embolectomy in acute ischemic stroke: results of the MERCI trial. Stroke 2005;36(7):1439–40.

[75] Flint AC, Duckwiler GR, Budzik RF, et al. Mechanical thrombectomy of intracranial internal carotid occlusion: pooled results of the MERCI and Multi MERCI Part I trials. Stroke 2007;38(4):1274–80.

ELSEVIER
SAUNDERS

Cardiol Clin 26 (2008) 267–275

CARDIOLOGY
CLINICS

Reducing the Risk for Stroke in Patients Who Have Atrial Fibrillation

David A. Garcia, MD[a],*, Elaine Hylek, MD, MPH[b]

[a]Department of Internal Medicine, 1 University of New Mexico, MSC10 5550, Albuquerque, NM 87131, USA
[b]Department of Medicine, General Internal Medicine Research Unit, Boston University School of Medicine,
91 East Concord Street, Suite 200, Boston, MA 02118, USA

Atrial fibrillation (AF) is a common dysrhythmia, and its prevalence, especially among the elderly, is expected to increase significantly in the coming decades [1]. For men and women 40 years of age and older, the lifetime risk for developing AF is one in four [2]. Because disorganized electromechanical activity can lead to thrombosis within the left atrium, patients who have AF at any age have a fivefold increased risk for stroke. An estimated 15% of all strokes occur in individuals who have AF [3]. Cerebrovascular accidents related to AF have a 25% 30-day mortality rate and are more likely to result in significant disability than are noncardioembolic strokes [4–6]. Warfarin has been shown to reduce the risk for stroke in patients who have AF. Despite its proved efficacy, warfarin continues to be underused, particularly among elderly patients who are at the highest risk for stroke.

Efficacy of warfarin

During the late 1980s and early 1990s, five primary prevention trials and one secondary prevention study yielded consistent results supporting the hypothesis that warfarin can reduce the risk for stroke among patients who have AF [7–12]. In a meta-analysis of these studies, Hart and colleagues [13] determined that compared with placebo, anticoagulation with a vitamin K

antagonist, such as warfarin, can effect a 62% reduction in the relative risk for stroke among patients who have AF. A significant proportion of the strokes reported among the patients assigned to receive warfarin in these trials occurred among patients whose anticoagulation was subtherapeutic. Thus, because trial results are derived from intention-to-treat analyses, it is likely that the relative risk reduction calculated by Hart and colleagues [13] underestimates the power of warfarin to protect patients who have AF from stroke.

Safety of warfarin

Pooled analysis of the primary stroke prevention trials demonstrates that the annual rate of major hemorrhage among patients who have AF treated with warfarin is 2.3% (annual rate of intracranial hemorrhage [ICH] is 0.3%) [14]. Major hemorrhage was defined slightly differently in these trials and could be represented by a bleeding event that required a blood transfusion or an emergency procedure, led to admission, involved the central nervous system, or resulted in prominent residual impairment. ICH, because it produces sequelae that are often at least as devastating as ischemic stroke, may be a more important clinical end point. A recent meta-analysis of six randomized clinical trials indicates that compared with placebo, oral anticoagulation is associated with an absolute risk increase of 0.3% per year for ICH [13]. This is consistent with the report from a large observational cohort study that the rate of ICH (per 100 person-years) increased from 0.23 among patients not taking warfarin to 0.46 among patients who were taking warfarin

A version of this article originally appeared in *Clinics in Geriatric Medicine*, volume 22, issue 1.

* Corresponding author.
  E-mail address: davgarcia@salud.unm.edu
(D.A. Garcia).

[15]. These findings (ie, that 1 year of warfarin therapy produces an estimated one to two additional ICHs per 1000 patients) have strongly supported the hypothesis that for most patients who have AF, the benefits of warfarin substantially outweigh the risks.

Translating the results of randomized trials into clinical practice

Despite the proved benefit of warfarin and low rates of major hemorrhage, warfarin therapy remains underused in clinical practice [16–21]. The authors of a study assessing the quality of care received by Medicare beneficiaries during the period from 1998 to 1999 reported that warfarin is prescribed at hospital discharge to only 42% to 65% of patients who have documented AF [22]. There may be several reasons why high-quality evidence of the efficacy of warfarin has not had a more widespread impact on clinical practice; concerns have been raised about whether the findings of randomized controlled trials (which enrolled highly selected patients who were closely monitored) can be generalized [23]. Indeed, the relatively low enrollment rate among patients screened for the landmark primary prevention

studies raises concerns about the external validity of the results (Table 1). The paucity of elderly participants included in placebo-controlled studies of vitamin K antagonists (see Table 1) is also important, because older age has repeatedly been shown to be an independent risk factor for major bleeding on warfarin [14,24–29]. Some reassurance is provided by the low rates of hemorrhagic stroke (0.1% and 0.4%, respectively) reported among the patients assigned to receive warfarin in two large clinical trials designed to evaluate ximelagatran: Stroke Prevention using an Oral Thrombin Inhibitor in Atrial Fibrillation (SPORTIF V and SPORTIF III) [30,31]. In SPORTIF V, 42% (n = 820) of patients randomized to warfarin were aged 75 years or older, and 33% (n = 565) were in this age range in SPORTIF III. It is important to point out that for SPORTIF V and III, 84% and 74% of patients, respectively, had been taking an oral vitamin K antagonist at the time of randomization. Thus, most of the patients included in these trials were already proved to be at low risk for hemorrhage.

Like the randomized controlled trials, many observational studies of AF populations have included relatively few patients older than the age of 80 years. A notable exception is the

Table 1

Randomized controlled trials evaluating primary stroke prevention in atrial fibrillation

Study	Design	Randomized/screened	Age comment
AFASAK	Warfarin versus ASA versus placebo	1007 of 2546 patients	Median age = 74.2 years
BAATAF	Warfarin versus no warfarin (ASA permitted)	n.r.	32 of 420 patients >80 years old
Canadian Atrial Fibrillation Anticoagulation (CAFA)	Warfarin versus placebo	n.r.	Mean age = 68 years (warfarin), mean age = 67.4 (placebo)
Stroke Prevention in Atrial Fibrillation (SPAF)	Group 1: warfarin versus ASA versus placebo Group 2: ASA versus placebo	1330 of 18,376 patients	278 of 1330 patients >75 years old
SPINAF	Warfarin versus placebo	538 of 7982 patients	88 of 538 patients >75 years old
Stroke Prevention using an Oral Thrombin Inhibitor in Atrial Fibrillation (SPORTIF) III	Warfarin versus ximelagatran (open label)	3410 of 5188 patients	1146 of 3410 patients ≥75 years old
SPORTIF V	Warfarin versus ximelagatran (double blind)	3922 of 4763 patients	1658 of 3922 patients ≥75 years old

The five primary prevention studies that established the efficacy and safety of warfarin and two recent "noninferiority" studies (SPORTIF III and V) comparing warfarin with ximelagatran are shown.

Abbreviations: AFASAK, atrial fibrillation, aspirin, anticoagulation; ASA, aspirin; BAATAF, Boston area anticoagulation trial for atrial fibrillation; n.r., not reported; SPINAF, stroke prevention in nonrheumatic atrial fibrillation.

Anticoagulation and Risk Factors in Atrial Fibrillation (ATRIA) study, an observational cohort study involving more than 11,500 adults who had nonvalvular AF. The mean age of enrolled patients was 71 years, and 2211 patients taking warfarin were aged 75 years or older. Treatment with warfarin was associated with a 51% lower risk for thromboembolism compared with no warfarin therapy (no antithrombotic therapy or aspirin), and the rate of ICH was 0.46% [15].

Although reassuring, studies of prevalent warfarin use may underestimate the rate of major hemorrhage, because the early phase of therapy, which is reported to convey the highest risk, is often not included. A recent observational cohort study of individuals starting warfarin for the first time highlights the complexity of this issue. In a consecutive series of 472 patients aged 65 years or older, 7% had a major hemorrhage during the first year of warfarin treatment [32]. This relatively high rate of bleeding was likely attributable to the advanced age of the participants (153 were aged 80 years or older), the restriction of the cohort of patients newly starting warfarin, and the not infrequent use of concomitant antiplatelet therapy. In summary, further studies are needed to optimize the benefits of "real-world" anticoagulation therapy among patients older than the age of 80 years.

Antiplatelet agents

Aspirin is an inexpensive, widely available, and relatively safe medication that has several advantages over warfarin: substantially less potential for drug-drug or drug-diet interactions, a wider therapeutic index, and no need for coagulation monitoring. Although a meta-analysis of six randomized controlled trials suggests that aspirin therapy does reduce the risk for ischemic stroke among patients who have AF, the protective effect associated with aspirin use is substantially less powerful than that observed with full-intensity warfarin therapy (pooled relative risk reductions for warfarin and aspirin, compared with placebo, are 22% and 62% respectively) [33]. All six of the individual trials included in the meta-analysis demonstrated a trend favoring aspirin over placebo, but only one of these studies (the Stroke Prevention in Atrial Fibrillation [SPAF] study) [9] reported a statistically significant difference. It is noteworthy that in the SPAF study, 52% of the strokes were nondisabling. When only the 12 patients who had more severe stroke are considered, the difference between aspirin and placebo in the SPAF study is not statistically

significant. The recently published Birmingham Atrial Fibrillation Treatment of the Aged (BAFTA) trial reaffirms that warfarin is superior to aspirin as a stroke prevention strategy among patients who have AF [34].

The thienopyridine derivative clopidogrel inhibits platelet function by a mechanism different from that of aspirin; the combination of clopidogrel plus aspirin has been shown to be of significant benefit for patients who have ischemic heart disease. This strategy of combining antiplatelet therapy was less effective at preventing stroke when compared with warfarin in the Atrial Fibrillation Clopidogrel trial with Irbesartan for prevention of Vascular Events (ACTIVE-W), however [35]. The ACTIVE-A study, a clinical trial designed to determine whether clopidogrel plus aspirin is more effective than aspirin alone (among warfarin-ineligible patients who have AF), is currently near completion.

Restoring sinus rhythm

Several nonpharmacologic strategies to prevent stroke in patients who have AF have been proposed; a comprehensive discussion of these is beyond the scope of this article, but important results from trials that examined the utility of a strategy to restore and maintain sinus rhythm in patients who have AF are worthy of mention. Cardioversion for patients who have AF has several theoretic benefits, one of which is the possibility that if normal atrial electromechanical activity can be re-established, the risk for cardioembolism might be eliminated and antithrombotic therapy would be unnecessary. The strategy of rhythm control has now been directly compared with simple rate control in several randomized clinical trials that enrolled patients who had AF and were at risk for stroke [36–40]. In a pooled analysis that included three of these trials, the frequency of ischemic stroke in patients assigned to rate control versus the frequency among patients assigned to rhythm control was comparable (3.5% versus 3.9%, respectively; odds ratio [OR] = 0.50, 95% confidence interval [CI]: 0.14–1.83; $P = .30$) [41]. Based on these results, the hope that restoring sinus rhythm might obviate the need to anticoagulate patients who have AF has greatly diminished.

Optimal target international normalized ratio range

The currently recommended anticoagulation intensity for stroke prevention in AF is an international normalized ratio (INR) of 2.0 to 3.0 [42,43]. Numerous studies have documented an increased risk for bleeding with an INR of 4.0 or greater (Fig. 1) [5,44]. Compared with patients whose INR is greater than 2, patients who have AF whose INR value is less than 2 are at increased risk to have a stroke; furthermore, the strokes experienced by patients who have AF with INR values less than 2 are more likely to result in death or disability (Fig. 2) [5].

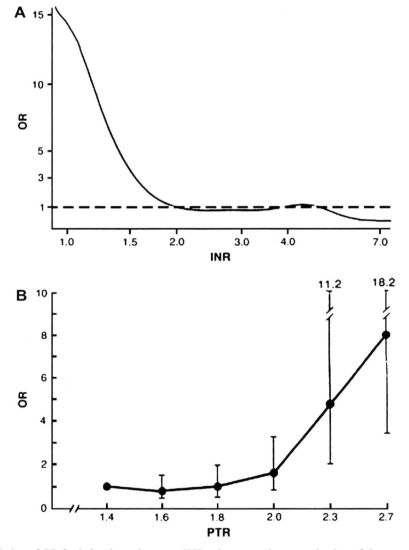

Fig. 1. (*A*) Relation of OR for ischemic stroke versus INR value at, or closest to, the time of the event. The reference value is an INR of 2.0. The dashed line corresponds to an OR of 1.0. All cases and controls had AF and were treated with warfarin. (*From* Hylek EM, Skates SJ, Sheehan MA, et al. An analysis of the lowest effective intensity of prophylactic anticoagulation for patients with nonrheumatic atrial fibrillation. N Engl J Med 1996;335:544; with permission. Copyright © 1996, Massachusetts Medical Society.) (*B*) Relation of OR for ICH versus prothrombin time ratio (PTR) value at, or closest to, the time of the event. In this display, the PTR values for the data points are the median values for the following intervals: 1.0 to 1.5, 1.6 to 1.7, 1.8 to 1.9, 2.0 to 2.1, 2.2 to 2.3, and 2.4 to 3.5. The reference interval is 1.0 to 1.5 (median PTR = 1.4). All cases and controls were taking warfarin. The INR equivalent can be roughly approximated as the square of the PTR value. (*From* Hylek EM, Singer DE. Risk factors for intracranial hemorrhage in outpatients taking warfarin. Ann Intern Med 1994;120:900; with permission.)

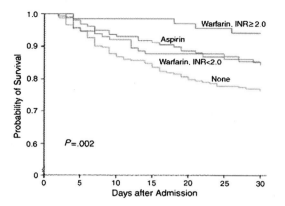

Fig. 2. Kaplan-Meier estimate of survival among non-valvular patients who have AF during the 30 days after an ischemic stroke. The patient groups are separated according to medication status at the time of admission. (*From* Hylek EM, Go AS, Chang Y, et al. Effect of intensity of oral anticoagulation on stroke severity and mortality in atrial fibrillation. N Engl J Med 2003;349:1024; with permission. Copyright © 2003 Massachusetts Medical Society.

Stroke risk assessment for individual patients

Several factors should be considered when determining whether a particular patient who has AF should receive warfarin therapy to prevent stroke: his or her baseline risk for stroke, his or her risk for bleeding on warfarin therapy, the overall burden of INR monitoring for him or her, and the patient's personal preferences. Several models and risk classification schemes are now available to assist clinicians in estimating an individual patient's annual risk for stroke [45–49]. Although these models were derived or validated in different populations, they have consistently identified important risk factors that are independently associated with an increased risk for stroke in patients who have AF. Advancing age, prior stroke, hypertension, heart failure, diabetes, and female gender are examples of such risk factors. A useful resource for estimating an individual patient's risk for stroke was derived by Wang and colleagues [49] from the Framingham Heart Study. The tool is easy to use and can be found on the Internet [50]. An adapted "point-based risk estimate" for the 5-year risk for stroke is reproduced in Fig. 3. Using this model, an 84-year-old woman with a history of diabetes and prior ischemic stroke would have an estimated 5-year risk for stroke of 48%. In contrast, a 70-year-old man with well-controlled hypertension would have a 5-year stroke risk closer to 7%.

Another often used risk classification scheme, congestive heart failure, hypertension, age > 75, diabetes mellitus, stroke ($CHADS_2$) estimates the annual risk for stroke of a patient who has AF based on the presence or absence of five risk factors (Table 2) [46]. The external validity of the $CHADS_2$ scheme is good, because the scoring system was derived from a cohort of 1733 Medicare patients who had AF. Although the simplicity of the mnemonic makes it easy to remember, the $CHADS_2$ scoring system may provide less precise risk estimates, because some factors, such as age and blood pressure, are treated as dichotomous (rather than continuous) variables.

Improving the safety margin of anticoagulant therapy

Older age is associated with lower maintenance doses of warfarin [51]. Large initiating doses of warfarin should be avoided in older patients. The warfarin dose schedule should be kept as consistent as possible to minimize dosing confusion. Clinicians should warn patients about (and remain vigilant for) medications known to interact with warfarin, especially amiodarone. Circumstantial evidence suggests that for warfarin-treated patients who must take concomitant aspirin, doses of 100 mg or less may have the most acceptable bleeding risk [52]. Anticoagulated patients who require analgesia should be counseled about the risks related to combining certain pain-relieving medications with warfarin. Nonsteroidal anti-inflammatory medications, regardless of their selectivity for cyclooxygenase inhibition, seem to increase the risk for hemorrhage among warfarin users—this association is probably related to some combination of these drugs' effects on the gastric mucosa and platelet function [53–55]. In the case of acetaminophen, augmentation of warfarin's anticoagulant effect through interference with the enzymes of the vitamin K cycle has been reported [56,57]. Aggressive blood pressure control is known to decrease the risk for ischemic and hemorrhagic stroke; appropriate antihypertensive therapy is especially important among patients taking anticoagulants [58]. Finally, it is important to warn patients about the risk for falling while taking warfarin; measures to minimize the risk of this complication should be instituted when possible.

Newer antithrombotic strategies

Because warfarin has many negative attributes (eg, narrow therapeutic window, drug-diet interactions, the need for INR monitoring), several

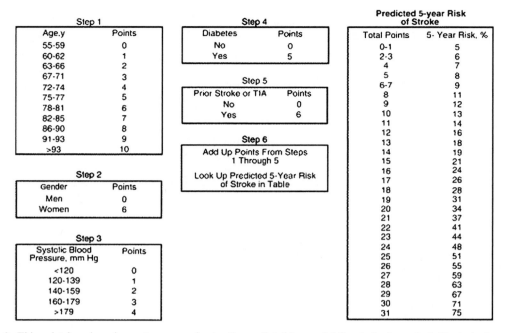

Step 1

Age.y	Points
55-59	0
60-62	1
63-66	2
67-71	3
72-74	4
75-77	5
78-81	6
82-85	7
86-90	8
91-93	9
>93	10

Step 2

Gender	Points
Men	0
Women	6

Step 3

Systolic Blood Pressure, mm Hg	Points
<120	0
120-139	1
140-159	2
160-179	3
>179	4

Step 4

Diabetes	Points
No	0
Yes	5

Step 5

Prior Stroke or TIA	Points
No	0
Yes	6

Step 6

Add Up Points From Steps 1 Through 5

Look Up Predicted 5-Year Risk of Stroke in Table

Predicted 5-year Risk of Stroke

Total Points	5-Year Risk, %
0-1	5
2-3	6
4	7
5	8
6-7	9
8	11
9	12
10	13
11	14
12	16
13	18
14	19
15	21
16	24
17	26
18	28
19	31
20	34
21	37
22	41
23	44
24	48
25	51
26	55
27	59
28	63
29	67
30	71
31	75

Fig. 3. This point-based scoring system approximates the predicted 5-year risk for stroke for an individual who has non-valvular AF. A more precise risk function is available at [50]. (*From* Wang TJ, Massaro JM, Levy D, et al. A risk score for predicting stroke or death in individuals with new-onset atrial fibrillation in the community: the Framingham Heart Study. JAMA 2003;290:1052; with permission.)

clinical trials examining alternative pharmacologic agents have been undertaken in recent years. Ximelagatran, an oral anticoagulant (direct thrombin inhibitor) that does not require coagulation monitoring, has been compared with warfarin therapy (target INR range: 2.0–3.0) for the prevention of stroke in patients who have AF. In two large randomized controlled trials (SPORTIF III and SPORTIF V) involving 7329 patients, ximelagatran proved to be at least as effective as warfarin in the prevention of stroke [30,31]. A pre-specified pooled analysis of the two studies (one was open label and one was blind) yielded annual rates of stroke or systemic embolism equal to 1.65% and 1.62% in the warfarin and ximelagatran groups, respectively ($P = .941$) [59]. Although no difference in the risk for major bleeding was observed, ximelagatran is not available because of other safety concerns that arose during review by regulatory agencies. Dabigatran, another oral direct thrombin inhibitor, is being compared with warfarin as a stroke prevention agent in a phase III trial that is nearly complete.

Idraparinux, an injectable indirect inhibitor of factor Xa, is another anticoagulant recently studied among patients who have AF. Its prolonged half-life permits once-weekly administration, and its highly predicable bioavailability precludes coagulation monitoring. A large phase III study comparing this drug with warfarin was stopped early because of excessive bleeding in the idraparinux arm. Several oral direct factor Xa inhibitors are currently in development; at the time of this writing, two of these (apixaban and rivoroxaban) are being studied in phase III AF stroke prevention trials.

Nonpharmacologic approaches

Other nonpharmacologic strategies for protecting patients who have AF from stroke (eg, the "maze" procedure, pulmonary vein isolation, occlusion or removal of the left atrial appendage, deployment of a polytetrafluoroethylene membrane) are being studied and have been described elsewhere [60–64]. At least one center has reported remarkably high rates of restoring (and maintaining) sinus rhythm using electrical ablation techniques [65]. To the authors' knowledge, however, there is no published high-quality evidence

Table 2
Risk for stroke in the National Registry of Atrial Fibrillation participants, stratified by CHADS$_2$ Score[a]

CHADS$_2$ score	No. patients (N = 1733)	No. strokes (N = 94)	NRAF crude stroke rate per 100 patient-years	NRAF adjusted stroke rate (95% CI)[b]
0	120	2	1.2	1.9 (1.2–3)
1	463	17	2.8	2.8 (2–3.8)
2	523	23	3.6	4 (3.1–5.1)
3	337	25	6.4	5.9 (4.6–7.3)
4	220	19	8	8.5 (6.3–11.1)
5	65	6	7.7	12.5 (8.2–17.5)
6	5	2	44	18.2 (10.5–27.4)

Abbreviation: NRAF, National Registry of Atrial Fibrillation.

[a] CHADS$_2$ score is calculated by adding 1 point for recent congestive heart failure, hypertension, age at least 75 years, or diabetes mellitus, and adding 2 points for having had a prior stroke or transient ischemic attack.

[b] The adjusted stroke rate is the expected stroke rate per 100 patient-years from the exponential survival model, assuring that aspirin was not taken.

From Gage BF, Waterman AD, Shannon W, et al. Validation of clinical classification schemes for predicting stroke: results from the National Registry of Atrial Fibrillation. JAMA 2001;285:2867; with permission.

demonstrating that any of these approaches reduce the risk for stroke in an unselected population that has AF.

Summary

Warfarin is highly effective at reducing the risk for stroke in AF. The benefit of oral anticoagulant therapy strongly outweighs the risk in most patients who have AF. More data are needed to define the overall risk-to-benefit ratio better for patients aged 80 years and older. Because a significant proportion of elderly individuals may not be optimal candidates for anticoagulant therapy, we must continue to evaluate alternative stroke prevention strategies while redoubling our efforts to understand the mechanisms underlying AF and thrombogenesis.

References

[1] Miyasaka Y, Barnes ME, Gersh BJ, et al. Secular trends in incidence of atrial fibrillation in Olmsted County, Minnesota, 1980 to 2000, and implications on the projections for future prevalence. Circulation 2006;114(2):119–25.

[2] Lloyd-Jones DM, Wang TJ, Leip EP, et al. Lifetime risk for development of atrial fibrillation: the Framingham Heart Study. Circulation 2004;110(9): 1042–6.

[3] Wolf PA, Abbott RD, Kannel WB. Atrial fibrillation as an independent risk factor for stroke: the Framingham Study. Stroke 1991;22(8):983–8.

[4] Lin HJ, Wolf PA, Kelly-Hayes M, et al. Stroke severity in atrial fibrillation. The Framingham Study. Stroke 1996;27(10):1760–4.

[5] Hylek EM, Go AS, Chang Y, et al. Effect of intensity of oral anticoagulation on stroke severity and mortality in atrial fibrillation. N Engl J Med 2003; 349(11):1019–26.

[6] Spratt N, Wang Y, Levi C, et al. A prospective study of predictors of prolonged hospital stay and disability after stroke. J Clin Neurosci 2003;10(6):665–9.

[7] Optimal oral anticoagulant therapy in patients with nonrheumatic atrial fibrillation and recent cerebral ischemia. The European Atrial Fibrillation Trial Study Group. N Engl J Med 1995;333(1):5–10.

[8] The effect of low-dose warfarin on the risk of stroke in patients with nonrheumatic atrial fibrillation. The Boston Area Anticoagulation Trial for Atrial Fibrillation Investigators. N Engl J Med 1990;323(22): 1505–11.

[9] Stroke Prevention in Atrial Fibrillation study. Final results. Circulation 1991;84(2):527–39.

[10] Connolly SJ, Laupacis A, Gent M, et al. Canadian Atrial Fibrillation Anticoagulation (CAFA) Study. J Am Coll Cardiol 1991;18:349–55.

[11] Ezekowitz MD, Bridgers SL, James KE, et al. Warfarin in the prevention of stroke associated with nonrheumatic atrial fibrillation. Veterans Affairs Stroke Prevention in Nonrheumatic Atrial Fibrillation Investigators. N Engl J Med 1992;327:1406–12.

[12] Petersen P, Boysen G, Godtfredsen J, et al. Placebo-controlled, randomised trial of warfarin and aspirin for prevention of thromboembolic complications in chronic atrial fibrillation. The Copenhagen AFASAK study. Lancet 1989;1:175–9.

[13] Hart RG, Pearce LA, Aguilar MI. Meta-analysis: antithrombotic therapy to prevent stroke in patients who have nonvalvular atrial fibrillation. Ann Intern Med 2007;146(12):857–67.

[14] Bleeding during antithrombotic therapy in patients with atrial fibrillation. The Stroke Prevention in Atrial Fibrillation Investigators. Arch Intern Med 1996;156(4):409–16.

[15] Go AS, Hylek EM, Chang Y, et al. Anticoagulation therapy for stroke prevention in atrial fibrillation: how well do randomized trials translate into clinical practice? JAMA 2003;290(20):2685–92.

[16] Gage BF, Boechler M, Doggette AL, et al. Adverse outcomes and predictors of underuse of antithrombotic therapy in Medicare beneficiaries with chronic atrial fibrillation. Stroke 2000;31(4):822–7.

[17] Fang MC, Stafford RS, Ruskin JN, et al. National trends in antiarrhythmic and antithrombotic

medication use in atrial fibrillation. Arch Intern Med 2004;164(1):55–60.

[18] Waldo AL, Becker RC, Tapson VF, et al. Hospitalized patients with atrial fibrillation and a high risk of stroke are not being provided with adequate anticoagulation. J Am Coll Cardiol 2005;46(9): 1729–36.

[19] Cohen N, Almoznino-Sarafian D, Alon I, et al. Warfarin for stroke prevention still underused in atrial fibrillation: patterns of omission. Stroke 2000;31(6):1217–22.

[20] Bungard TJ, Ghali WA, Teo KK, et al. Why do patients with atrial fibrillation not receive warfarin? Arch Intern Med 2000;160(1):41–6.

[21] Partington SL, Abid S, Teo K, et al. Pre-admission warfarin use in patients with acute ischemic stroke and atrial fibrillation: the appropriate use and barriers to oral anticoagulant therapy. Thromb Res 2007;120(5):663–9.

[22] Jencks SF, Cuerdon T, Burwen DR, et al. Quality of medical care delivered to Medicare beneficiaries: a profile at state and national levels. JAMA 2000; 284(13):1670–6.

[23] Hylek EM, D'Antonio J, Evans-Molina C, et al. Translating the results of randomized trials into clinical practice: the challenge of warfarin candidacy among hospitalized elderly patients with atrial fibrillation. Stroke 2006;37(4):1075–80.

[24] Warfarin versus aspirin for prevention of thromboembolism in atrial fibrillation: Stroke Prevention in Atrial Fibrillation II Study. Lancet 1994;343(8899): 687–91.

[25] Pengo V, Legnani C, Noventa F, et al. Oral anticoagulant therapy in patients with nonrheumatic atrial fibrillation and risk of bleeding. A Multicenter Inception Cohort Study. Thromb Haemost 2001; 85(3):418–22.

[26] Hylek EM, Singer DE. Risk factors for intracranial hemorrhage in outpatients taking warfarin. Ann Intern Med 1994;120:897–902.

[27] Steffensen FH, Kristensen K, Ejlersen E, et al. Major haemorrhagic complications during oral anticoagulant therapy in a Danish population-based cohort. J Intern Med 1997;242(6):497–503.

[28] van der Meer FJ, Rosendaal FR, Vandenbroucke JP, et al. Bleeding complications in oral anticoagulant therapy. An analysis of risk factors. Arch Intern Med 1993;153(13):1557–62.

[29] Landefeld CS, Rosenblatt MW, Goldman L. Bleeding in outpatients treated with warfarin: relation to the prothrombin time and important remediable lesions. Am J Med 1989;87(2):153–9.

[30] Albers GW, Diener HC, Frison L, et al. Ximelagatran vs warfarin for stroke prevention in patients with nonvalvular atrial fibrillation: a randomized trial. JAMA 2005;293(6):690–8.

[31] Olsson SB. Stroke prevention with the oral direct thrombin inhibitor ximelagatran compared with warfarin in patients with non-valvular atrial

fibrillation (SPORTIF III): randomised controlled trial. Lancet 2003;362(9397):1691–8.

[32] Hylek EM, Evans-Molina C, Shea C, et al. Major hemorrhage and tolerability of warfarin in the first year of therapy among elderly patients with atrial fibrillation. Circulation 2007;115(21):2689–96.

[33] Hart RG, Benavente O, McBride R, et al. Antithrombotic therapy to prevent stroke in patients with atrial fibrillation: a meta-analysis. Ann Intern Med 1999;131(7):492–501.

[34] Mant J, Hobbs FD, Fletcher K, et al. Warfarin versus aspirin for stroke prevention in an elderly community population with atrial fibrillation (the Birmingham Atrial Fibrillation Treatment of the Aged Study, BAFTA): a randomised controlled trial. Lancet 2007;370(9586):493–503.

[35] Connolly S, Pogue J, Hart R, et al. Clopidogrel plus aspirin versus oral anticoagulation for atrial fibrillation in the Atrial Fibrillation Clopidogrel Trial with Irbesartan for Prevention of Vascular Events (ACTIVE W): a randomised controlled trial. Lancet 2006;367(9526):1903–12.

[36] Opolski G, Torbicki A, Kosior DA, et al. Rate control vs rhythm control in patients with nonvalvular persistent atrial fibrillation: the results of the Polish How to Treat Chronic Atrial Fibrillation (HOT CAFE) Study. Chest 2004;126(2):476–86.

[37] Wyse DG, Waldo AL, DiMarco JP, et al. A comparison of rate control and rhythm control in patients with atrial fibrillation. N Engl J Med 2002;347(23): 1825–33.

[38] Van Gelder IC, Hagens VE, Bosker HA, et al. A comparison of rate control and rhythm control in patients with recurrent persistent atrial fibrillation. N Engl J Med 2002;347(23):1834–40.

[39] Hohnloser SH, Kuck KH, Lilienthal J. Rhythm or rate control in atrial fibrillation—Pharmacological Intervention in Atrial Fibrillation (PIAF): a randomised trial. Lancet 2000;356(9244):1789–94.

[40] Carlsson J, Miketic S, Windeler J, et al. Randomized trial of rate-control versus rhythm-control in persistent atrial fibrillation: the Strategies of Treatment of Atrial Fibrillation (STAF) study. J Am Coll Cardiol 2003;41(10):1690–6.

[41] de Denus S, Sanoski CA, Carlsson J, et al. Rate vs rhythm control in patients with atrial fibrillation: a meta-analysis. Arch Intern Med 2005;165(3): 258–62.

[42] Fuster V, Ryden LE, Cannom DS, et al. ACC/AHA/ ESC 2006 guidelines for the management of patients with atrial fibrillation: a report of the American College of Cardiology/American Heart Association Task Force on Practice Guidelines and the European Society of Cardiology Committee for Practice Guidelines (writing committee to revise the 2001 guidelines for the management of patients with atrial fibrillation): developed in collaboration with the European Heart Rhythm Association and the Heart Rhythm Society. Circulation 2006;114(7):e257–354.

[43] Singer DE, Albers GW, Dalen JE, et al. Antithrombotic therapy in atrial fibrillation: the Seventh ACCP Conference on Antithrombotic and Thrombolytic Therapy. Chest 2004;126(3 Suppl):429S–56S.

[44] Palareti G, Leali N, Coccheri S, et al. Bleeding complications of oral anticoagulant treatment: an inception-cohort, prospective collaborative study (ISCOAT). Italian Study on Complications of Oral Anticoagulant Therapy. Lancet 1996;348(9025): 423–8.

[45] Hart RG, Pearce LA, McBride R, et al. Factors associated with ischemic stroke during aspirin therapy in atrial fibrillation: analysis of 2012 participants in the SPAF I-III clinical trials. The Stroke Prevention in Atrial Fibrillation (SPAF) Investigators. Stroke 1999;30(6):1223–9.

[46] Gage BF, Waterman AD, Shannon W, et al. Validation of clinical classification schemes for predicting stroke: results from the National Registry of Atrial Fibrillation. JAMA 2001;285(22):2864–70.

[47] Risk factors for stroke and efficacy of antithrombotic therapy in atrial fibrillation. Analysis of pooled data from five randomized controlled trials. Arch Intern Med 1994;154(13):1449–57.

[48] van Walraven C, Hart RG, Wells GA, et al. A clinical prediction rule to identify patients with atrial fibrillation and a low risk for stroke while taking aspirin. Arch Intern Med 2003;163(8):936–43.

[49] Wang TJ, Massaro JM, Levy D, et al. A risk score for predicting stroke or death in individuals with new-onset atrial fibrillation in the community: the Framingham Heart Study. JAMA 2003;290(8):1049–56.

[50] Available at: http://www.nhlbi.nih.gov/about/framingham/stroke.htm. Accessed February 20, 2008.

[51] Garcia D, Regan S, Crowther M, et al. Warfarin maintenance dosing patterns in clinical practice: implications for safer anticoagulation in the elderly population. Chest 2005;127(6):2049–56.

[52] Massel D, Little SH. Risks and benefits of adding anti-platelet therapy to warfarin among patients with prosthetic heart valves: a meta-analysis. J Am Coll Cardiol 2001;37(2):569–78.

[53] Battistella M, Mamdami MM, Juurlink DN, et al. Risk of upper gastrointestinal hemorrhage in warfarin users treated with nonselective NSAIDs or COX-2 inhibitors. Arch Intern Med 2005;165(2): 189–92.

[54] Wolfe MM, Lichtenstein DR, Singh G. Gastrointestinal toxicity of nonsteroidal antiinflammatory drugs. N Engl J Med 1999;340(24):1888–99.

[55] Delaney JA, Opatrny L, Brophy JM, et al. Drug-drug interactions between antithrombotic medications and the risk of gastrointestinal bleeding. CMAJ 2007;177(4):347–51.

[56] Mahe I, Bertrand N, Drouet L, et al. Paracetamol: a haemorrhagic risk factor in patients on warfarin. Br J Clin Pharmacol 2005;59(3):371–4.

[57] Thijssen HH, Soute BA, Vervoort LM, et al. Paracetamol (acetaminophen) warfarin interaction: NAPQI, the toxic metabolite of paracetamol, is an inhibitor of enzymes in the vitamin K cycle. Thromb Haemost 2004;92(4):797–802.

[58] Arima H, Hart RG, Colman S, et al. Perindopril-based blood pressure-lowering reduces major vascular events in patients with atrial fibrillation and prior stroke or transient ischemic attack. Stroke 2005; 36(10):2164–9.

[59] Albers GW. Stroke prevention in atrial fibrillation: pooled analysis of SPORTIF III and V trials. Am J Manag Care 2004;10(14 Suppl):S462–9 [discussion: S9–73].

[60] Kosakai Y, Kawaguchi AT, Isobe F, et al. Modified maze procedure for patients with atrial fibrillation undergoing simultaneous open heart surgery. Circulation 1995;92(9 Suppl):II359–64.

[61] Blackshear JL, Odell JA. Appendage obliteration to reduce stroke in cardiac surgical patients with atrial fibrillation. Ann Thorac Surg 1996;61(2):755–9.

[62] Sueda T, Imai K, Ishii O, et al. Efficacy of pulmonary vein isolation for the elimination of chronic atrial fibrillation in cardiac valvular surgery. Ann Thorac Surg 2001;71(4):1189–93.

[63] Oral H, Pappone C, Chugh A, et al. Circumferential pulmonary-vein ablation for chronic atrial fibrillation. N Engl J Med 2006;354(9):934–41.

[64] Sievert H, Lesh MD, Trepels T, et al. Percutaneous left atrial appendage transcatheter occlusion to prevent stroke in high-risk patients with atrial fibrillation: early clinical experience. Circulation 2002; 105(16):1887–9.

[65] Pappone C, Augello G, Sala S, et al. A randomized trial of circumferential pulmonary vein ablation versus antiarrhythmic drug therapy in paroxysmal atrial fibrillation: the APAF Study. J Am Coll Cardiol 2006;48(11):2340–7.

ELSEVIER
SAUNDERS

Cardiol Clin 26 (2008) 277–288

CARDIOLOGY
CLINICS

Chronic Antithrombotic Therapy in Post–Myocardial Infarction Patients

Rangadham Nagarakanti, MD[a], Sandeep Sodhi, MD[b],
Robert Lee, MD[c], Michael Ezekowitz, MB ChB, PhD[a],*

[a]Lankenau Institute for Medical Research, Clinical Research Center, Suite G-36, 100 Lancaster Avenue,
Wynnewood, PA 19096-3425, USA
[b]Drexel University College of Medicine, Academic Office, Mail Stop 470, Suite 6608, NCB,
245 North 15th Street, Philadelphia, PA 19102, USA
[c]Department of Medicine, Harbor-UCLA Medical Center, 1000 West Carson Street, Torrance, CA 90502, USA

Despite encouraging trends during the past 3 decades, coronary heart disease remains the leading cause of death in the United States and other industrialized countries. Data from the National Center for Health Statistics and the National Heart, Lung, and Blood Institute [1] emphasize the full dimensions of this health problem, revealing that nearly 13 million Americans have coronary heart disease and that 7.5 million have had a myocardial infarction (MI). Because 1.1 million MIs occur in the United States alone each year, and because 450,000 of them are recurrent infarctions, which carry an inherently greater risk of death and disability than first events, the importance of secondary prevention strategies that can be implemented widely is unparalleled in health care. Antithrombotic therapies, both antiplatelet and anticoagulant, have become the mainstays of these strategies. This article covers the use of chronic antiplatelet and anticoagulation agents after MI. It does not include the management of these patients in the acute phase.

Pathogenesis

Rupture of an atherosclerotic plaque is the usual initiating event in an acute coronary syndrome (ACS), leading to subsequent thrombus formation. Persistent thrombotic occlusion results in acute MI [2]. Platelets play an important role in this process. Intimal injury caused by plaque rupture exposes collagen and von Willebrand's factor to which circulating platelets adhere [3]. Following adhesion, multiple metabolic pathways are stimulated within the platelet, resulting in the production and release of thromboxane A2, ADP, and other substances from platelet granules. These platelet products stimulate further platelet recruitment, activation, and vasoconstriction; they also lead to platelet aggregation by activating the glycoprotein IIb-IIIa (GP IIb-IIIa) complex, which binds platelets to one another through linkage with fibrinogen molecules [4]. Aggregating platelets form the core of the growing thrombotic mass, with upstream or downstream propagation of fibrin and red blood cell–rich clot [5]. Platelet-rich thrombi are more resistant to clot lysis than red blood cell–rich thrombi, and, if lysis occurs, platelet-rich thrombi promote the development of reocclusion [6]. Even after successful reperfusion, the ruptured plaque remains supportive of additional platelet activation and aggregation, predisposing to cyclical coronary flow [7] or frank thrombotic reocclusion [8]. Changes in platelet function also have been observed after primary percutaneous coronary intervention in patients who have an acute ST-segment elevation MI (STEMI) [9]. There is a transient reduction in platelet activity 8 hours after angioplasty associated with a fall in the platelet count that probably is caused by

---

A version of this article originally appeared in *Clinics in Geriatric Medicine*, volume 22, issue 1.

* Corresponding author.

E-mail address: ezekowitzM@mlhs.org
(M. Ezekowitz).

sequestration of hyperactive platelets. Twenty-four to 48 hours after angioplasty, however, there is an increase in platelet activation with in vitro evidence of hyperaggregability and enhanced adherence to endothelial cells. It is possible that these changes increase the risk of thrombotic reocclusion of the recanalized infarct-related artery. They also constitute part of the rationale for aggressive antiplatelet therapy in such patients.

Treatment

Antithrombotic therapies, both antiplatelet and anticoagulant, have become the mainstays of strategies for preventing reocclusion in patients who have had an MI. This article discusses the studies of antiplatelet agents, in particular aspirin and clopidogrel, and anticoagulants, in particular vitamin K antagonists (VKAs) and oral direct thrombin inhibitors.

Antiplatelet agents

Antiplatelet agents interfere with a number of platelet functions, including aggregation, release of granule contents, and platelet-mediated vascular constriction. They can be classified according to their mechanism of action (Box 1) (Fig. 1).

Aspirin

Aspirin has been used in primary and secondary prevention of coronary heart disease, transient ischemic attack, and stroke and in the acute therapy of patients who have an ACS. The antiplatelet activity of aspirin is mediated by inhibition of the synthesis of thromboxane A2 [10]. Thromboxane A2 is released by platelets in response to a number of agonists, amplifying the platelet response that leads to aggregation. Aspirin irreversibly acetylates and inactivates cyclo-oxygenase, which catalyzes the first step of the conversion of arachidonic acid to thromboxane A2 [11,12]. The functional defect induced by aspirin persists for the life of the platelet. An increase in arterial wall shear stress, however, as may occur with an acute hypertensive episode or plaque rupture, can reverse the antithrombotic effect of aspirin [13].

Clinical trials

The Antithrombotic Trialists' Collaboration reviewed the effect of antiplatelet therapy, mostly aspirin, in 12 trials of more than 5000 patients who had a non–ST elevation ACS [14]. Antiplatelet therapy produced a significant 46% reduction

---

> **Box 1. Classification of antiplatelet agents**
>
> 1. Aspirin and related compounds (nonsteroidal anti-inflammatory drugs and sulfinpyrazone) block cyclo-oxygenase (prostaglandin H synthase), the enzyme that mediates the first step in the biosynthesis of prostaglandins and thromboxanes (including thromboxane A2) from arachidonic acid [10].
> 2. The thienopyridines clopidogrel and ticlopidine achieve their antiplatelet effect by blocking the binding of ADP to a specific platelet receptor, thereby inhibiting the activation of the GP IIb-IIIa complex and platelet aggregation [11].
> 3. GP IIb-IIIa antibodies and receptor antagonists inhibit the final common pathway of platelet aggregation (the cross-bridging of platelets by fibrinogen binding to the GP IIb-IIIa receptor) and also may prevent initial adhesion to the vessel wall [12].
>
> GP IIb-IIIa antibodies and receptor antagonists are used in the acute management of MI. This article does not discuss GP IIb-IIIa antibodies and receptor antagonists any further, because the focus is on chronic antithrombotic therapy in post-MI patients.

---

in the combined end point of subsequent nonfatal MI, nonfatal stroke, or vascular death (8% versus 13.3%). The range of findings is illustrated by the following clinical trials that evaluated different types of therapy.

The VA Cooperative Study was a multicenter, double-blind, randomized trial that compared aspirin (75–325 mg/d) with placebo in 1266 men who had a non–ST elevation ACS (rest angina or new-onset angina occurring with minimal physical activity). Aspirin lowered the incidence of death or acute MI by 51% (5% versus 10.1%) [15]. Although therapy was discontinued after 12 weeks, the mortality rate remained 43% lower after 1-year follow-up in the aspirin group.

A double-blind, randomized Canadian multicenter trial compared four regimens in 555 patients

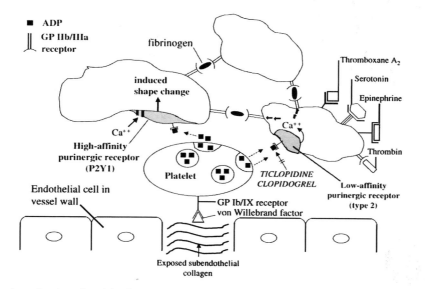

Fig. 1. Mechanism of action of antiplatelet agents. Clopidogrel and ticlopidine block the binding of ADP to the type 2 purinergic receptor and subsequently prevent platelet aggregation. (*From* Sharis PJ, Cannon CP, Loscalzo J. The antiplatelet effects of ticlopidine and clopidogrel. Ann Intern Med 1998;129:395; with permission.)

who had a non–ST elevation ACS (rest or crescendo angina): aspirin (325 mg/d); sulfinpyrazone (200 mg four times per day); combination therapy; or placebo [16]. Treatment was initiated within 8 days after hospitalization and continued for 18 months. Aspirin administration resulted in a 9% benefit when compared with placebo and a 71% reduction in mortality and a 51% reduction in the combined end point of death or nonfatal MI when compared with placebo. There was no observable benefit with sulfinpyrazone, given alone or in combination with aspirin.

The Research Group on Instability in Coronary Artery Disease in Southwest Sweden (RISC) trial randomly assigned 796 patients who had a non–ST elevation ACS to low-dose aspirin (75 mg/d), heparin (5 days of intermittent intravenous infusion), or placebo [17]. Compared with placebo, aspirin was associated with a highly significant reduction in the combined end point of acute MI or death at 5, 30, and 90 days of treatment. The absolute benefit at 90 days was approximately 12% (6.8% versus 18.8%); one of every eight treated patients avoided a cardiovascular event at 90 days. Prolonged follow-up showed that the benefit of low-dose aspirin was maintained after 1 year of therapy [17].

Dose and duration of aspirin therapy

In the Antithrombotic Trialists' Collaboration, the most widely tested regimen in the secondary prevention trials was medium-dose aspirin (75–325 mg/d). Neither higher aspirin doses nor other antiplatelet drugs were more effective than daily aspirin in this dose range [14]. There was insufficient evidence to confirm the efficacy of doses below 75 mg/d. A dose of 75 to 150 mg/d may provide optimal efficacy while limiting toxicity. In the Antithrombotic Trialists' Collaboration overview, aspirin at a dose of 75 to 150 mg/d was as effective as a dose of 150 to 325 mg/d [14]. Optimal duration of therapy has not been tested in a prospective, randomized fashion. The benefit in patients who had unstable angina was even greater (8% versus 13.3%) [14]. Prolonged therapy seems to be warranted.

Clopidogrel

Clopidogrel has been studied more extensively than ticlopidine in patients who had a non–ST elevation ACS. Clopidogrel blocks the binding of ADP to a specific platelet receptor, thereby inhibiting the activation of the GP IIb-IIIa complex and platelet aggregation [10].

The efficacy of clopidogrel was evaluated in the *C*lopidogrel in *U*nstable Angina to Prevent *R*ecurrent *E*vents (CURE) trial, which randomly assigned 12,562 patients who presented within 24 hours after the onset of a non–ST elevation ACS to aspirin alone (75–325 mg/d) or to clopidogrel (300-mg loading dose followed immediately by 75 mg/d) and aspirin (75–325 mg/d); most were at increased risk because of ECG changes (mostly ST depression of 1 mm or T wave inversion of 2 mm) or elevated cardiac enzymes [18]. The primary end point was cardiovascular death, MI, or stroke. At an average follow-up of 9 months, combination therapy was associated with reductions in the primary end point (9.3% versus 11.4% for aspirin alone), largely caused by fewer nonfatal MIs (5.2% versus 6.7%).

Clopidogrel was associated with modest reductions in the incidence of severe or refractory in-hospital ischemia, in-hospital heart failure, and need for a revascularization procedure and with a significant increase in major bleeding (3.7% versus 2.7%) but not in life-threatening bleeding or hemorrhagic stroke.

A subsequent analysis from the CURE trial evaluated the time course of benefit of clopidogrel [19]. Evidence of benefit began to emerge within 24 hours and gradually increased in magnitude during the first 30 days (4.3% versus 5.4% incidence of the primary end point; relative risk 0.79). The benefit continued to increase from 31 days to 1 year (5.2% versus 6.3% incidence of new events; relative risk 0.82). There was no significant excess of late life-threatening bleeding, but there was a small excess of major bleeds (5/1000) that was much smaller than the total cardiovascular benefit at 1 year (22/1000) (Box 2).

Anticoagulants

This section reviews the role of VKAs and oral direct thrombin inhibitors in secondary prevention of coronary artery disease.

Vitamin K antagonists

Pharmacology

Coagulation factors II, VII, IX, and X require γ-carboxylation of glutamate residues to transform them into their active, procoagulant forms [20]. This modification is performed directly by the enzyme vitamin K–dependent carboxylase. Two other enzymes, vitamin K reductase and vitamin K epoxide reductase, supply the reduced form of vitamin K (vitamin KH2) necessary for the γ-carboxylation reaction. Both enzymes are sensitive to the inhibitory actions of VKAs, with vitamin K epoxide reductase more so than vitamin K reductase. The anticoagulation produced with VKAs derives from this indirect inhibition of the γ-carboxylation of coagulation factors II, VII, IX, and X. The result is the hepatic

---

Box 2. Recommendations

- In most health care settings, for moderate and low-risk patients who have had an MI, the authors recommend aspirin alone at a dose of 75 to 150 mg once a day for an indefinite duration.
- The combination of aspirin and clopidogrel might be more beneficial than aspirin alone, but it might not be a good option in geriatric patients, who are already at increased risk of bleeding.
- Clopidogrel should be administered to patients who cannot take aspirin because of hypersensitivity or gastrointestinal intolerance.

---

production of these coagulation factors with greatly reduced activity. Proteins C and S, which have anticoagulant properties, require similar γ-carboxylation to transform into their active forms and are inhibited by VKAs. Anticoagulation through the inhibition of the coagulation pathway is the overall clinical manifestation of VKA administration.

Treatment

Several studies have been conducted in recent years to establish the clinical benefits of VKAs for chronic anticoagulation in patients after MI, either in addition to or instead of traditional treatment with aspirin. The most widely studied VKA has been warfarin. Although the theoretic benefits of warfarin in the patient who has had a MI have been largely recognized, successful translation to clinical practice has been somewhat indeterminate. Because of the complex pharmacokinetics and pharmacodynamics of warfarin, maintaining international normalized ratios (INRs) in the therapeutic range has proved relatively troublesome. Studies have shown that variations in the expression of genes for enzyme complexes such as vitamin K epoxide reductase are responsible for the variations in dose response in different warfarin-treated patients [21]. In addition to genetic variations that predispose certain patients to increased sensitivity or resistance, numerous environmental factors affect the biologic activity of warfarin [20]. When combined with warfarin, many drugs, including herbal medicines, increase or decrease the level of anticoagulation drastically by altering either the absorption of warfarin or its metabolism and clearance from the body. Also, drugs that affect platelet activity, such as aspirin and nonsteroidal anti-inflammatory drugs, can potentiate the already increased risk of bleeding in patients receiving warfarin. Other environmental factors that may affect the biologic activity of warfarin include changes in disease states, including hepatic dysfunction or hypermetabolic conditions; changes in dietary intake of vitamin K; and noncompliance or dosing errors. The cause of over- and underanticoagulation in patients receiving warfarin often cannot be determined, as outlined by a recent study that undertook extensive evaluation of this matter [22].

The difficulties with warfarin treatment are exacerbated in the geriatric population. The elderly generally are more likely to be taking multiple prescription drugs and herbal medicines, increasing the risk of interactions with warfarin [23]. The elderly also are more likely to have concomitant diseases (eg, reduced metabolic clearance from hepatic dysfunction) that may alter the pharmacokinetics of warfarin. Other possible ways in which increasing age indirectly may create more problems when administering warfarin are inconsistency of diet and activity, decreased cognitive abilities leading to increased risk of noncompliance or dosing errors, and overall lower body weights. Wittkowsky and coworkers [24] showed that patients aged 65 years or older experience warfarin-related major bleeding events at a mean INR of 1.1 units lower than patients younger than 65 years. The recently published Birmingham Atrial Fibrillation Treatment of the Aged (BAFTA) study in high-risk elderly patients (mean age, 81.5 years), however, showed that the frequency of major stroke, arterial embolism, and intracranial hemorrhage was significantly lower (1.8% versus 3.8%) in patients taking warfarin than in those treated with aspirin [25].

The Coumadin Aspirin Reinfarction Study (CARS) proposed that warfarin at a low fixed dose in addition to aspirin would give more clinical benefit than aspirin monotherapy in the prevention of nonfatal MI, nonfatal ischemic stroke, and cardiovascular death in patients who had had MI [26]. A total of 8803 patients who had had either non-STEMI or STEMI were assigned randomly to three groups: (1) 160 mg aspirin, (2) 80 mg aspirin plus 1 mg warfarin, or (3) 80 mg aspirin plus 3 mg warfarin. Median time of follow-up was 14 months. Although there was no age exclusion in CARS, the mean age of the study population was relatively young, 59 ± 11 years. The results showed no significant differences in the rates of these primary events among the three groups. Median INRs in the 1-mg warfarin group were 1.06, 1.05, and 1.04 at weeks 1 and 4 and month 6, respectively. Median INRs in the 3-mg warfarin group were 1.51, 1.27, and 1.19 at weeks 1 and 4 and month 6, respectively. This study showed low rates of major bleeding events in all three groups, although there were significantly more events in the 3-mg warfarin group than in the aspirin monotherapy group. The CARS investigators concluded that the addition of low fixed doses of warfarin, either 1 mg or 3 mg, to aspirin provided no clinical benefit for patients after MI.

In the Organization to Assess Strategies for Ischemic Syndromes study, a two-phase substudy was performed to examine the effect of adding warfarin to standard therapy in patients who had had either an episode of unstable angina or non-STEMI [27]. The first phase compared standard therapy versus 3 mg of warfarin (mean INR, 1.48) plus standard therapy in 309 patients. A total of 87% of patients in each group received aspirin as part of the standard therapy. In this study the mean age was slightly older than in the CARS: 65 ± 12 years in the standard therapy group , and 63 ± 10 years in the warfarin group. Follow-up time was 6 months. Similar to CARS, this study showed no significant differences in the composite primary outcome of cardiovascular death, new MI, and refractory angina in the two groups. This study also showed a low rate of major bleeding events in both groups, although there was a trend toward increased major bleeding events in the warfarin group. A significantly higher rate of minor bleeding events was reported in the warfarin group. Twenty-nine percent of the patients assigned to the warfarin group discontinued therapy during the study for a variety of reasons.

In the second phase, the protocol was modified to target an increase in INR with the belief that this increase could provide a clinical difference. Standard therapy was compared with moderate-intensity dose-adjusted warfarin (mean INR, 2.3) plus standard therapy in 197 patients, with 85% of patients in each group receiving aspirin as part of the standard therapy. The mean age in both groups was 64 ± 12 years. Follow-up time was 3 months. The results of the second phase showed a trend toward decreasing rates of the composite primary outcome of cardiovascular death, new

MI, and refractory angina in the warfarin group. Again, low rates of major bleeding events were reported in both groups; this time there were no significant differences in major bleeding events in the two groups. There was a significantly higher rate of minor bleeding events in the warfarin group. Fifty-two percent of the patients assigned to the warfarin group discontinued therapy during the study for a variety of reasons. Pertinent to the focus of this article, follow-up time in both phases of the Organization to Assess Strategies for Ischemic Syndromes study was relatively short, with the first phase lasting only 6 months and the second phase lasting only 3 months. The application of these results to a more chronic clinical setting is somewhat indeterminate.

The next major trial that investigated the clinical benefits of warfarin was the Combined Hemotherapy and Mortality Prevention (CHAMP) study. A total of 162 mg of aspirin was compared with 81 mg of aspirin plus dose-adjusted warfarin (mean INR, 1.8) in 5059 patients who had had either non-STEMI or STEMI [28]. The median age was 62 years, and the median follow-up time was 2.7 years. This study found no significant difference between the two groups in the primary outcome of all-cause mortality. Furthermore, there was no significant difference in a composite secondary outcome of cardiovascular events (vascular mortality, recurrent MI, or stroke). Similar to the previous studies, rates of major bleeding events were low, but significantly higher rates of both major and minor bleeding events were recorded in the combination group. Also, 25.3% of the patients initially assigned to the combination group discontinued warfarin therapy during the study for unspecified reasons, as compared with 12.6% in the aspirin monotherapy group. The CHAMP investigators concluded that no clinical benefits were observed in patients receiving warfarin titrated to a mean INR of 1.8 in addition to aspirin when compared with those receiving aspirin monotherapy.

The results reported in both CARS and the CHAMP study, that warfarin therapy provided no added clinical benefit to the standard post-MI regimen of aspirin, were speculated to be based on the relatively low doses of warfarin used in those trials. In CARS, the group receiving 3 mg of warfarin reached a maximum median INR of 1.51; in the CHAMP study the mean INR in the warfarin group was 1.8.

The Antithrombotics in the Secondary Prevention of Events in Coronary Thrombosis (ASPECT-2) study examined the possibility that higher doses of warfarin might confer significant clinical benefit. The protocol stratified 999 patients who had had either non-STEMI or STEMI into three groups The first group received aspirin monotherapy (80 mg), the second group received acetylsalicylic acid (80 mg) plus dose-adjusted warfarin, and the third group received dose-adjusted warfarin alone [29]. In the combination group, the mean INR was 2.4 and was designated as moderate intensity; in the warfarin group, the mean INR was 3.2 and was designated as high intensity. The mean ages in all three groups were comparable, ranging from 61 ± 11 to 62 ± 11 years. The median follow-up time was 12 months. In ASPECT-2, results showed a significant decrease in composite primary outcome (death, MI, or stroke) in both the combination group and the warfarin group when compared with the aspirin monotherapy group. When each primary outcome was examined independently, however, there were no significant differences among the three groups [30]. There was no significant difference in the rate of major bleeding events, with all groups reporting a low rate of 1% to 2%, but there was a significant increase in the rate of minor bleeding events in the combination group. Sixty-two of the 330 patients (18.8%) initially assigned to warfarin discontinued therapy during the trial, as did 68 of 333 patients (20.4%) initially assigned to combination therapy. In comparison, only 34 of 336 patients (10.1%) initially assigned to aspirin monotherapy discontinued therapy during the trial. The ASPECT-2 study concluded that either high-intensity warfarin therapy or moderate-intensity warfarin therapy in combination with aspirin was more effective in reducing cardiovascular events and death than aspirin alone in patients after MI.

The Antithrombotics in the Prevention of Reocclusion in Coronary Thrombosis (APRICOT-2) study examined a slightly different aspect than the previous studies. The investigators compared 80 mg of aspirin monotherapy versus moderate-intensity dose-adjusted warfarin (mean INR, 2.6) plus 80 mg of aspirin; however, the patient population consisted of 308 patients who had had STEMI and who had been treated with thrombolytics with restoration of thrombolysis in MI grade 3 flow [31]. The primary outcome for this study was reocclusion of the infarct-related artery at 3-month angiographic follow-up. Mean age was 58 ± 10 years in the aspirin group and 57 ± 11 years in the combination group. Of importance with respect to the geriatric population is that patients age

75 years and older were excluded from APRICOT-2. This study reported a significant decrease in the rate of reocclusion and a significant increase in event-free survival (death, reinfarction, or revascularization) in the combination group. No significant differences in rates of major or minor bleeding events were noted. Only 11 of 135 patients (8.1%) initially assigned to combination therapy discontinued warfarin therapy during the trial; however, the duration of the study was only 3 months, considerably shorter than the follow-up time of similar studies. It was concluded that post-STEMI patients benefited from moderate-intensity warfarin in addition to aspirin with significantly reduced rates of reocclusion of the infarct-related artery and reduced rates of recurrent events after successful fibrinolysis. Again, with such a short follow-up time, the clinical benefits seen in APRICOT-2 are more difficult to apply to a more chronic time course.

One of the most recent studies, the Warfarin-Aspirin Reinfarction Study (WARIS-2), compared 160 mg of acetylsalicylic acid monotherapy versus moderate-intensity dose-adjusted warfarin plus 75 mg of acetylsalicylic acid versus high-intensity dose-adjusted warfarin alone in 3630 patients who had had either non-STEMI or STEMI [32]. The mean INR was 2.2 in the moderate-intensity combination group and 2.8 in the high-intensity warfarin-alone group. Mean ages in all three groups were similar, ranging from 60 ± 10 to 61 ± 10 years; however, a limitation in this trial when considering the geriatric population is that patients age 75 years and older were excluded. A strength of the WARIS-2 was its relatively long mean follow-up time of approximately 4 years. This study reported a significant decrease in the rate of composite primary outcome (death, MI, or stroke) in both the high-intensity warfarin-alone group and the moderate-intensity combination group when compared with the aspirin monotherapy group. Of note, the significance was restricted to the rates of MI and stroke; there was no significant difference in death among the groups. Significant increases in both major and minor bleeding events were reported in the warfarin group and the combination group, although the rates were relatively low in all three groups. A total of 387 of 1216 patients (31.8%) initially assigned to high-intensity warfarin and 480 (39.7%) of 1208 patients initially assigned to combination therapy discontinued the assigned medication during the course of the study, compared with 191 of 1206 patients (15.8%) initially assigned to aspirin

monotherapy. The WARIS-2 investigators concluded that moderate-intensity warfarin in addition to aspirin or high-intensity warfarin alone resulted in reduced risk of reinfarction and ischemic stroke in patients after MI but also entailed a higher risk of bleeding.

Despite the advances made by recent studies, there continue to be areas of uncertainty concerning the role of VKAs in chronic anticoagulation in patients who have had either non-STEMI or STEMI. High-intensity oral VKAs (target INR, 3–4) alone or moderate-intensity oral VKAs (target INR, 2–3) with aspirin in patients after MI, with meticulous INR monitoring, was given a 2B recommendation from the Seventh American College of Chest Physicians Conference on Antithrombotics and Thrombolytic Therapy [33]. In the geriatric population, however, the areas of uncertainty become even less clear. There have not been any major trials targeting this population, and certain major trials excluded patients 75 years and older. Furthermore, there are issues concerning VKAs, such as risk of bleeding and drug–drug interactions, which typically are magnified in older patients. A recent trial in high-risk elderly patients (mean age, 81.5 years) who had atrial fibrillation, however, demonstrated that oral anticoagulation is more effective than aspirin in prevention of stroke and found no difference in bleeding [25]. The unique clinical situation of chronic anticoagulation in elderly patients needs to be addressed specifically before stronger recommendations can be made concerning appropriate therapy in the post-MI setting.

Oral direct thrombin inhibitors

Data from WARIS-II and ASPECT-II have led to increased use of aspirin or oral VKAs in secondary prevention. The use of oral VKAs after MI is restricted because of the many food–drug and drug–drug interactions needing regular coagulation monitoring and subsequent dose adjustments and because of the risk of bleeding, especially when combined with acetylsalicylic acid. Such limitations have prompted the development of new oral anticoagulants that are safer and more effective. Ximelagatran is the most widely studied oral direct thrombin inhibitor and is the drug of focus here.

Ximelagatran

Ximelagatran is the first in a new class of oral direct thrombin inhibitors. Ximelagatran inhibits

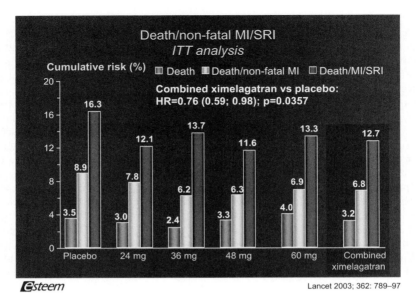

Fig. 2. Patients who had had recent myocardial infarction were assigned randomly to ximelagatran at one of four doses or to placebo, with all participants receiving 160 mg/d of aspirin. ITT, intention to treat; SRI, severe recurrent ischemia. (*From* Wallentin L, Wilcox RG, Weaver WD, et al. Oral ximelagatran for secondary prophylaxis after myocardial infarction: the ESTEEM randomized controlled trial. Lancet 2003;362:789–97; with permission.)

the action of thrombin in the coagulation cascade. It also inhibits fibrin-bound thrombin.

After oral administration, ximelagatran is metabolized rapidly to its active form, melagatran [34], which is excreted mainly through the kidneys. Melagatran is stable over time, and its metabolism is unaffected by age [35], sex, body weight [36], or ethnic origin [37]. The bioconversion of

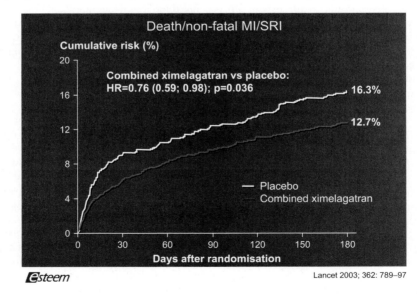

Fig. 3. Oral ximelagatran significantly reduced the risk for the primary end point compared with placebo from 16.3% (102 of 638) to 12.7% (154 of 1245) (hazard ratio [HR], 0.76; 95% confidence interval, 0.59–0.98; P = .036) for the combined ximelagatran groups versus placebo. ITT, intention to treat; SRI, severe recurrent ischemia. (*From* Wallentin L, Wilcox RG, Weaver WD, et al. Oral ximelagatran for secondary prophylaxis after myocardial infarction: the ESTEEM randomized controlled trial. Lancet 2003;362:793; with permission.)

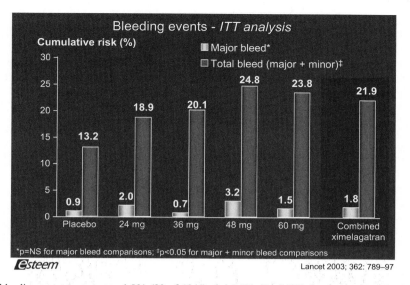

Fig. 4. Major bleeding events were rare, 1.8% (23 of 1245) and 0.9% (6 of 638) (hazard ratio, 1.97; 95% confidence interval, 0.80–4.84) in the combined ximelagatran and placebo groups, respectively. ITT, intention to treat; NS, not significant. (*From* Wallentin L, Wilcox RG, Weaver WD, et al. Oral ximelagatran for secondary prophylaxis after myocardial infarction: the ESTEEM randomized controlled trial. Lancet 2003;362:789–97; with permission.)

ximelagatran and the elimination of melagatran are independent of the hepatic cytochrome P-450 enzyme system, providing a low potential for drug–drug interactions [38], and there are no known clinically relevant food or alcohol interactions [39]. Melagatran's pharmacokinetics are unchanged, and its pharmacodynamic properties show only minor additive effects when oral ximelagatran and acetylsalicylic acid are given concomitantly [40].

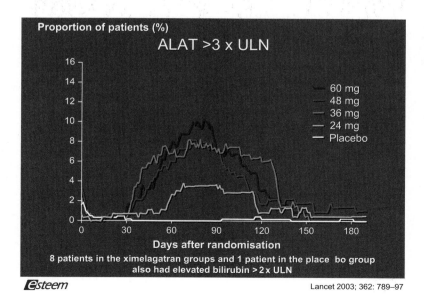

Fig. 5. Proportion of patients having rise of transaminases in different groups. ALAT, alanine amito transferase; ULN, upper limit of normal. (*From* Wallentin L, Wilcox RG, Weaver WD, et al. Oral ximelagatran for secondary prophylaxis after myocardial infarction: the ESTEEM randomized controlled trial. Lancet 2003;362:789–97; with permission.)

Data on the use of oral direct thrombin inhibition with ximelagatran have been provided recently in the ESTEEM trial [41]. In this study, 1883 patients who had had recent MI were assigned randomly to ximelagatran at one of four doses or to placebo, with all participants receiving 160 mg/d of aspirin (Fig. 2). Compared with aspirin alone, those receiving any dose of ximelagatran had a 24% relative risk reduction (95% confidence interval, 0.59–0.98) in the combined end point of nonfatal MI, severe recurrent ischemia, or death (Figs. 3 and 4). The mean age of patients was 69 years (46–84 years).

The benefit of ximelagatran given twice daily came at an increased risk of liver function test abnormalities, a finding consistent across ximelagatran trials (Fig. 5).

Dabigatran

Dabigatran is another novel oral direct thrombin inhibitor. It is a potent, competitive, and reversible direct inhibitor of thrombin. Like ximelagatran, dabigatran produces a predictable anticoagulant response with no known drug or food interactions and reduces the need for laboratory monitoring. The half-life of dabigatran is approximately 8 hours after single-dose administration and up to 14 to 17 hours after multiple doses. It usually is given twice daily [42]. It currently is under investigation for prevention and treatment of thromboembolic events. The first evaluation of dabigatran in patients who had atrial fibrillation in phase II trial has been completed [43]. Two doses of dabigatran (150 mg and 110 mg twice daily) currently are undergoing testing in comparison with warfarin (INR 2–3) in a very large, ongoing, phase III, noninferiority, randomized, controlled trial, the Randomized Evaluation of Long-Term Anticoagulant Therapy (RELY) study.

Although oral direct thrombin inhibitors show considerable promise, further evaluation is needed to determine the effectiveness and safety of direct thrombin inhibitors in secondary prophylaxis after MI. Ongoing studies comparing dabigatran with warfarin will evaluate this novel therapeutic approach fully.

Summary

After MI, all patients should be put on daily low-dose aspirin irrespective of their age. The combination of aspirin and clopidogrel should be avoided in the geriatric population because the risk of bleeding overweighs the benefit.

Clopidogrel should be reserved for patients who have hypersensitivity or gastrointestinal intolerance to aspirin. Using high-intensity oral VKAs (target INR, 3–4) alone or moderate-intensity oral VKAs (target INR, 2–3) with aspirin is not recommended in geriatric patients who have had MI. In the future, oral direct thrombin inhibitors may replace oral VKAs; however, more studies are needed before one consider oral direct thrombin inhibitors as better agents than oral VKAs for anticoagulation in patients after MI.

References

[1] Morbidity and mortality: 2002 chart book on cardiovascular, lung, and blood diseases. Bethesda (MD): National Heart, Lung, and Blood Institute; 2002.

[2] Fuster V, Badimon L, Badimon JJ, et al. The pathogenesis of coronary artery disease and the acute coronary syndromes. N Engl J Med 1992;326: 242–50.

[3] Coller BS, Scudder LE, Beer J, et al. Monoclonal antibodies to platelet glycoprotein IIb/IIIa as antithrombotic agents. Ann N Y Acad Sci 1991;614: 193–213.

[4] Lefkovits J, Plow E, Topol E. Platelet glycoprotein IIb/IIIa receptors in cardiovascular medicine. N Engl J Med 1995;332:1553–9.

[5] Sherman CT, Litvack F, Grundfest W, et al. Coronary angioscopy in patients with unstable angina pectoris. N Engl J Med 1986;315:913–9.

[6] Jang IK, Gold HK, Ziskind AA, et al. Differential sensitivity of erythrocyte-rich and platelet-rich arterial thrombi to lyse with recombinant tissue-type plasminogen activator: a possible explanation for resistance to coronary thrombolysis. Circulation 1989;79:920–8.

[7] Golino P, Ashton JH, Glas-Greenwalt P, et al. Mediation of reocclusion by thromboxane A2 and serotonin after thrombolysis with tissue-type plasminogen activator in a canine preparation of coronary thrombosis. Circulation 1988;77:678–84.

[8] Gash AK, Spann JF, Sherry S, et al. Factors influencing reocclusion after coronary thrombolysis for acute myocardial infarction. Am J Cardiol 1986;57: 175–7.

[9] Gawaz M, Neumann FJ, Ott I, et al. Platelet function in acute myocardial infarction treated with direct angioplasty. Circulation 1996;93:229–37.

[10] Patrono C. Aspirin as an antiplatelet drug. N Engl J Med 1994;330:1287–94.

[11] Foster CJ, Prosser DM, Agans JM, et al. Molecular identification and characterization of the platelet ADP receptor targeted by thienopyridine antithrombotic drugs. J Clin Invest 2001;107:1591–8.

[12] Faulds D, Sorkin EM. Abciximab (c7E3 Fab): a review of its pharmacology and therapeutic

potential in ischemic heart disease. Drugs 1994;48: 583–98.

[13] Maalej N, Folts JD. Increased shear stress overcomes the antithrombotic platelet inhibitory effect of aspirin in stenosed dog coronary arteries. Circulation 1996;93:1201–5.

[14] Antithrombotic Trialists' Collaboration. Collaborative meta-analysis of randomised trials of antiplatelet therapy for prevention of death, myocardial infarction, and stroke in high risk patients. BMJ 2002;324:71–86.

[15] Lewis HD, Davis JW, Archibald DG, et al. Protective effects of aspirin against acute myocardial infarction and death in men with unstable angina: results of a Veterans Administration Cooperative Study. N Engl J Med 1983;309:396–403.

[16] Cairns JA, Gent M, Singer J, et al. Aspirin, sulfinpyrazone, or both in unstable angina: results of a Canadian multicenter trial. N Engl J Med 1985;313:1369–75.

[17] Risk of myocardial infarction and death during treatment with low dose aspirin and intravenous heparin in men with unstable coronary artery disease. The RISC Group. Lancet 1990;336:827–30.

[18] Yusuf S, Zhao F, Mehta SR, et al. Effects of clopidogrel in addition to aspirin in patients with acute coronary syndromes without ST-segment elevation. N Engl J Med 2001;345:494–502.

[19] Mehta SR, Yusuf S, Peters RJ, et al, for the Clopidogrel in Unstable angina to prevent Recurrent Events trial (CURE) Investigators. Effects of pretreatment with clopidogrel and aspirin followed by long-term therapy in patients undergoing percutaneous coronary intervention: the PCI-CURE study. Lancet 2001;358:527–33.

[20] Takahashi H, Wilkinson GR, Nutescu EA, et al. Different contributions of polymorphisms in VKORC1 and CYP2C9 to intra- and inter-population differences in maintenance doses of warfarin in Japanese, Caucasians and African Americans. Pharmacogenet Genomics 2006;16:101–10.

[21] Ansell J, Hirsh J, Poller L, et al. The pharmacology and management of the vitamin K antagonists: the Seventh ACCP Conference on Antithrombotics and Thrombolytic Therapy. Chest 2004;126(3 Suppl): 204S–33S.

[22] Wittkowsky AK, Devine EB. Frequency and causes of overanticoagulation and underanticoagulation in patients treated with warfarin. Pharmacotherapy 2004;24:1311–6.

[23] Fitzmaurice DA, Blann AD, Lip GY. Bleeding risks of antithrombotic therapy. BMJ 2002;325:828–31.

[24] Wittkowsky AK, Whitely KS, Devine EB, et al. Effect of age on international normalized ratio at the time of major bleeding in patients treated with warfarin. Pharmacotherapy 2004;24:600–5.

[25] Mant J, Hobbs FDR, Fletcher K, et al, on behalf of the BAFTA investigators. Warfarin versus aspirin for stroke prevention in an elderly community population with atrial fibrillation (the Birmingham Atrial Fibrillation Treatment of the Aged Study, BAFTA): a randomised controlled trial. Lancet 2007;370:493–503.

[26] Randomised double-blind trial of fixed low-dose warfarin with aspirin after myocardial infarction. Coumadin Aspirin Reinfarction Study (CARS) Investigators [abstract]. Lancet 1997;350:389–96.

[27] Anand SS, Yusuf S, Pogue J, et al. Long-term oral anticoagulant therapy in patients with unstable angina or suspected non-Q-wave myocardial infarction: Organization to Assess Strategies for Ischemic Syndromes (OASIS) pilot study results. Circulation 1998;98:1064–70.

[28] Fiore LD, Ezekowitz MD, Brophy MT, et al. Department of Veterans Affairs Cooperative Studies Program clinical trial comparing combined warfarin and aspirin with aspirin alone in survivors of acute myocardial infarction: primary results of the CHAMP study. Circulation 2002;105:557–63.

[29] van Es RF, Jonker JJ, Verheugt FW, et al. Aspirin and Coumadin after acute coronary syndromes (the ASPECT-2 study): a randomized controlled trial. Lancet 2002;360:109–13.

[30] Jeddy AS, Gleason BL. Aspirin and warfarin versus aspirin monotherapy after myocardial infarction. Ann Pharmacother 2003;37:1502–5.

[31] Brouwer MA, van den Bergh PJ, Aengevaeren WR, et al. Aspirin plus Coumarin versus aspirin alone in the prevention of reocclusion after fibrinolysis for acute myocardial infarction: results of the Antithrombotics in the Prevention of Reocclusion in Coronary Thrombolysis (APRICOT-2). Trial Circulation 2002;106:659–65.

[32] Hurlen M, Abdelnoor M, Smith P, et al. Warfarin, aspirin, or both after myocardial infarction. N Engl J Med 2002;347:969–74.

[33] Harrington RA, Becker RC, Ezekowitz M, et al. Antithrombotic therapy for coronary artery disease: the Seventh ACCP Conference on Antithrombotic and Thrombolytic Therapy. Chest 2004;126(3 Suppl): 513S–48S.

[34] Eriksson UG, Bredberg U, Hoffmann K-J, et al. Absorption, distribution, metabolism, and excretion of ximelagatran, an oral direct thrombin inhibitor, in rats, dogs, and humans. Drug Metab Dispos 2003; 31:294–305.

[35] Johansson LC, Frison L, Lofgren U, et al. Influence of age on the pharmacokinetics and pharmacodynamics of ximelagatran, an oral direct thrombin inhibitor. Clin Pharmacokinet 2003;42:381–92.

[36] Sarich TC, Peters GR, Wollbratt M, et al. No influence of obesity on the pharmacokinetics and pharmacodynamics of melagatran, the active form of the oral direct thrombin inhibitor, ximelagatran. Clin Pharmacokinet 2003;42:485–92.

[37] Johansson LC, Andersson M, Fager G, et al. No influence of ethnic origin on the pharmacokinetics and pharmacodynamics of melagatran, following oral administration of ximelagatran, a novel, oral

direct thrombin inhibitor, to healthy male volunteers. Clin Pharmacokinet 2003;42:475–84.

[38] Eriksson-Lepkowska M, Thuresson A, Johansson S, et al. The oral direct thrombin inhibitor ximelagatran has no effect on the pharmacokinetics of P450-metabolized drugs. Pathophysiol Haemost Thromb 2002;32:130.

[39] Eriksson UG, Bredberg U, Gislén K, et al. Pharmacokinetics and pharmacodynamics of ximelagatran, a novel oral direct thrombin inhibitor, in young, healthy male subjects. Eur J Clin Pharmacol 2003;59:35–43.

[40] Fager G, Eriksson-Lepkowska M, Frison L, et al. Influence of acetylsalicylic acid on the pharmacodynamics and pharmacokinetics of melagatran, the active form of the oral direct thrombin inhibitor H 376/95. Eur Heart J 2000;21:441.

[41] Wallentin L, Wilcox RG, Weaver WD, et al. Oral ximelagatran for secondary prophylaxis after myocardial infarction: the ESTEEM randomized controlled trial. Lancet 2003;362:789–97.

[42] Stangier J, Rathgen K, Stahle H, et al. The pharmacokinetics, pharmacodynamics and tolerability of dabigatran etexilate, a new oral direct thrombin inhibitor, in healthy male subjects. Br J Clin Pharmacol 2007;64(3):292–303.

[43] Ezekowitz MD, Reilly PA, Nehmizn G, et al. A dose exploration pilot study of dabigatran, a novel oral direct thrombin inhibitor, with and without concomitant acetylsalicylic acid, in comparison to warfarin in patients with non-valvular atrial fibrillation (PETRO Study). Am J Cardiol 2007;100: 1419–26.

Cardiol Clin 26 (2008) 289–298

Antithrombotic Therapy in Peripheral Arterial Disease

Evan C. Lipsitz, MD, FACS[a],*, Soo Kim, MD[b]

[a]Division of Vascular and Endovascular Surgery, Vascular Diagnostic Laboratory Services, Montefiore Medical Center and the Albert Einstein College of Medicine, 111 East 210th Street, Bronx, NY 10467, USA
[b]University of Medicine and Dentistry New Jersey, New Jersey Medical School, Newark, NJ, USA

Lower-extremity occlusive disease represents a significant health problem not only by its direct impact but also by virtue of the systemic nature of the disease process. Peripheral atherosclerosis is associated with varying degrees of involvement elsewhere in the body, potentially affecting all organ systems. With the aging population one can only expect that the problem will increase both in number and complexity over the next few decades. Antithrombotic agents are prescribed for use in individuals with atherosclerotic disease of the arteries in the lower extremity to prevent ischemia and gangrene. They are also used to improve the durability of interventions performed to treat this atherosclerotic disease, including angioplasty with or without stents, and surgical bypass using autologous vein or prosthetic material. Although these agents have been shown to have significant benefit in patients with peripheral arterial disease (PAD) their use must be tempered by consideration of their risks, many of which may be increased in the elderly population. These include the increased risks of falls with associated trauma, potential difficulties with self-administration of medication, decreases in renal function or hepatic metabolism, gastrointestinal bleeding, and interactions with other medications that are commonly used in this population. Equally important is the fact that in many cases these medications are prescribed for the remainder of the patient's lifetime. Because many older patients have

complex arterial pathology, however, this population stands to gain major benefit from the use of these antithrombotic agents. The goals of medical therapy for patients with PAD are to prevent progression of atherosclerotic disease, minimize the occurrence of cardiovascular events, improve functional status in patients with claudication, and prevent limb loss. This article reviews the pathophysiology of PAD, and data regarding the use of antiplatelet and anticoagulant agents.

Peripheral arterial disease

PAD is a common manifestation of atherosclerosis presenting as obstructive arterial disease interfering with blood flow to the extremities. Physicians may mistake PAD for musculoskeletal or neurologic disorders because symptomatology can mimic nonvascular etiology. An understanding of PAD risk factors, clinical presentation, differential diagnosis, stages, progression, physical examination, and diagnostic work-up is important for the guidance of medical therapy.

Risk factors

Age

PAD is largely but not exclusively a disease of the elderly. The development of early atherosclerotic changes can be seen even in children and manifest as an increase in intimal macrophages with foam cells. Because atherosclerosis is a continual process and the development of symptoms is generally a late manifestation of this process, elderly people are afflicted more commonly than the younger population. The prevalence of PAD

A version of this article originally appeared in *Clinics in Geriatric Medicine,* volume 22, issue 1.

* Corresponding author

E-mail address: elipsitz@aol.com (E.C. Lipsitz).

increases sharply with age, from 3% in patients younger than 60 years of age to 20% in patients older than 75 years of age [1].

Hypertension

The Framingham Offspring study found that hypertension is a major risk factor for the development and progression of PAD [2]. Although there are no reports that definitively show that antihypertensive therapy alters the progression of disease, aggressive antihypertensive therapy is supported by the Joint National Committee on the detection, evaluation, and treatment of hypertension, which concluded that PAD is considered to be equivalent in risk to ischemic heart disease [3].

β-Blockers are frequently used for antihypertensive therapy mainly for their cardioprotective effects. There is no adverse effect on symptoms of claudication caused by β-blockers and they may be used safely for patients with PAD unless there are other contraindications [4]. The angiotensin-converting enzyme inhibitors were shown to be cardioprotective in patients with PAD by the HOPE trial [5]. Of note is the fact that the benefit of the angiotensin-converting enzyme inhibitors was independent of blood pressure because blood pressure difference between the placebo group and ramipril group was not statistically significant. Although antihypertensive therapy has no, as yet, proven benefit for directly inhibiting PAD progression, it does improve mortality rates in these patients, whose demise is usually secondary to cardiovascular event, justifying therapy.

Smoking

There is no debate that smoking is the single most modifiable risk factor for the development and progression of atherosclerosis. Multiple factors, such as activation of the sympathetic nervous system with resultant vasoconstriction, oxidation of low-density lipoprotein (LDL) cholesterol, inhibition of tissue plasminogen activator release from the endothelium, increased blood fibrinogen concentration, increased platelet activity, increased expression of plaque tissue factor, and endothelial dysfunction, are involved in the process [6]. The Reykjavik study showed the risk of developing intermittent claudication increased in smokers by a factor of 8 to 10 [7]. One study compared groups of patients who quit smoking and who did not quit with a baseline intermittent claudication and found that no patients from the smoking cessation group developed rest pain,

whereas 16% of smokers did develop rest pain [8]. For patients requiring arterial reconstructive surgery, patients who quit smoking show improved postoperative graft patency rates [9]. Patients should be strongly advised to quit smoking because continuing to do so increases the progression of their pre-existing disease and makes any interventions that are required more likely to fail. One recent study showed that the enhanced platelet aggregation and intraplatelet redox imbalance in long-term smokers can be significantly improved after as little as 2 weeks of smoking cessation [10]. According to the US Public Health Service guideline, it is important to identify, document, and treat every tobacco user at every office visit [11].

Diabetes mellitus

Diabetes increases the risk for atherogenesis by deleterious effects on the vessel wall, blood cells, and rheology [12]. The cardiovascular health study found that diabetes was associated with an almost fourfold increased prevalence of PAD in patients older than 65 years of age [13]. Given the increased prevalence of PAD in patients with diabetes, the effect of glycemic control on the progression of disease is of the utmost importance. The benefits of glycemic control on microvascular pathology, such as retinopathy, neuropathy, and nephropathy, have been shown in several studies [14,15]. The benefit of tight glycemic control on macrovascular disease, however, is less clearly defined. A surrogate marker of large artery atherosclerosis, the thickness of carotid intima-media, was used as an end point in the Diabetes Control and Complications Trial in long-term follow-up. They found statistically significant reduction in thickness with aggressive glycemic control [16]. Tight glycemic control can be recommended based on a subgroup analysis of the UK Prospective Diabetes Study, which showed reduction in the hemoglobin A_{1c} by 1% resulting in an 18% reduction in myocardial infarction, a 15% reduction in stroke, and a 42% reduction in episodes of PAD [15]. A review article by Stoyioglou and Jaff [17] concerning medical treatment of PAD also recommends aggressive glycemic control with a target hemoglobin A_{1c} of 7 or less in patients with PAD.

Hyperlipidemia

The increased risk of PAD caused by elevated cholesterol is similar to the elevated risk of coronary artery disease [18]. Reduction in LDL cholesterol level has been associated with reduction in cardiovascular events including myocardial infarction, stroke, and vascular death. There are multiple studies demonstrating that hydroxymethylglutaryl-CoA reductase inhibitors (ie, statins) may actually improve walking distance and pain-free walking time, and lower the rate of new or worsening intermittent claudication [19–21]. Stains have also recently been shown to improve the patency of peripheral bypass procedures [22]. Based on these studies, patients with PAD should be started on statin therapy if possible. The Heart Protection Study in the UK enrolled more than 20,000 patients randomized to receive simvastatin in addition to existing cardiovascular therapy. They showed statistically significant benefits in a group who received simvastatin regardless of the initial cholesterol level. The target LDL level set forth by the National Cholesterol Education Program is less than 100 mg/dL [18]. Recent data suggest lower target LDL level may be beneficial [23].

Recent studies have focused on the importance of C-reactive protein and the anti-inflammatory effects of statins as the most important benefit of statin therapy [24]. Ridker and coworkers [24] examined the C-reactive protein level and LDL level before the initiation of statin therapy and evaluated event-free survival. They found that regardless of LDL level, C-reactive protein level of less than 2 mg/L was associated with increased event-free survival. The authors recommended that when using statins to reduce cardiovascular risk, monitoring of C-reactive protein and cholesterol levels should be performed. In the REVERSAL study over 500 patients with documented coronary artery disease were randomized to receive moderate treatment (40 mg pravastatin per day) or intensive treatment (80 mg atorvastatin per day) and had intravascular ultrasound performed at baseline and 18 months following the initiation of treatment in addition to LDL and C-reactive protein levels. The study found that patients with reductions in both LDL and C-reactive protein that were greater than the median reduction in the study also had significantly slower progression of atherosclerosis than patients in whom reduction in LDL and C-reactive protein were less than the median reduction in the study [25].

Diagnosis

Diagnosis of PAD begins with a thorough history and physical examination. The initial assessment should include the patient's body habitus including the presence of contracture and ambulatory status. The pulse examination should include auscultation for carotid bruit and abdominal bruits and palpation for any palpable abdominal mass. The lower extremities are inspected with special attention to differences between the limbs regarding color, temperature, swelling, and general appearance. A careful pulse examination includes grading of the pulse quality and confirming that the pulse is in fact present and does not represent the examiner's own pulse or muscular twitches from the patient. The level of an occlusive or stenotic lesion can often be identified with history and physical examination alone.

Ankle-brachial index (ABI) can be a useful adjunct for the diagnosis. The ABI is a ratio of systolic blood pressure in the dorsalis pedis or posterior tibial arteries of the lower extremity to systolic blood pressure in the brachial arteries in the upper extremity. Normally, the ratio is 1 or a bit greater. This examination requires only blood pressure cuff and a Doppler device and can be performed in an office setting. ABI has been validated against angiographic evaluation for PAD and found to be almost 100% specific and 95% sensitive [26]. Calcified arteries can lead to a falsely elevated ABI because of incompressibility of the vessels. Similarly, subclavian stenosis can lead to a falsely lowered ABI on the basis of a brachial artery pressure that is lower than systemic pressure.

Improvements in duplex ultrasound technology have made arterial duplex mapping an effective, noninvasive method for delineating the arterial anatomy of the extremities. This modality can be used as a first-line measure to assess the therapy that may be required to treat a given patient's symptoms. Angiography and other invasive imaging modalities should be reserved for definitive treatment or for planning a surgical procedure.

Clinical presentation and staging

Patients with PAD may be asymptomatic or symptomatic, presenting with claudication or critical limb ischemia manifest as rest pain, ulceration, or gangrene. In one study, 14% of the patients from a general internal medical practice without a history of PVD were found to have abnormal ABI (<0.9) [27]. Another report evaluated a patient group with risk factors for PVD and found that 29% of patients had PVD by ABI criteria, although only 11% presented with symptoms [28]. In this situation treatment is not required for the majority of patients, although close follow-up and perhaps alteration of the patient's medical regimen may be in order.

Claudication is caused by insufficient oxygen supply to meet the demands of muscular activity as in the case of exertional angina. The clinical presentation is of reproducible pain or discomfort in a muscle group that is induced by exertion and relieved by rest. Claudication is generally divided into two categories based on a somewhat arbitrary walking distance. Those patients able to walk more than 1 block are described as having mild claudication, whereas those unable to walk 1 block are described as having disabling claudication [1].

The absence or degree of symptomatology may not correlate with the patient's anatomy, because several other factors need to be considered. These include the patient's exercise tolerance, which may be limited because of a number of factors including cardiopulmonary limitations or generalized weakness and level of activity. The impact of the symptoms on the patient's lifestyle should dictate therapy. For example, a relatively active patient who lives independently and presents with rest pain or a nonhealing ulcer may benefit from arterial reconstructive surgery, whereas a patient who is bed-bound in a nursing facility with the same symptoms will not realize the same benefits and may be better served with a primary amputation.

Elderly patients may develop nocturnal leg cramps, which are thought to be neuromuscular in origin. This cramping is frequently mistaken for vascular insufficiency, even in the absence of symptoms with exertion [1]. Patients who have spinal stenosis may present with similar symptoms but with intact peripheral pulses. This is shown as pseudoclaudication and warrants evaluation of the patient's spine.

The most common site for claudication is in the calf, usually attributable to disease in the superficial femoral artery. Thigh claudication can be attributed to iliac or common femoral artery disease. Leriche syndrome consists of impotence, buttock claudication, and gluteus muscle atrophy secondary to occlusive disease of the aortoiliac segment. It should be remembered that most patients presenting with claudication do not experience any worsening of their symptoms and that only a small minority progress to limb threat.

Patients presenting with rest pain may have a vascular etiology but other causes need to be ruled out. Patients with peripheral neuropathy, sciatica, lumbosacral disk disease, spinal stenosis, and arthritis may all complain of pain at rest. True rest pain is manifest by the absence of pulses and relief with dependency of the affected limb. Most patients describe sleeping with the affected leg in a dependent position to prevent symptoms. These patients show compromised circulation on noninvasive testing.

Because of the enormous capacity of the arterial system to compensate for arterial narrowing or occlusion by its collateral reserve when patients develop limb-threatening ischemia, the disease process is usually advanced with multiple, sequential occlusions or stenoses. It takes approximately five times the oxygen supply to heal an ischemic lesion than it does to maintain the resting state. Many patients with underlying PAD may only manifest and come to treatment when a lesion develops, following minor trauma for example. Such patients require intervention for limb salvage.

An additional complicating factor arises in patients with mixed arterial and venous disease. These patients can be difficult to treat because they are not candidates for compressive therapy as a result of their arterial insufficiency and because arterial interventions often increase swelling. The benefits of antiplatelet or anticoagulant medications are seen in this group of patients and may be of increased importance because of the limited therapeutic options.

Patients with PAD may be classified into one of five stages depending on symptoms as shown in Table 1. Surgical intervention is usually reserved for stages III and IV disease; however, all patients may benefit from antithrombotic therapy.

Treatment

The presence of arterial stenoses or occlusions does not in and of itself indicate a need for intervention. Patients with PAD, however, should be on a maximally cardiovascular protective regimen. Additionally, patients undergoing therapy with angioplasty and stenting, atherectomy, or bypass warrant close follow-up in conjunction with maximal medical therapy. The goals of therapy for patients with PAD should be prevention of both cardiovascular events and progression of the atherosclerotic disease process. In many cases intervention may actually accelerate the progression of atherosclerotic disease and substitute a good short term result for a poor long term outcome.

Table 1
Staging of infrainguinal arteriosclerosis with hemodynamically significant stenosis or occlusions

Stage	Presentation	Invasive diagnostic and therapeutic intervention
0	No signs or symptoms	Never justified
I	Intermittent claudication(<1 block); no physical changes	Usually unjustified for surgical intervention
II	Severe claudication (<1/2 block); dependent rubor; decreased temperature	Sometimes justified, not always necessary, may remain stable
III	Rest pain, atrophy, cyanosis, dependent rubor	Usually indicated but may do well for long periods without revascularization
IV	Nonhealing ischemic ulcer or gangrene	Usually indicated

Antiplatelet agents

Aspirin

Aspirin exerts its antithrombotic effect by inhibiting platelet aggregation. This effect is irreversible and lasts for the lifespan of platelets, or approximately 7 to 10 days. It also inhibits prostaglandin synthesis and acts as analgesic, antipyretic, and antirheumatic. The antiplatelet Trialists Analysis [29] is a meta-analysis of randomized trials on the prevention of myocardial infarction, ischemic stroke, and death with antiplatelet therapy. Patients defined as having PAD include those with intermittent claudication, and those who have undergone peripheral arterial reconstructive surgery or angioplasty. The study found an odds reduction of 23% in serious vascular events including ischemic stroke, myocardial infarction, and vascular death in patients in the aspirin group. Physician's Health Study [30] found that taking aspirin, 325 mg every other day, decreased the need for peripheral arterial surgery, although there was no difference in the development of claudication between the aspirin and placebo groups. The report of the Seventh ACCP Conference on Antithrombotic and Thrombolytic Therapy recommends for lifelong aspirin therapy (75–325 mg/d) compared with no antiplatelet therapy in patients with chronic limb ischemia [31]. This recommendation is based on the fact that most patients with PAD and no clinical manifestations of coronary or cerebrovascular disease do have occult coronary or cerebrovascular disease and stand to benefit from this therapy. The recommendation is also based on the fact that although ticlopidine and clopidogrel show a minimally greater benefit, aspirin is much less expensive. The Trans-Atlantic Consensus Conference also recommends "all patients with peripheral arterial disease (whether symptomatic or asymptomatic) should be considered for treatment with low-dose aspirin, or other approved antiplatelet (unless contraindicated), to reduce the risk of cardiovascular morbidity and mortality" [32].

Ticlopidine

Ticlopidine is a thienopyridine derivative that interferes with platelet membrane function by inhibiting ADP-induced platelet-fibrinogen binding and platelet-platelet interactions. This leads to inhibition of both platelet aggregation and release of platelet granule contents. As is the case for aspirin, these effects are irreversible and last for the lifespan of the platelet. Ticlopidine has been shown to reduce cardiovascular events in patients and to improve walking distance and lower-extremity ABI in patients with intermittent claudication [33,34]. In comparing ticlopidine, aspirin, and clopidogrel, a meta-analysis of randomized studies found that ticlopidine was the most effective in improving walking distance and improvement in mortality [35]. Ticlopidine is associated with a risk of thrombocytopenia and leukopenia, however, requiring close hematologic monitoring for at least 3 months. There is a reported risk of thrombocytopenic purpura in 1 in 2000 to 4000 patients [36]. Because of these possible side effects the Seventh ACCP Conference on Antithrombotic and Thrombolytic Therapy recommends clopidogrel over ticlopidine [31].

Clopidogrel

Clopidogrel is another thienopyridine derivative, but without hematologic side effects of ticlopidine. Clopidogrel inhibits ADP-induced platelet aggregation by direct inhibition of ADP receptor binding and ADP-mediated activation of the glycoprotein IIb-IIIa complex. The ADP receptor site is irreversibly modified and again, aggregation is inhibited for the platelet's lifespan. The CAPRIE trial is a randomized, blinded, international trial designed to assess the relative efficacy of clopidogrel and aspirin in reducing the risk of a composite outcome cluster of ischemic stroke, myocardial infarction, or vascular death [37]. Relative safety was also assessed in the study. The study population included patients with atherosclerotic vascular disease manifested as recent ischemic stroke, myocardial infarction, or symptomatic PAD followed for 1 to 3 years. More than 19,000 patients were randomized to receive aspirin (325 mg/d) or clopidogrel (75 mg/d). The study showed an overall relative risk reduction of 8.7% in favor of clopidogrel. In subgroup analysis, the patients taking clopidogrel had a relative risk reduction of 24% compared with patients on aspirin (Fig. 1). More recently, in a study of high-risk patients with recent ischemic stroke or transient ischemic attack, the MATCH trial found that the addition of aspirin to clopidogrel was associated with a nonsignificant difference in reduction of major vascular events. There was, however, an increased risk of life-threatening or major bleeding with the addition of aspirin [38].

Pentoxifylline

Pentoxifylline is a methylxanthine derivative and a weak antithrombotic agent that exerts its effect by lowering blood viscosity, improving erythrocyte flexibility, lowering fibrinogen levels, and retarding platelet aggregation [39,40]. It also increases leukocyte deformability and inhibits neutrophil adhesion

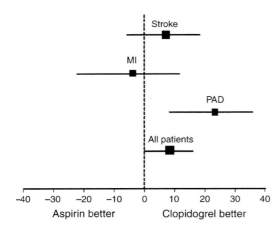

Fig. 1. Relative-risk reduction by subgroup in the CAPRIE trial. MI, myocardial infarction; PAD, peripheral arterial disease. (*From* CAPRIE Steering Committee. A randomized, blinded, trial of clopidogrel versus aspirin in patients at risk of ischemic events (CAPRIE). Lancet 1996;348:1329–39; with permission.)

and activation. Pentoxifylline is the first medication approved by the Food and Drug Administration for the symptomatic relief of intermittent claudication in 1984 [2]. A review of multiple trials concluded that the actual improvement in walking distance attributable to pentoxifylline is unpredictable and may not be clinically important when compared with the effects of placebo [41]. Pentoxifylline is generally very well tolerated with a low incidence of side effects. It is, however, not recommended in patients with recent cerebral or retinal hemorrhage or with a history of sensitivity to methylxanthines, such as caffeine, theophylline, and theobromine. Although pentoxifylline is recommended for the treatment of intermittent claudication, a meaningful response is seen only in a minority of patients.

Cilostazol

Cilostazol is a quinolinone derivative that inhibits cellular phosphodiesterase, most specifically phosphodiesterase III. Although its exact mechanisms are not fully understood, it suppresses platelet aggregation and is a direct arterial vasodilator. Cilostazol produces greater dilation in femoral beds than in vertebral, carotid, or visceral arteries. It also affects cardiovascular function. Because other medications that inhibit phosphodiesterase have shown decreased survival compared with placebo in patients with class III to IV congestive heart failure, cilostazol is not recommended for patients with congestive heart failure. Cilostazol may also decrease triglycerides and increase high-density lipoprotein. It is the second drug approved by the Food and Drug Administration for the treatment of intermittent claudication. The mechanism by which cilostazol improves walking distance in patients with claudication is not fully understood. The efficacy of cilostazol as an agent for improving walking distance is well demonstrated in multiple trials. In one study patients were randomly assigned to either placebo or cilostazol and completed a 16-week course of therapy. Differences in absolute claudication distance were then compared. Patients in the cilostazol group improved their absolute claudication distance by 47%, whereas the placebo group improved only 13% ($P < .001$) [42]. A similar study found improvement of absolute claudication distance in the cilostazol group by 31% and a drop of 9% in placebo group ($P < .01$) [43]. Another study looked at the effect of withdrawal of cilostazol [44]. Patients with intermittent claudication were randomized into one of three groups: (1) cilostazol, (2) pentoxifylline, or (3) placebo. After completing a 24-week course, cilostazol and pentoxifylline were changed to placebo and the patients were followed for 6 more weeks. They found that there was a more significant decrease in absolute claudication distance for the cilostazol group than the pentoxifylline or placebo group.

Side effects include headache, diarrhea, palpitation, and dizziness. Patients may take cilostazol with aspirin or clopidogrel without additional increase in bleeding time [45]. Cilostazol should be taken one-half hour before or 2 hours after eating because high-fat meals increase absorption. Concurrent administration of several drugs, such as diltiazem and omeprazole, and grapefruit juice can increase serum concentrations of cilostazol [46]. Cilostazol is indicated for the treatment of claudication and many patients experience an increase in walking distance, although it is not as well tolerated overall as pentoxifylline.

Anticoagulants

Heparin, low-molecular-weight heparin, vitamin K antagonist

There is no role for heparin, warfarin, or other formal anticoagulation in the management of intermittent claudication. A Cochrane review studied the effects of anticoagulant drugs, namely, unfractionated heparin, low-molecular-weight heparin, and vitamin K antagonists [47]. The review considered multiple trials and found no benefit with anticoagulation in either pain-free walking distance or maximum walking distance. There was also no benefit in mortality or incidence of cardiovascular events. The only significant finding was an increased risk of bleeding in patients on anticoagulation. Based on these findings, the Cochrane review recommended against the use of anticoagulation for intermittent claudication. Similarly, anticoagulation should not be used as a primary modality in the treatment of chronic limb-threatening ischemia. In some patients who have undergone revascularization with a bypass and who have a compromised outflow tract warfarin anticoagulation is recommended. This is frequently the case in patients who have undergone a below-knee popliteal or tibial bypass with a prosthetic conduit. Finally, in patients with microembolization, also referred to as the "blue toe" syndrome, in addition to treating the underlying cause and occasionally performing thrombolysis, these patients also receive anticoagulation to prevent further thrombosis of the microvasculature.

There is a role for formal anticoagulation, usually heparin, in treatment of acute limb ischemia. The Seventh ACCP conference on Antithrombotic and Thrombolytic Therapy recommends systemic anticoagulation with heparin to prevent thrombotic propagation in patients presenting with acute arterial emboli or in situ thrombosis [31]. The purpose of heparin anticoagulation in this setting is to prevent propagation of an acute thrombus or embolus and to prevent thrombosis of the now compromised outflow tract. An additional advantage is that the body's own fibrinolytic mechanisms may be given enough competitive advantage to lyse the clot. Finally, the patient may be stabilized while other diagnostic work-up and therapeutic options are considered.

Heparin-induced thrombocytopenia is a potential side effect of heparin therapy discussed in detail elsewhere in this issue. Heparin-induced thrombocytopenia is an antibody-associated thrombocytopenia that develops 5 to 10 days following the initiation of heparin therapy, but which may occur within 24 hours in cases of repeat exposure. This thrombocytopenia is generally defined as a decrease in platelet count of greater than 50% from baseline or a platelet count of less than 150,000/μL [48]. The syndrome is associated with a greatly increased risk of venous or arterial thrombosis and has a high morbidity. It is caused by antibodies to heparin and platelet factor 4 complex, which leads to platelet activation. Heparin-induced thrombocytopenia antibodies can be tested to confirm the diagnosis. When heparin-induced thrombocytopenia is suspected, all heparin including heparin flush for intravenous and intrarterial catheters must be discontinued because the syndrome is dose independent and even a small amount can cause thrombosis. A patient is then started on a nonheparin alternative anticoagulant, generally direct thrombin inhibitors, such as lepirudin or argatroban. Warfarin is avoided until platelet count recovery is achieved because warfarin may predispose to microvascular thrombosis and can cause venous limb gangrene and skin necrosis. More extensive discussion on heparin and heparin-induced thrombocytopenia can be found elsewhere in this issue.

Thrombolysis

The use of thrombolytics, such as urokinase or recombinant tissue-type plasminogen activator, is an alternative for the treatment of acute in situ thrombosis or embolus and acute limb ischemia. In 1960s and 1970s, thrombolytics were given intravenously (ie, systemically), but the practice has been largely abandoned with the introduction of catheter-directed thrombolysis. A catheter is positioned in or at the area of thrombosis over a guidewire and used to deliver thrombolytics locally. This enables the lysis to be performed with a reduced overall dose thereby minimizing systemic side effects of the thrombolytic agents. There have been several randomized studies comparing the various thrombolytic agents, most of which have not found a significant difference between the agents. The Surgery vs Thrombolysis for Ischemia of the Lower Extremity (STILE) study included a comparison of recombinant tissue-type plasminogen activator and urokinase and concluded that both drugs had similar efficacy and safety [49]. Another study comparing recombinant tissue-type plasminogen activator and urokinase demonstrated a higher successful lysis rate with recombinant tissue-type plasminogen activator ($P < .05$), but also a greater incidence of bleeding complications [50].

Thrombolysis provides an alternative to surgical thrombectomy in the setting of acute ischemia. Its advantages are that it can be performed using a minimally invasive approach and that in most cases angiography is required before undertaking surgical thrombectomy, so that the diagnosis and therapy can be accomplished in the same setting. Its major drawbacks are the local and systemic hemorrhagic complications. More recently, suction thrombectomy has also been used with or without thrombolysis. Finally, other analyses have evaluated the use of antiplatelet agents, such as the platelet IIb-IIIa complex inhibitor abciximab, in conjunction with thrombolysis [51]. Although thrombolysis occurred faster, there was a higher incidence of bleeding complications. There are several prospective randomized studies comparing surgical intervention with catheter-based thrombolysis. Overall, there is no clear answer to which therapy is superior based on these studies. Ouriel and coworkers [52] compared patients with acute limb ischemia of less than 7 days undergoing thrombolysis with angioplasty with those undergoing immediate surgery. The authors found that the limb salvage rates were similar in the two groups, but that 1-year survival was improved in patients randomized to thrombolysis on the basis of fewer cardiopulmonary complications (84% versus 58%; $P = .01$). In comparing patients with acute (≤ 14 days) versus chronic

(> 14 days) ischemia the STILE trial found that thrombolysis resulted in improved amputation-free survival at 6 months and shorter hospital stay in patients with acutely ischemic limbs, whereas surgical intervention was more effective for more chronic ischemia [49]. Further analysis of STILE trial data revealed that factors predictive of a poor outcome with lysis were femoropopliteal occlusion, diabetes, and critical ischemia [53,54]. Another trial, the Thrombolysis or Peripheral Arterial Surgery (TOPAS), compared recombinant urokinase versus surgery in acute arterial occlusion, again defined as ≤ 14 days. The authors found no statistically significant difference in amputation-free survival rate at 6 months and 1 year between the urokinase group and the surgery group. The most concerning complication of thrombolysis therapy is intracranial bleeding. The intracranial bleeding rate was found to be 1% to 2% in STILE and TOPAS. Recently, a working party reached a consensus on the use of thrombolysis in the management of acute lower-extremity native artery occlusion [55]. In patients with ischemia of less than 14 days thrombolysis followed by correction of the causative lesion is proposed as the preferred therapy. Immediate surgical intervention is preferred when thrombolysis leads to an unacceptable delay in restoring perfusion. Primary amputation is indicated for patients with irreversible ischemia and those who are nonreconstructible.

For patients presenting with occluded infrainguinal bypass grafts, surgical thrombectomy with or without revision, thrombolytic therapy with or without revision, or creation of a new bypass graft are options. The risks and benefits must be carefully considered in choosing which therapy to use because no clear benefit has been established for either strategy.

Summary

The management of patients with PAD requires a multidisciplinary and individualized approach, especially for patients requiring intervention and for those on antithrombotic therapy. Communication between the patient's primary physician, consulting medical specialists, and vascular surgeon is essential because all may contribute synergistically to deliver optimal care to the patient.

References

[1] Criqi MH, Denenber JO, Langer RD, et al. The epidemiology of peripheral arterial disease:

importance of identifying the population at risk. Vasc Med 1997;2:221–6.

[2] Murabito JM, Evans JC, Nieto K, et al. Prevalence and clinical correlates of peripheral arterial disease in the Framingham Offspring Study. Am Heart J 2002;143:961–5.

[3] Chobanian AV, Bakris GL, Black HR, et al. The seventh report of the joint national committee on prevention, detection, evaluation, and treatment of high blood pressure. JAMA 2003;289:2560–72.

[4] Radack K, Deck C. Beta-adrenergic blocker therapy does not worsen intermittent claudication in subjects with peripheral arterial disease: a meta-analysis of randomized controlled trials. Arch Intern Med 1991;151:1769–76.

[5] The Heart Outcomes Prevention Evaluation Study Investigators. Effects of an angiotensin-converting-enzyme inhibitor, ramipril, on cardiovascular events in high-risk patients. N Engl J Med 2000;342:145.

[6] Newby DE, Wright RA, Labinjoh C, et al. Endothe-lial dysfunction, impaired endogenous fibrinolysis, and cigarette smoking: a mechanism for arterial thrombosis and myocardial infarction. Circulation 1999;99:1411–5.

[7] Ingolfsson IO, Sigurdsson G, Sigvaldason H, et al. Marked decline in the prevalence and incidence of intermittent claudication in Icelandic men 1968–1986: a strong relationship to smoking and serum cholesterol-the Reykjavik Study. J Clin Epidemiol 1994;47:1237–43.

[8] Jonason T, Bergstrom R. Cessation of smoking in patients with intermittent claudication. Br J Surg 1982;69:S24.

[9] Aemli FM, Stein M, Provan JL, et al. The effect of postoperative smoking on femoropopliteal bypass grafts. Ann Vasc Surg 1999;3:20–5.

[10] Morita H, Ikeda H, Haramaki N, et al. Only two-week smoking cessation improves platelet aggreg-ability and intraplatelet redox imbalance of long-term Smokers. J Am Coll Cardiol 2005;45:589–94.

[11] The Tobacco Use and Dependence Clinical Practice Guideline Panel. Staff, and Consortium Representa-tives. A clinical practice guideline for treating to-bacco use and dependence: a US public health service report. JAMA 2000;283:3244–54.

[12] American Diabetes Association. Peripheral arterial disease in people with diabetes. Diabetes Care 2003;26:3333–41.

[13] Newman AB, Siscovick DS, Manolio TA, et al. An-kle-arm index as a marker of atherosclerosis in the Cardiovascular Health Study. Cardiovascular Heart Study (CHS) Collaborative Research Group. Circu-lation 1993;88:837–45.

[14] The Diabetes Control and Complications Trial In-vestigators. Effect of intensive diabetes management on macrovascular events and risk factors in the Dia-betes Control and Complications Trial. Am J Cardi-ol 1995;75:894–903.

[15] UK Prospective Diabetes Study (UKPDS) Group. Intensive blood glucose control with sulphonylureas or insulin compared with conventional treatment and risk of complications in patients with type 2 di-abetes (UKPDS 33). Lancet 1998;352:837–53.

[16] Nathan DM, Lachin J, Cleary P, et al. Intensive di-abetes therapy and carotid intima-media thickness in type 1 diabetes mellitus. Diabetes Control and Com-plications Trial; Epidemiology of Diabetes Interven-tions and Complications Research Group. N Engl J Med 2003;348:2294–303.

[17] Stoyioglou A, Jaff MR. Medical treatment of pe-ripheral arterial disease: a comprehensive review. J Vasc Interv Radiol 2004;15:1197–207.

[18] National Cholesterol Education Program (NCEP) Expert Panel on Detection, Evaluation, and Treat-ment of High Blood Cholesterol in Adults (Adult Treatment Panel III). Third Report of the National Cholesterol Education Program (NCEP) expert Panel on Detection, Evaluation, and Treatment of High Blood Cholesterol in Adults (Adult Treatment Panel III) final report. Circulation 2002;106:3143–421.

[19] Mondillo S, Ballo P, Barbati R, et al. Effects of sim-vastatin on walking performance and symptoms of intermittent claudication in hypercholesterolemic patients with peripheral vascular disease. Am J Med 2003;114:359–64.

[20] Mohler ER III, Hiatt WR, Creager MA. Cholesterol reduction with atorvastatin improves walking dis-tance in patients with peripheral arterial disease. Cir-culation 2003;108:1481–6.

[21] Aronow WS, Nayak D, Woodworth S, et al. Effects of simvastatin versus placebo on treadmill exercise time until the onset of intermittent claudication in older patients with peripheral arterial disease at six months and at one year after treatment. Am J Cardiol 2003;92:711–2.

[22] Abbruzzese TA, Havens J, Belkin M, et al. Statin therapy is associated with improved patency of autogenous infrainguinal bypass grafts. J Vasc Surg 2004;39:1178–85.

[23] Cannon CP, Braunwald E, McCabe CH, et al, for the Pravastatin or Atorvastatin Evaluation and In-fection Therapy-Thrombolysis in Myocardial In-farction 22 Investigators. Intensive versus moderate lipid lowering with statins after acute cor-onary syndromes. N Engl J Med 2004;350:1495–502.

[24] Ridker CP, Cannon PM, Morrow D, et al. C-reac-tive protein levels and outcomes after statin therapy. N Engl J Med 2005;352:20–8.

[25] Nissen SE, Tuzcu EM, Schoenhagen P, et al. Statin therapy, LDL cholesterol, C-reactive protein, and coronary artery disease. N Engl J Med 2005;352:29–38.

[26] Bernstein EF, Fronek A. Current statues of non-invasive tests in the diagnosis of peripheral arterial disease. Surg Clin North Am 1982;62:473–87.

[27] McGrae McDermott M, Kerwin DR, Liu K, et al. Prevalence and significance of unrecognized lower

extremity peripheral arterial disease in general medicine practice. J Gen Intern Med 2001;16:384.

[28] Hirsch AT, Criqui MH, Treat-Jacobson D, et al. Peripheral arterial disease detection, awareness, and treatment in primary care. JAMA 2001;286:1317.

[29] Antithrombotic Trialists' Collaboration. Collaborative meta-analysis of randomised trials of antiplatelet therapy for prevention of death, myocardial infarction, and stroke in high risk patients. BMJ 2002;324:71–86.

[30] Goldhaber SZ, Manson JE, Stampfer MJ, et al. Low-dose aspirin and subsequent peripheral arterial surgery in the Physicians' Health Study. Lancet 1992;3450:143–5.

[31] Clagett GP, Sobel M, Jackson MR, et al. Antithrombotic therapy in peripheral arterial occlusive disease: the Seventh ACCP Conference on Antithrombotic and Thrombolytic Therapy. Chest 2004;126:609S–26S.

[32] Dormandy JA, Rutherford RB. Management of peripheral arterial disease (PAD). TASC Working Group. TransAtlantic Inter-Society Consensus (TASC). J Vasc Surg 2000;31:S1–296.

[33] Boissel JP, Peyrieux JC, Destors JM. Is it possible to reduce the risk of cardiovascular events in subjects suffering from intermittent claudication of the lower limbs? Thromb Haemost 1989;62:681–5.

[34] Arcan JC, Panak E. Ticlopidine in the treatment of peripheral occlusive arterial disease. Semin Thromb Hemost 1989;15:167–70.

[35] Girolami B, Bernardi E, Prins MH, et al. Antithrombotic drugs in the primary medical management of intermittent claudication: a meta-analysis. Thromb Haemost 1999;81:715.

[36] Bennett CL, Weinberg PD, Rozenberg-Ben-Dror K, et al. Thrombotic thrombocytopenic purpura associated with ticlopidine: a review of 60 cases. Ann Intern Med 1998;128:541–4.

[37] CAPRIE Steering Committee. A randomized, blinded, trial of clopidogrel versus aspirin in patients at risk of ischemic events (CAPRIE). Lancet 1996; 348:1329–39.

[38] Diener HC, Bogousslavsky J, Brass LM, et al, on behalf of the MATCH investigators. Aspirin and clopidogrel compared with clopidogrel alone after recent ischemic stroke or transient ischemic attack in high-risk patients (MATCH): randomised, double-blind, placebo-controlled trial. Lancet 2004;364:331–7.

[39] Angelkort B, Maurin N, Bouteng K. Influence of pentoxifylline on erythrocyte deformability in peripheral occlusive arterial disease. Curr Med Res Opin 1979;6:255–8.

[40] Johnson WC, Sentissi JM, Baldwin D, et al. Treatment of claudication with pentoxifylline: are benefits related to improvement in viscosity? J Vasc Surg 1987;6:211–6.

[41] Radack K, Wyderski RJ. Conservative management of intermittent claudication. Ann Intern Med 1990; 113:135–46.

[42] Money SR, Herd JA, Isaacsohn JL, et al. Effect of cilostazol on walking distances in patients with intermittent claudication caused by peripheral vascular disease. J Vasc Surg 1998;27:267–75.

[43] Dawson DL, Cutler BS, Messiner MH, et al. Cilostazol has beneficial effects in treatment of intermittent claudication: results from a multicenter, randomized, prospective, double-blind trial. Circulation 1998;98:678–86.

[44] Dawson DL, DeMaioribus CA, Hagino RT, et al. The effect of withdrawal of drugs treating intermittent claudication. Am J Surg 1999;178:141–6.

[45] Wilhite D, Comerota AJ, Schmieder FA, et al. Managing PAD with multiple platelet inhibitors: the effect of combination therapy on bleeding time. J Vasc Surg 2003;38:710.

[46] Drugs for intermittent claudication. Med Lett Drugs Ther 2004;46:13.

[47] Cosmi B, Conti E, Coccheri S. Anticoagulant (heparin, low molecular weight heparin and oral anticoagulants) for intermittent claudication. Cochrane Database Syst Rev 2001;2:CD001999.

[48] Lewis BE, Walenga JM, Wallis DE. Anticoagulation with Novastan (argatroban) in patients with heparin-induced thrombocytopenia and heparin-induced thrombocytopenia and thrombosis syndrome. Semin Thromb Hemost 1997;23:197.

[49] The STILE Investigators. Results of a prospective randomized trial evaluating surgery versus thrombolysis for ischemia of the lower extremity: the STILE trial. Ann Surg 1994;220:251–68.

[50] Schweizer J, Altmann E, Flor JH, et al. Comparison of tissue plasminogen activator and urokinase in the local infiltration thrombolysis of peripheral arterial occlusions. Eur J Radiol 1996;23:64–73.

[51] Duda SH, Tepe G, Luz O, et al. Peripheral artery occlusion: treatment with abciximab plus urokinase versus urokinase alone: a randomized pilot trial (the PROMPT study). Radiology 2001;221: 689–96.

[52] Ouriel K, Kendarpa K, Schuerr DM, et al. Prourokinase versus urokinase for recanalization of peripheral occlusions, safety and efficacy: the PURPOSE trial. J Vasc Interv Radiol 1999;10: 1083–91.

[53] Weaver FA, Comerota AJ, Youngblood M, et al. Surgical revascularization versus thrombolysis for nonembolic lower extremity native artery occlusions: results of a prospective randomized trial. J Vasc Surg 1996;24:513–21.

[54] Comerota AJ, Weaver FA, Hosking JD, et al. Results of prospective, randomized trial of surgery versus thrombolysis for occluded lower extremity bypass grafts. Am J Surg 1996;172:105–12.

[55] Working Party on Thrombolysis in the Management of Limb Ischemia. Thrombolysis in the management of limb peripheral arterial occlusion: a consensus document. Am J Cardiol 1998;81:207–18.

**ELSEVIER
SAUNDERS**

Cardiol Clin 26 (2008) 299–309

**CARDIOLOGY
CLINICS**

Perioperative Management of Oral Anticoagulation

Martin O'Donnell, MB, MRCP(I),
Clive Kearon, MB, MRCP(I), FRCP(C), PhD*

*McMaster University and Henderson Research Centre, 711 Concession Street,
Hamilton, ON L8V 1C3, Canada*

Chronic anticoagulant therapy with vitamin K antagonists (eg, warfarin) requires temporary interruption before surgery because anticoagulation is associated with excessive operative bleeding [1–4]. Warfarin's antithrombotic effect takes days to recede after it is stopped and a similar length of time to re-establish after it is restarted [5]. During the period of anticoagulation cessation, patients are at increased risk of thromboembolism [1–4]. Elderly patients constitute a large proportion of patients who are treated with oral anticoagulants and present a greater than average risk of both thromboembolism and bleeding during this period [6]. Consequently, there is considerable uncertainty about the optimal approach to perioperative management of anticoagulation that maximizes patient safety with efficient health care delivery. Developing a rational approach requires the clinician to estimate the risks of thrombosis and bleeding associated with different approaches to management (Box 1) [1]. The risk of venous and arterial thromboembolism associated with different conditions, and the relative risk reduction for thromboembolism achieved by anticoagulation, are summarized in Table 1 [1]. In general, arterial thromboembolism is associated with far greater mortality (about 40% of events) and major disability (about 20% of events) [1] than recurrent venous thromboembolism, which has an estimated mortality of 6% [7] and estimated major disability of 5% or less in treated patients. In addition, because the risk of

thromboembolism and bleeding are often influenced by the surgical procedure, it is helpful to consider anticoagulant management separately for the preoperative and postoperative periods.

Accordingly, based on an individual assessment of risk factors for arterial or venous thrombosis and the risk of postoperative bleeding, this article outlines the preoperative and postoperative approach to anticoagulant management, following a brief description of the therapies most commonly used in the perioperative period. The prevention of arterial thromboembolism is considered separately from those whose indication is the prevention of venous thrombosis (Fig. 1).

Perioperative bridging therapy

In this article, the term "bridging therapy" refers to the use of therapeutic-dose unfractionated heparin (UFH) or low-molecular-weight-heparin (LMWH) and does not include lower doses of UFH and LMWH that are used to prevent venous thromboembolism [8]. Based on the predicted decline in the International Normalized Ratio (INR) (starts to fall at approximately 29 hours after the last dose of warfarin, and then decreases with a half-life of approximately 22 hours) it is reasonable to start bridging therapy approximately 60 hours after the last dose of warfarin (eg, third morning after last evening dose) [9–13]. Historically, intravenous UFH was used as bridging therapy because it has a short half-life (60 minutes) and is readily reversed [8]. Intravenous administration necessitates hospitalization before surgery, however, making intravenous UFH inconvenient and expensive. More recently, the use of subcutaneous LMWH has allowed

A version of this article originally appeared in Clinics in Geriatric Medicine, Volume 22, issue 1.

* Corresponding author.

E-mail address: kearonc@mcmaster.ca (C. Kearon)

Box 1. Factors influencing perioperative anticoagulant management

Risk of thromboembolism without
    anticoagulation
        During the preoperative period
        During the postoperative period
Risk reduction for thromboembolism with
    Oral anticoagulation
    Unfractionated or low-molecular-
        weight heparin
Incremental risk of bleeding with
    unfractionated or low-molecular-
        weight heparin bridging therapy
        During the preoperative period
        During the intraoperative period
        During the postoperative period
Consequences of thromboembolism
    (venous or arterial)
Consequences of bleeding
Patient preference (eg, fear of
    thromboembolism or bleeding)
Cost of unfractionated or low-molecular-
    weight heparin bridging therapy

Table 1
Rates of thromboembolism associated with different indications for oral anticoagulation and risk reduction with anticoagulation

Indication	% Control rate	% Risk reduction
Venous thromboembolism		
Acute venous thromboembolism		
0–1 mo	40/mo[a]	80
1–3 mo	10/2 mo[a]	90
Recurrent venous thromboembolism[b]	15/y[a]	90
Arterial thromboembolism		
NVAF	4.5/y	75[c]
NVAF and previous embolism	12/y	75[c]
Mechanical heart valve	8/y	75[c]
Acute arterial embolism		
0–1 mo	15/mo	75[c]

Abbreviation: NVAF, nonvalvular atrial fibrillation.

[a] An increase in the risk of venous thromboembolism associated with surgery (estimated to be 100-fold) is not included in these rates.

[b] Last episode of venous thromboembolism more than 3 months previously, but require long-term anticoagulation because of high risk of recurrence.

[c] Risk reduction with oral anticoagulation; risk reduction with bridging therapy is uncertain but expected to be less (see discussion).

Adapted from Kearon C, Hirsch J. Management of anticoagulation before and after elective surgery. N Engl J Med 1997;336:1506–11. Copyright © 1997, Massachusetts Medical Society.

bridging therapy to be administered to outpatients. Outpatient therapy seems to be feasible and safe in elderly patients provided they have no contraindication, such as significant renal impairment [14]. With this approach, doses of LMWH that are recommended for treatment of venous thromboembolism are administered once [1,11,13,15] or twice [12,16] daily, generally for 3 days before surgery. The authors' group completed a prospective cohort study that measured anti-Xa LMWH heparin levels shortly before surgery or invasive procedure in 80 patients receiving a standardized regimen of preoperative LMWH (enoxaparin, 1 mg/kg twice daily, last dose given ≥ 12 hours before surgery). It was observed that residual anticoagulant activity was present in most patients. Importantly, in two thirds, the anti-Xa level was within therapeutic range (≥ 0.5 IU/mL) [17]. Based on this observation and others [18,19], the authors' practice is to administer a twice-daily regimen with the last dose (eg, approximately 100 U/kg of LMWH) given more than 24 hours before surgery or invasive procedure.

Perioperative bridging LMWH therapy has not been evaluated in randomized trials. At least three large cohort studies, however, have studied the safety and feasibility of bridging therapy with a standardized regimen of LMWH [11–13]. Kovacs and coworkers [11] recruited 224 patients at risk of arterial embolism (112 with prosthetic valves and 112 with atrial fibrillation; mean age, 70 years), who required temporary interruption of warfarin, to receive a standardized regimen of perioperative LMWH. In this prospective cohort study, LMWH was started 3 days before surgery (dalteparin, 200 units/kg once daily on the third and second days before surgery and 100 units/kg on the morning before surgery); was not given on the day of surgery; was restarted the day after surgery (dalteparin, 200 units/kg daily or fixed low-dose 5000 units daily if patient was judged to be at high risk of postoperative bleeding); and was given for at least 4 days postoperatively and until the INR was higher than 1.9. During the 5-day preoperative and 90-day postoperative period, there were eight episodes of thromboembolism, of which two were considered cardioembolic and occurred on postoperative days 14 (transient ischemic attack) and 42 (ischemic stroke). Importantly, six of the eight episodes occurred in patients

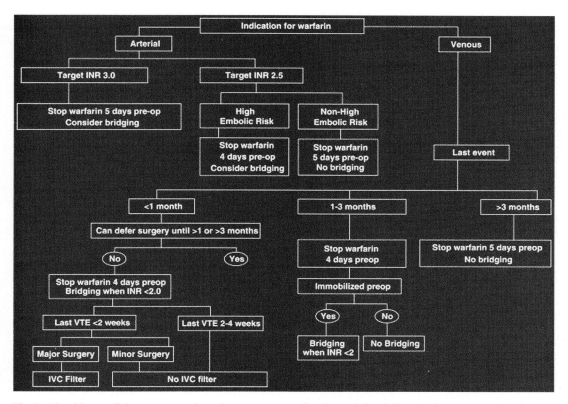

Fig. 1. Algorithm outlining an approach to the management of anticoagulation before elective surgery. INR, international normalized ratio; IVC, inferior vena cava; VTE, venous thromboembolism.

who had postoperative warfarin therapy withheld or deferred because of bleeding. Fifteen episodes of major bleeding were reported, of which eight occurred during or within 6 hours after surgery. There were no episodes of thromboembolism or major bleeding preoperatively [11].

Douketis and colleagues [12] reported the frequency of thromboembolism and major bleeding in a registry of 650 consecutive patients at risk of arterial embolism (215 with mechanical valves, 346 with atrial fibrillation, 89 with other indication; mean age, 68 years) who required temporary interruption of warfarin. Warfarin was discontinued 5 days (INR target 2–3) or 6 days (INR target 2.5–3.5) before surgery. The INR was measured on the third or fourth day before the procedure and preoperative LMWH (dalteparin, 100 units/kg twice daily) was started if the INR was less than 2.5, with last dose given greater than or equal to 12 hours before surgery. LMWH was restarted the day after surgery (dalteparin, 100 units/kg twice daily) in those considered not to be at high risk of postoperative bleeding (surgical procedure

considered to be associated with a low risk of bleeding and primary hemostasis established postoperatively). During the study period (5 days preoperatively and approximately 2 weeks after surgery), there were four episodes of thromboembolism, of which two were cardiac arrests, one was a systemic embolism, and one was a transient ischemic attack; all occurred in the postoperative period. Six episodes of major bleeding occurred, all in the postoperative period [12].

Dunn and colleagues [13] treated 260 patients (176 with atrial fibrillation; mean age, 68 years) who required temporary interruption of warfarin with once-daily enoxaparin (1.5 mg/kg) for 3 days before the procedure, followed by the same regimen restarted the morning after the procedure and continued until the INR was therapeutic. In this prospective cohort study there were four episodes of thromboembolism in the atrial fibrillation group during 28 days of follow-up, of which two were transient ischemic attacks and two were peripheral arterial thromboembolism (no episodes of ischemic stroke). In the entire cohort, the incidence of major bleeding during the period of bridging enoxaparin therapy was 3.5%, with almost all episodes of major bleeding occurring in the 40 patients who had undergone major surgery (eight episodes; 20% incidence) [13].

Although these studies [11–13] support the feasibility of bridging therapy with LMWH, clinical trials are required to determine whether the benefit of bridging therapy outweighs the associated risks of bleeding. Currently, it is generally recommended that patients with the highest risk of arterial or venous thromboembolism who require interruption of oral anticoagulant therapy for surgery should receive therapeutic-dose heparin therapy (UFH or LMWH) during much of the interval when the INR is subtherapeutic [2–5].

Preoperative management of anticoagulation

Certain surgical procedures are associated with a low risk of bleeding. Consequently, there is uncertainty about the need to reverse anticoagulation for some invasive procedures. For example, it does not seem to be necessary for dental extractions [5,20] (a local hemostatic agent may be used with more extensive dental surgery [21]) or for extracapsular cataract removal under local anaesthetic [22]. Similarly, the American Society for Gastrointestinal Endoscopy recommends that, because of a low associated risk of bleeding, diagnostic endoscopy (upper endoscopy, colonoscopy, and flexible sigmoidoscopy) with or without biopsy (but not polypectomy), diagnostic endoscopic retrograde cholangiopancreatography, and biliary stent implantation (without sphincterotomy) can be performed with an INR of up to 2.5 [23]. In general, it is more acceptable to perform surgical procedures while on anticoagulant therapy if the site of potential bleeding is accessible (eg, mouth or skin) rather than remote (eg, percutaneous biopsy of internal organs).

For surgery and invasive procedures associated with a moderate or high risk of bleeding, vitamin K antagonists are stopped 4 to 5 days before surgery, depending on the targeted anticoagulant intensity (see Fig. 1). In patients whose INR is 2 to 3 (ie, target INR of 2.5), it takes about 4 days for the INR spontaneously to fall to 1.5 or less in most (approximately 95%) patients [9], an intensity of anticoagulation that is not expected to be associated with an increase in intraoperative bleeding [9,24–28]. If the INR is 2.5 to 3.5 (ie, target INR of 3), this is expected to take 5 days. There is evidence that the rate of decline

in INR is slower in elderly patients [29]. Although the authors usually recommend that the INR be measured on the day before surgery, they take particular care to ensure it is measured in elderly patients (≥ 75 years), to determine if it has decreased adequately. If on the morning before surgery the INR is 1.6 or 1.7 they generally give 1 mg, and if the INR is 1.8 or higher they generally give 2 mg of vitamin K orally to accelerate the reversal of anticoagulation and then repeat the INR the day of surgery [30]. In general, fresh frozen plasma should be avoided for elective surgery.

Another approach to management in this setting is to shorten the interval when the INR is subtherapeutic by withholding fewer doses of warfarin preoperatively while giving a small dose of oral vitamin K (eg, 1 mg) to accelerate reversal of anticoagulation. The safety of this approach is not known, and although it seems reasonable for most patients if surgery needs to be performed before the INR can spontaneously decrease to an acceptable level, unless accompanied by bridging therapy, this practice is discouraged for patients with mechanical heart valves [31,32].

Arterial thromboembolism

Prevention of systemic embolism with oral anticoagulation (vitamin K antagonists) is most commonly used in patients with atrial fibrillation or another cardiac source of arterial thromboembolism (eg, valvular heart disease, native or prosthetic) [5]. Patients with nonvalvular atrial fibrillation have an average risk of systemic embolism of about 4.5% per year in the absence of antithrombotic therapy [33]. In individual patients, this risk varies from about 1% to 20%, depending on the prevalence of risk factors (ie, previous embolism, hypertension, age ≥ 75 years, left ventricular dysfunction, diabetes, mitral stenosis) [33–36]. The average rate of major thromboembolism in nonanticoagulated patients with mechanical heart valves is estimated to be 8%, with the risk in individuals also varying widely according to the prevalence of risk factors (ie, caged ball or disk valves, mitral position, atrial fibrillation, previous embolism, age ≥ 70 years) [37–40]. Previous thromboembolism is the single most important risk factor for stroke in patients with atrial fibrillation [33,35,36,41] and it is also an important risk factor in patients with prosthetic heart valves [39,40]. Consequently, the period of subtherapeutic oral anticoagulation should be kept to a minimum in patients with previous embolism, and in others who are at highest risk for embolism (see Fig. 1).

Efficacy of heparins in prevention of systemic thromboembolism

Although there is good evidence that UFH and LMWH are effective at preventing venous thromboembolism [8,42], this is less certain for the prevention of cardioembolism, particularly with the use of LMWH. In the only trial to evaluate the efficacy of LMWH for the reduction of early recurrent stroke in patients with atrial fibrillation exclusively, dalteparin, 100 IU/kg twice daily, was not shown to be superior to aspirin therapy (odds ratio = 1.1 in favor of aspirin; 95% confidence interval, 0.6–2.2) [43]. Similarly, subgroup analyses of other studies that have evaluated LMWH in acute ischemic stroke and subsequent meta-analyses have also failed to demonstrate a benefit in reduction of systemic embolism over aspirin [44–46]. In the International Stroke Trial, however, UFH (5000 or 12,500 IU subcutaneously twice daily) was more effective than aspirin at preventing early recurrent stroke (within 14 days) in the subgroup of patients with atrial fibrillation (N = 3169) [47]. Rates of recurrent ischemic stroke were 4.9%, 3.4%, and 2.3% in the non-UFH, UFH 5000 IU, and UFH 12,500 IU groups, respectively (P = .001) [47]. In addition, therapeutic or near-therapeutic doses of UFH approximately halves the frequency of stroke associated with acute myocardial infarction in the absence of treatment with thrombolytic therapy and aspirin (but not with such therapy), supporting that UFH can reduce cardioembolism [48].

There are less data relating to the efficacy of UFH and LMWH for the prevention of embolism in patients with mechanical heart valves. Indirect comparisons suggest that subcutaneous UFH is substantially less effective than oral anticoagulants at preventing thromboembolic complications in pregnant women with mechanical heart valves; however, less than currently recommended therapeutic doses of UFH were often used in these patients [49,50]. Although one cannot conclude that LMWH does not reduce the risk of thromboembolism in patients with mechanical heart valves when oral anticoagulation is interrupted [51], taken together these data suggest that UFH, and particularly LMWH, are less effective than warfarin at preventing cardioembolism.

Bridging therapy with heparin

Despite uncertainty about efficacy, most authorities recommend use of bridging therapy for patients with the highest risk of embolism [2–4,8,52–54]. With mechanical heart valves, this includes those for which a higher (eg, target INR 3; range, 2.5–3.5) intensity of anticoagulation is recommended (ie, tilting disk and bileaflet mitral valves, bileaflet aortic valves with atrial fibrillation, caged ball or caged disk valves, any valve with previous embolism) [40]. With atrial fibrillation, this includes those with a history of embolism or multiple risk factors [33,35,36,41]. To support withholding bridging heparin therapy in patients at low or intermediate risk of arterial thromboembolism, Garcia and colleagues [55] reported a low frequency of arterial thromboembolism (0.75%) in 535 patients with atrial fibrillation undergoing temporary interruption of warfarin without bridging therapy (four episodes [0.7%]; two occurred in patients with previous stroke). In addition, because current evidence suggests that therapeutic dose LMWH is not effective at preventing ischemic stroke in patients with atrial fibrillation [43,44], the authors rarely use bridging LMWH therapy in such patients.

Patient and physician preference

After a discussion of the risks and benefits of bridging therapy in patients with mechanical heart valve or atrial fibrillation, some patients express a preference either to receive or not receive such therapy. Their decision may be influenced by previous good or bad experience with bridging therapy; aversion to subcutaneous injections (self-administered, or by another); fear of stroke; or cost implications. Similarly, referring physicians (eg, cardiologists, cardiac surgeons) may have a strong preference that their patients receive bridging therapy. Because preoperative bridging therapy may reduce embolism and is associated with a low risk of major bleeding, the authors do not discourage its use, particularly in patients with prosthetic heart valves where there is less evidence challenging the efficacy of bridging therapy than there is for those with atrial fibrillation [43,44,56].

Venous thromboembolism

Oral anticoagulation with vitamin K antagonists, is indicated for the prevention of recurrent venous thromboembolism, a risk that declines rapidly during the 3 months after an acute episode [57,58]. It is estimated that stopping anticoagulation within 1 month of an acute event is associated with a very high risk of recurrent venous thromboembolism (ie, 40% over a 1-month period) (see Table 1) and that this risk is intermediate if anticoagulants are stopped during the second and third months of treatment (ie, 10% over a 2-month period [1]).

If feasible, surgery should be deferred following an acute episode of venous thromboembolism until patients have received at least 1 month, and preferably 3 months, of anticoagulation (see Fig. 1). If this is not feasible and surgery is performed within 1 month of an acute event, bridging therapy should be used while the INR is less than 2. If it is necessary to perform surgery within 2 weeks of an acute episode of venous thromboembolism, the risk of pulmonary embolism is probably acceptable if bridging therapy is withheld for 18 hours or less (eg, with intravenous UFH, 6 hours preoperatively and 12 hours postoperatively) and the duration of surgery is short (eg, 1 hour or less). Consequently, patients who do not have major surgery and do not have a high risk of postoperative bleeding can be managed with bridging therapy. Patients who have major surgery within 2 weeks of an acute episode of proximal deep vein thrombosis or pulmonary embolism, however, should have a vena caval filter inserted preoperatively or intraoperatively [1]. Currently available temporary filters allow removal of the filter in the postoperative period, when it becomes safe to re-establish oral anticoagulation.

If the most recent episode of venous thromboembolism occurred between 1 and 3 months previously, warfarin should only be withheld for four doses to minimize the period of thrombotic risk; however, unless patients are immobilized (ie, already hospitalized) neither bridging therapy nor prophylactic doses of UFH or LMWH are necessary preoperatively. If patients are immobilized in hospital before surgery, they should receive prophylactic doses of UFH or LMWH when the INR decreases to less than 1.6. The INR of outpatients can be checked the day before surgery and, depending on its value, a single dose of oral vitamin K or subcutaneous LMWH can be considered at that time. Three months or greater of anticoagulation is usually reserved for patients with multiple episodes of venous thromboembolism; a single episode of unprovoked thrombosis; or thrombosis in association with a persistent risk factor, such as active malignancy. Interruption of warfarin therapy during this phase of treatment is estimated to be associated with a much lower risk of thromboembolism than if it is stopped during the first 3 months of therapy (eg, 10%–15% per year). Consequently, it is reasonable to withhold five doses of warfarin before surgery in patients who have already been treated with 3 or more months of anticoagulation and not use bridging therapy.

Postoperative management of anticoagulation

Major surgery is associated with a marked increase in the risk of venous thromboembolism; in the short term, this is estimated to be a 100-fold increase in risk [1]. Unlike venous thromboembolism, however, the increase in arterial embolism associated with nonvascular surgery has not been adequately quantified.

Recent surgery is a major risk factor for anticoagulant-induced bleeding [1]. Whereas bleeding is uncommon when warfarin is started after major surgery [8,28,59–61], bleeding is expected to be substantial if therapeutic doses of UFH or LMWH are administered within days of operation [59]. For example, when both are started within 24 hours of major orthopedic surgery, prophylactic doses of LMWH (ie, less than half the dose used for bridging therapy) are associated with more bleeding than warfarin [8,59,60]. Although the consequences of an episode of major bleeding in the postoperative period (eg, case fatality estimated at 3%) [62,63] are generally less severe than those of an episode of thromboembolism, because the absolute risk of thromboembolism before re-establishing oral anticoagulation is often extremely low, administration of bridging therapy has the potential to do more harm than good during this interval (see the section on perioperative bridging) [1]. Because there is a delay of about 12 to 24 hours after warfarin administration before the INR begins to increase, warfarin should be restarted as soon as possible after surgery unless patients have additional invasive procedures planned or are actively bleeding (Fig. 2).

Arterial thromboembolism

In patients with the highest risk of arterial embolism (see previously), it is reasonable to use bridging therapy after surgery provided the risk of bleeding is minimal (eg, minor surgical or diagnostic procedures) (see Fig. 2).

If intravenous UFH is being used for postoperative bridging therapy, it should be started without a loading bolus dose, no sooner than 12 hours after surgery, at a rate of no more than 18 units/kg/h [64]. In the absence of a loading dose, the first activated partial thromboplastin time measurement should be deferred for 12 hours

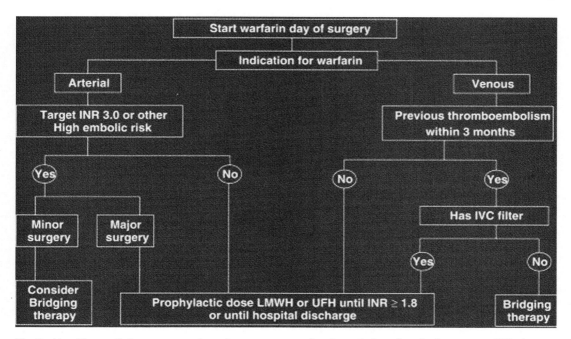

Fig. 2. Algorithm outlining an approach to the management of anticoagulation after elective surgery. INR, international normalized ratio; IVC, inferior vena cava; LMWH, low-molecular-weight heparin; UFH, unfractionated heparin.

for a stable anticoagulant response to have been attained. Compared with therapeutic-dose subcutaneous LMWH, intravenous UFH has the advantage that it is rapidly eliminated when stopped, and can be effectively reversed by protamine sulfate if bleeding occurs [65]. If therapeutic-dose subcutaneous LMWH is being used, it should probably not be started until approximately 24 hours after surgery. With hospitalized patients, the LMWH dose can be increased in a step-wise fashion over 36 hours, starting with a prophylactic dose within 12 hours of surgery. Twice-daily dosing may be preferable to once-daily dosing in the early postoperative period because lower peaks of anticoagulant effect are induced, and the smaller twice-daily dose is expected to be eliminated sooner if bleeding occurs close to the time of injection; however, once-daily and twice-daily regimens have been used postoperatively [10–13].

Bridging therapy is not recommended after surgery that is associated with a moderate or higher risk for bleeding, even if patients are considered to have a high risk of arterial embolism [1,13,55]. Instead, subcutaneous UFH or LMWH, in doses recommended for thromboembolism prophylaxis of high-risk patients, should

be given to hospitalized patients until the INR reaches 1.8 [8].

Venous thromboembolism

Because surgery is a major risk factor for venous thromboembolism, the need for antithrombotic prophylaxis is much greater postoperatively than it is preoperatively. Patients who have had an episode of venous thromboembolism within 3 months of surgery are expected to have a very high risk of recurrence postoperatively. Consequently, bridging therapy is recommended in this setting until the INR is 2 or greater, provided the surgeon does not believe that the patient is at high risk for bleeding [1]. Although patients who have a vena caval filter remain at high risk of recurrent venous thrombosis, they are at least partially protected from pulmonary embolism [66] and, consequently, bridging therapy can be avoided in these patients in the early postoperative period.

Provided there have been no previous episodes of thromboembolism within 3 months before surgery, postoperative bridging therapy is not indicated. Subcutaneous UFH or LMWH is recommended in doses used for venous thromboembolism prophylaxis of high-risk patients while the INR is less than 1.8 and patients are hospitalized. Because there is a concern that restarting warfarin may induce a transient hypercoagulable state in patients with protein C or protein S deficiency [67], patients with these conditions should restart warfarin slowly, at no more than the expected maintenance dose, and should receive at least prophylactic doses of UFH or LMWH until the INR is at 2 for 2 days.

Qualifying remarks

The recommendations outlined are strongly influenced by a number of assumptions, some of which are considered in greater detail. It is proposed that, for most patients, warfarin is withheld preoperatively long enough for the INR to fall spontaneously to a value of 1.5 or lower before surgery without the need for bridging therapy. Because the INR is prolonged to some extent for much of this time, it is estimated that this interruption of warfarin exposes patients to a small risk of thromboembolism preoperatively (ie, equivalent to the thromboembolic risk associated with 1 day of "no anticoagulation") [68–70]. For the same reason, provided warfarin is restarted the day of surgery, it is estimated that patients are exposed to a similar small risk of thromboembolism postoperatively while oral anticoagulant therapy is being re-established. It has also been assumed that the risk of thromboembolism associated with a day without anticoagulation is one 365th part of the risk associated with a year without therapy. Hence, a 10% per year risk of thromboembolism translates to a daily risk of approximately 0.03%, or a 1 in 3650 probability of an event. If stopping oral anticoagulation induces a transient rebound hypercoagulable state [1,4,71], or starting anticoagulation induces a transient paradoxical hypercoagulable state [67], the daily risk of thromboembolism may be underestimated. There is no convincing clinical evidence, however, to support either of these phenomena in unselected patients [71].

It is concluded that warfarin should be interrupted for as short a time as possible (usually 4 or 5 days) when it is necessary to reverse oral anticoagulant therapy. Most patients can then have invasive procedures performed without the need for bridging therapy and, because of the associated risk of bleeding, bridging therapy should generally be avoided within 2 days of major surgery. Because this assessment is based on an interpretation of mostly indirect data, however, and because these data are open to different interpretations, uncertainty as to the optimal management of such patients is acknowledged.

Finally, perioperative management of anticoagulation can cause anxiety for patients, surgeons, anesthetists, and those that manage long-term anticoagulant therapy. Good communication between all of these parties is essential to ensure that an optimal management strategy is identified, that this strategy is then successfully executed, and that the potential for recrimination is minimized in the unlikely event of a serious thrombotic or hemorrhagic complication.

References

[1] Kearon C, Hirsh J. Management of anticoagulation before and after elective surgery. N Engl J Med 1997; 336(21):1506–11.

[2] Heit JA. Perioperative management of the chronically anticoagulated patient. J Thromb Thrombolysis 2002;12:81–7.

[3] Ansell JE. The perioperative management of warfarin therapy. Arch Intern Med 2003;163:881–3.

[4] Dunn AS, Turpie AG. Perioperative management of patients receiving oral anticoagulants: a systematic review. Arch Intern Med 2003;163:901–8.

[5] Ansell J, Hirsh J, Dalen J, et al. Managing oral anticoagulant therapy. Chest 2001;119:22S–38S.

[6] Halperin JL. Anticoagulation for atrial fibrillation in the elderly. Am J Geriatr Cardiol 2005;14(2): 81–6. Review.

[7] Douketis JD, Kearon C, Bates S, et al. Risk of fatal pulmonary embolism in patients with treated venous thromboembolism. JAMA 1998;279:458–62.

[8] Geerts WH, Pineo G, Heit JA, et al. Prevention of venous thromboembolism. Chest 2004;126: 338S–400S.

[9] White RH, McKittrick T, Hutchinson R, et al. Temporary discontinuation of warfarin therapy: changes in the international normalized ratio. Ann Intern Med 1995;122:40–2.

[10] Tinmouth AH, Morrow BH, Cruickshank MK, et al. Dalteparin as periprocedure anticoagulation for patients on warfarin and at high risk of thrombosis. Ann Pharmacother 2001;35:669–74.

[11] Kovacs M, Kearon C, Rodger M, et al. Single-arm study of bridging therapy with low-molecular-weight heparin for patients at risk of arterial embolism who require temporary interruption of warfarin. Circulation 2004;110(12):1658–63.

[12] Douketis JD, Johnson JA, Turpie AG. Low-molecular-weight heparin as bridging anticoagulation during interruption of warfarin: assessment of

a standardized periprocedural anticoagulation regimen. Arch Intern Med 2004;164(12):1319–26.

[13] Dunn AS, Spyropoulos AC, Turpie AG. Bridging therapy in patients with long-term oral anticoagulants who require surgery: the Prospective Perioperative Enoxaparin Cohort trial (PROSPECT). J Thromb Haemost 2007;5(11):2211–8.

[14] Wells PS, Kovacs MJ, Bormanis J, et al. Expanding eligibility for outpatient treatment of deep venous thrombosis and pulmonary embolism with low-molecular-weight heparin: a comparison of patient self-injection with homecare injection. Arch Intern Med 1998;158(16):1809–12.

[15] Spandorfer JM, Lynch S, Weitz HH, et al. Use of enoxaparin for the chronically anticoagulated patient before and after procedures. Am J Cardiol 1999;84:478–80, A10.

[16] Turpie AGG, Johnson J. Temporary discontinuation of oral anticoagulants: role of low molecular weight heparin (Dalteparin). Circulation 2002;102: II-826 (abstract 3983).

[17] O'Donnell M, Kearon C, Johnson J, et al. Prevalence of residual anticoagulant activity following bridging low molecular weight heparin. Ann Intern Med 2007;146(3):184–7.

[18] Becker RC, Spencer FA, Gibson M, et al. Influence of patient characteristics and renal function on factor Xa inhibition pharmacokinetics and pharmacodynamics after enoxaparin administration in non-ST-segment elevation acute coronary syndromes. Am Heart J 2002;143:753–9.

[19] Douketis JD, Kinnon K, Crowther MA. Thromboprophylaxis with twice-daily but not with once-daily low-molecular-weight heparin is associated with a detectable anticoagulant effect at time of epidural catheter removal in patients receiving co-administered continuous epidural analgesia. Thromb Haemost 2002;88(1):37–40.

[20] Wahl MJ. Dental surgery in anticoagulated patients. Arch Intern Med 1998;158:1610–6.

[21] Sindet-Pederson S, Ramstrom G, Bernvil S, et al. Hemostatic effect of tranexamic acid mouthwash in anticoagulant-treated patients undergoing oral surgery. N Engl J Med 1989;320:840–3.

[22] McCormack P, Simcock PR, Tullo AB. Management of the anticoagulated patient for ophthalmic surgery. Eye 1993;7(Pt 6):749–50.

[23] Guideline on the management of anticoagulation and antiplatelet therapy for endoscopic procedures. American Society for Gastrointestinal Endoscopy. Gastrointest Endosc 1998;48:672–5.

[24] Tinker JH, Tarhan S. Discontinuing anticoagulant therapy in surgical patients with cardiac valve prostheses: observations in 180 operations [abstract]. JAMA 1978;239:738–9.

[25] Francis CW, Marder VJ, Evarts CM, et al. Two-step warfarin therapy: prevention of postoperative venous thrombosis without excessive bleeding. JAMA 1983;249:374–8.

[26] Taberner DA, Poller L, Burslem RW, et al. Oral anticoagulants controlled by the British comparative thromboplastin versus low-dose heparin in prophylaxis of deep vein thrombosis. Br Med J 1978;1: 272–4.

[27] Rustad H, Myhre E. Surgery during anticoagulant treatment: the risk of increased bleeding in patients on oral anticoagulant treatment [abstract]. Acta Med Scand 1963;173:115–9.

[28] Francis CW, Pellegrini VD Jr, Leibert KM, et al. Comparison of two warfarin regimens in the prevention of venous thrombosis following total knee replacement. Thromb Haemost 1996;75:706–11.

[29] Hylek EM, Regan S, Go AS, et al. Clinical predictors of prolonged delay in return of the international normalized ratio to within the therapeutic range after excessive anticoagulation with warfarin. Ann Intern Med 2001;135(6):393–400.

[30] Crowther MA, Julian J, McCarty D, et al. Treatment of warfarin-associated coagulopathy with oral vitamin K: a randomised controlled trial. Lancet 2000;356:1551–3.

[31] Shields RC, McBane RD, Kuiper JD, et al. Efficacy and safety of intravenous phytonadione (vitamin K1) in patients on long-term oral anticoagulant therapy. Mayo Clin Proc 2001;76:260–6.

[32] Bonow RO, Carabello B, de LA Jr, et al. Guidelines for the management of patients with valvular heart disease: executive summary. A report of the American College of Cardiology/American Heart Association Task Force on Practice Guidelines (Committee on Management of Patients with Valvular Heart Disease). Circulation 1998;98:1949–84.

[33] Atrial Fibrillation Investigators. Risk factors for stroke and efficacy of antithrombotic therapy in atrial fibrillation analysis of pooled data from five randomized trials. Arch Intern Med 1994;154: 1449–57.

[34] Atrial Fibrillation Investigators. Echocardiographic predictors of stroke in patients with atrial fibrillation. Arch Intern Med 1998;158:1316–20.

[35] Hart RG, Halperin JL. Atrial fibrillation and thromboembolism: a decade of progress in stroke prevention. Ann Intern Med 1999;131:688–95.

[36] Singer DE, Albers GW, Dalen JE, et al. Antithrombotic therapy in atrial fibrillation. Chest 2004;126: 429S–56S.

[37] Mok CK, Boey J, Wang R, et al. Warfarin versus dipyridamole-aspirin and pentoxifylline-aspirin for the prevention of prosthetic heart valve thromboembolism: a prospective randomized clinical trial. Circulation 1985;72:1059–63.

[38] Cannegieter SC, Rosendaal FR, Briet E. Thromboembolic and bleeding complications in patients with mechanical heart valve prostheses. Circulation 1994; 89(2):635–41.

[39] Horstkotte D, Scharf RE, Schultheiss HP. Intracardiac thrombosis: patient-related and device-related factors. J Heart Valve Dis 1995;4:114–20.

[40] Salem DN, Stein PD, Al-Ahmad A, et al. Antithrombotic therapy in patients with mechanical and biological prosthetic heart valves. Chest 2004;126: 457S–82S.

[41] European Atrial Fibrillation Trial Study Group. Secondary prevention in non-rheumatic atrial fibrillation after transient ischaemic attack or minor stroke. Lancet 1993;342:1255–62.

[42] Buller HR, Agnelli G, Hull RD, et al. Antithrombotic therapy for venous thromboembolic disease. Chest 2004;126:401S–28S.

[43] Berge E, Abdelnoor M, Nakstad PH, et al. Low molecular-weight heparin versus aspirin in patients with acute ischaemic stroke and atrial fibrillation: a double-blind randomised study. HAEST Study Group. Heparin in Acute Embolic Stroke Trial. Lancet 2000;355:1205–10.

[44] Hart RG, Palacio S, Pearce LA. Atrial fibrillation, stroke, and acute antithrombotic therapy: analysis of randomized clinical trials. Stroke 2002;33:2722–7.

[45] Bath PM, Lindenstrom E, Boysen G, et al. Tinzaparin in acute ischaemic stroke (TAIST): a randomised aspirin-controlled trial. Lancet 2001;358:702–10.

[46] Bath PM, Iddenden R, Bath FJ. Low-molecular-weight heparins and heparinoids in acute ischemic stroke: a meta-analysis of randomized controlled trials. Stroke 2000;31:1770–8.

[47] Saxena R, Lewis S, Berge E, et al. Risk of early death and recurrent stroke and effect of heparin in 3169 patients with accute ischemic stroke and atrial fibrillation in the International Stroke Trial. Stroke 2001; 32(10):2333–7.

[48] Collins R, Peto R, Baigent C, et al. Aspirin, heparin, and fibrinolytic therapy in suspected acute myocardial infarction. N Engl J Med 1997;336:847–60.

[49] Chan WS, Anand S, Ginsberg JS. Anticoagulation of pregnant women with mechanical heart valves: a systematic review of the literature. Arch Intern Med 2000;160:191–6.

[50] Salazar E, Izaguirre R, Verdejo J, et al. Failure of adjusted doses of subcutaneous heparin to prevent thromboembolic phenomena in pregnant patients with mechanical cardiac valve prostheses. J Am Coll Cardiol 1996;27:1698–703.

[51] Montalescot G, Polle V, Collet JP, et al. Low molecular weight heparin after mechanical heart valve replacement. Circulation 2000;101:1083–6.

[52] Douketis JD, Crowther MA, Cherian SS. Perioperative anticoagulation in patients with chronic atrial fibrillation who are undergoing elective surgery: results of a physician survey. Can J Cardiol 2000; 16:326–30.

[53] Douketis JD, Crowther MA, Cherian SS, et al. Physician preferences for perioperative anticoagulation in patients with a mechanical heart valve who are undergoing elective noncardiac surgery. Chest 1999; 116:1240–6.

[54] Garcia DA, Ageno W, Libby EN, et al. Perioperative anticoagulation for patients with mechanical heart valves: a survey of current practice. J Thromb Thrombolysis 2004;18(3):199–203.

[55] Garcia DA, Regan S, Henault LE, et al. Risk of thromboembolism with short-term interruption of warfarin therapy. Arch Intern Med 2008;168(1): 63–9.

[56] Ginsberg JS, Chan WS, Bates SM, et al. Anticoagulation of pregnant women with mechanical heart valves. Arch Intern Med 2003;163:694–8.

[57] Coon WW, Willis PW. Recurrence of venous thromboembolism. Surgery 1973;73:823–7.

[58] Heit JA, Mohr DN, Silverstein MD, et al. Predictors of recurrence after deep vein thrombosis and pulmonary embolism: a population-based cohort study. Arch Intern Med 2000;160:761–8.

[59] Hull R, Raskob G, Pineo G, et al. A comparison of subcutaneous low-molecular-weight heparin with warfarin sodium for prophylaxis against deep-vein thrombosis after hip or knee implantation. N Engl J Med 1993;329:1370–6.

[60] Colwell CW Jr, Collis DK, Paulson R, et al. Comparison of enoxaparin and warfarin for the prevention of venous thromboembolic disease after total hip arthroplasty. J Bone Joint Surg 1999;81-A: 932–40.

[61] Hull RD, Raskob GE, Rosenbloom D, et al. Heparin for 5 days as compared with 10 days in the initial treatment of proximal venous thrombosis. N Engl J Med 1990;322:1260–4.

[62] Collins R, Scrimgeour A, Yusuf S, et al. Reduction in fatal pulmonary embolism and venous thrombosis by perioperative administration of subcutaneous heparin. N Engl J Med 1988;318:1162–73.

[63] Kakkar VV, Cohen AT, Edmonson RA, et al. Low molecular weight versus standard heparin for prevention of venous thromboembolism after major abdominal surgery. Lancet 1993;341:259–65.

[64] Raschke RA, Reilly BM, Guidry JR, et al. The weight-based heparin dosing nomogram compared with a standard care nomogram. Ann Intern Med 1993;119:874–81.

[65] Hirsh J, Warkentin TE, Shaughnessy SG, et al. Heparin and low-molecular-weight heparin: mechanisms of action, pharmacokinetics, dosing, monitoring, efficacy, and safety. Chest 2001;119:64S–94S.

[66] Decousus H, Leizorovicz A, Parent F, et al. A clinical trial of vena caval filters in the prevention of pulmonary embolism in patients with proximal deep-vein thrombosis. N Engl J Med 1998;338: 409–15.

[67] Harrison L, Johnston M, Massicotte MP, et al. Comparison of 5-mg and 10-mg loading doses in initiation of warfarin therapy. Ann Intern Med 1997;126:133–6.

[68] Bern MM, Lokich JJ, Wallach SR, et al. Very low doses of warfarin can prevent thrombosis in central venous catheters. Ann Intern Med 1990;112(6):423–8.

[69] Ridker PM, Goldhaber SZ, Danielson E, et al. Long-term, low-intensity warfarin therapy for

prevention of recurrent venous thromboembolism. N Engl J Med 2003;348:1425–34.

[70] Blackshear JL, Baker VS, Rubino F, et al. Adjusted-dose warfarin versus low-intensity, fixed-dose warfarin plus aspirin for high-risk patients with atrial

fibrillation: stroke prevention in atrial fibrillation III randomised clinical trial. Lancet 1996;348:633–8.

[71] Palareti G, Legnani C. Warfarin withdrawal: pharmacokinetic-pharmacodynamic considerations. Clin Pharmacokinet 1996;30:300–13.

ELSEVIER
SAUNDERS

Cardiol Clin 26 (2008) 311–320

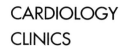
CARDIOLOGY
CLINICS

Index

Note: Page numbers of article titles are in **boldface** type.